SECOND EDITION

INTRODUCTION TO OCCUPATION

The Art and Science of Living

New multidisciplinary perspectives for understanding human occupation as a central feature of individual experience and social organization

Edited by
Charles H. Christiansen, EdD
American Occupational Therapy Foundation, Bethesda, Maryland

Elizabeth A. Townsend, PhD
Dalhousie University, Halifax, Nova Scotia

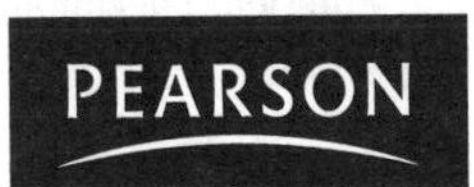

Upper Saddle River, New Jersey 07458

Library of Congress Cataloging-in-Publication Data
Introduction to occupation : the art and science of living : new multidisciplinary perspectives for understanding human occupation as a central feature of individual experience and social organization / edited by Charles H. Christiansen and Elizabeth A. Townsend. — 2nd ed.
p. cm.
ISBN-13: 978-0-13-199942-8
ISBN-10: 0-13-199942-7
1. Occupations—Psychological aspects. 2. Human behavior. I. Christiansen, Charles. II. Townsend, Elizabeth A.

BF481.I58 2010
158.6—dc22

2008045778

Notice: The authors and the publisher of this volume have taken care that the information and technical recommendations contained herein are based on research and expert consultation, and are accurate and compatible with the standards generally accepted at the time of publication. Nevertheless, as new information becomes available, changes in clinical and technical practices become necessary. The reader is advised to carefully consult manufacturers' instructions and information material for all supplies and equipment before use, and to consult with a healthcare professional as necessary. This advice is especially important when using new supplies or equipment for clinical purposes. The authors and publisher disclaim all responsibility for any liability, loss, injury, or damage incurred as a consequence, directly or indirectly, of the use and application of any of the contents of this volume.

Publisher: Julie Levin Alexander
Assistant to Publisher: Regina Bruno
Executive Editor: Mark Cohen
Development Editor: Melissa Kerian
Assistant Editor: Nicole Ragonese
Executive Marketing Manager: Katrin Beacom
Marketing Specialist: Michael Sirinides
Marketing Assistant: Judy Noh
Production Managing Editor: Patrick Walsh
Production Editor: Katherine Boilard, Pine Tree Composition, Inc.
Manufacturing Manager: Ilene Sanford
Manufacturing Buyer: Pat Brown
Senior Design Coordinator: Maria Guglielmo Walsh
Cover Design: Kevin Kall
Senior Media Editor: Amy Peltier
Media Project Manager: Lorena Cerisano
Composition: Laserwords Private Limited, Chennai, India
Printing & Binding: Edwards Brothers
Cover Printer: Phoenix Color

Pearson Education Ltd., London
Pearson Education Singapore, Pte. Ltd
Pearson Education Canada, Inc.
Pearson Education–Japan
Pearson Education Australia PTY, Limited
Pearson Education North Asia, Ltd., Hong Kong
Pearson Educación de Mexico, S.A. de C.V.
Pearson Education Malaysia, Pte. Ltd.
Pearson Education Upper Saddle River, New Jersey

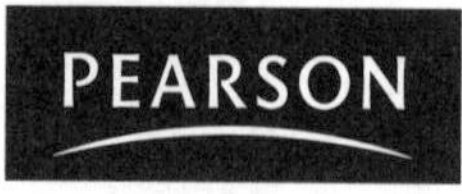

10 9 8 7 6 5 4 3 2 1
ISBN 10: 0-13-199942-7
ISBN 13: 978-0-13-199942-8

To Caren, Jim, Janet and Kim, who have always been there for me.

~Charles Christiansen

To my colleagues and family for persistent support, and to my good fortune in being a woman with many occupational possibilities.

~Elizabeth Townsend

Contents

Figures, Tables, and Boxes

FIGURES

TABLES

BOXES

Foreword

Carolyn Baum, PhD, OTR/L, FAOTA
Washington University, St. Louis, MO

Sometimes you find just the book you are looking for; this is it. I hold a firm belief in the power and value of occupation: In fact, I teach the theory and foundation course in our curriculum. I often find myself in faculty discussions about the science underpinning our occupational therapy curriculum model. There is a consensus that our curriculum model, which serves to prepare occupational therapy practitioners, is supported by neuroscience, environmental science, and occupational science. To date, we have not found a book for an entire course on the theories and science that support occupations' use in practice—this is it.

Occupational therapists are being asked to respond to and act on the needs of society through the healthcare system and the community systems that serve those with chronic health conditions and disability. Society expects occupational therapists and occupational therapy assistants to help people develop the skills and strategies to achieve personal goals and improve the quality of their everyday lives. Our method of helping is through enhancing capacity for occupational engagement and removing barriers that limit the ability of people to engage in the occupations that are meaningful and necessary to their everyday lives. All the developing areas of occupational therapy practice are centered on the needs of people to engage in occupations. I will review just a few. Because we recognize the importance of personal places and the memories of meaningful experiences imbued there, we can use our expertise in activity (occupation), performance, and environment to help people remain independent in their own homes and communities. Knowing who can safely drive (an occupation) to remain on the highways is important to individuals, to families, and to society. Helping children and youth achieve the capacity to be successful in school (learning and developmental occupations), be engaged with families and communities, and transition into adult roles, including employment, also is of vital importance. Helping workers prevent unnecessary disabilities, return to work after accidents, and have work and work stations that enable success in the world of work (what the public usually thinks about when we talk about occupations) is of unquestionable value. Therapy personnel can help older workers retain their ability to engage in productive work or civic engagement. They can help those with persistent mental health issues gain the skills to live in the least-restrictive environment, engage in meaningful occupations, and avoid social isolation. All these opportunities require the practitioner to have a rich understanding of the theories and science that support the individual's need, responsibility, and right to engage in occupation.

Many people come to the field of occupational therapy because they want to help people. By fully understanding occupation on an individual, community, and population level, practitioners in occupational therapy and other fields will be armed with the tools to make contributions to the health and well-being of the people they will serve.

Preface

The Latin phase *carpe diem* is a call for humans to be active and meditative about the possibilities that confront us as we literally harvest the day. Our occupations—how we harvest our days—present possibilities to perform, contemplate, make choices, exert control, develop habits, make meaning, connect with others, create communities, build societies, and otherwise seize our potential as humans, individually and collectively. The second edition of *Introduction to Occupation: The Art and Science of Living* presents the latest knowledge about occupation so that each of us around the world may understand how to seize and harvest our days for health, well-being, happiness, and the development of more just and peaceful societies.

***Introduction to Occupation* will appeal to any student, practitioner, researcher, or educator with an interest in everyday life.** We anticipate that *Introduction to Occupation* will be read by archeologists and anthropologists who study everyday life in the past and present; by sociologists and other social scientists who study employment, leisure, household work, family life, and other *occupational* concepts; by musicians and other artists who specialize in creative occupations; and by occupational scientists and occupational therapists, whose core domain of concern is occupation.

Nowadays, it is often said that the speed of change makes it difficult, if not impossible, to keep abreast of all the information needed to stay current in the world. Developments in information technology, reflected in the growth of the Internet, are helping people to cope, but paradoxically, new technologies are also making it easier for change to occur. Smart phones, lightweight notebook computers, and iPods with wireless capability and Internet connectivity are enabling people to stay connected nearly everywhere, to share their ideas and creativity, and to stay informed. These technologies also change what people do, how they use time, and how their use of time is influenced by others.

For millennia, philosophers have grappled with the conditions that define a good life. Socrates was convinced that there were no more important questions than those concerning how to live well and happily. Today's intense and widespread public interest in positive psychology (which, at its core, emphasizes finding ways to live happily) suggests that Socrates' questions continue to be as relevant now as they were in his time. Perhaps the profound changes of our time impel us to reflect on these questions as a way of seeking guidance.

Moreover, Socrates' assertion that values and meaning are more important to happiness than materialistic matters have tended to be confirmed by the modern research of psychologists who are studying the factors that contribute to "happiness" in everyday life. Time and again, these studies point to satisfying certain universal human needs as essential to positive feelings. Interestingly, those needs typically have components involving meaning and relationships. All of them are in some way embodied in human doing.

It seems a small step from identifying important needs essential for happiness and well-being to examining the means by which humans can create these conditions. The central question remains, How should people live their lives if they are to be happy? Yet, only recently have significant efforts been made in the context of science to examine what people do, where and how they do it, and how they feel about what they do as a means for providing informed advice to community planners, policy experts, and human service workers who seek guidance in helping people find better ways to live.

To put this second edition in context, knowledge of human occupation is elementary yet growing rapidly. There are articles, books, stories, and films and other materials on work-related occupations. The repertoire of knowledge of work-related occupations is enriched by wide-ranging research on subjects such as time use, leisure, occupational hazards and safety, occupational medicine, and occupational therapy. Still there is much to learn about occupation. Everyday occupations collectively define, organize, and influence all aspects of peoples' lives. This book takes the view that occupations include all meaningful acts that collectively define and give meaning to daily living.

For these reasons, understanding human occupations, with all the complexity that surrounds such understanding, has become a central concern to occupational scientists. As this book reveals, occupational scientists come from myriad disciplines, ranging from sociology and psychology to geography, public policy and the health sciences. Within this volume, one finds a collection of introductory chapters that discuss human occupation, from the standpoint of place, culture, time use, human development, social justice, deprivation, work and leisure, and health (to name a few). The intent is to provide a backdrop that introduces the reader to the breadth of the topic and to provide a context for those in the health and social sciences, including public health, health psychology, social work, and occupational therapy, to begin to understand the central importance of everyday activity to human existence, meaning, and yes, happiness and well-being.

This second edition includes updated chapters from the first volume and adds new topics and study materials to help the reader become exposed to the broad range of ideas and concerns of occupational science. Given the complexity and breadth of occupation, the book cannot be exhaustive, either in individual chapters or across the span of the book. We hope, however, that exposure to the ideas here will invite a further examination of one or more specific topic areas.

We are indebted to the contributors to this volume and its precursor, to our consultants, who provided expert review of the material to enhance study and learning, and to those editorial assistants who provided dependable and helpful assistance. In particular, we thank the publishers, especially Mark Cohen and Melissa Kerian for their continued support, Charles Hayden and Judy Wolf for their work in early parts of manuscript preparation, Sarah Gibson for reference support, and Linda Buxell, Katie Barrett, Kristine Haertl, and Julie Bass Haugen, who provided helpful and timely advice with study guide materials.

Charles Christiansen
Bethesda, Maryland

Elizabeth Townsend
Halifax, Nova Scotia

Contributing Authors

Eric Asaba, PhD, OTR
Assistant Professor and Postdoctoral Fellow, Karolinska Institutet
Stockholm, Sweden
Research Associate and Chief Occupational Therapist, Asaba Medical Research Foundation and affiliated Kohnan Hospital
Tamang City, Japan

Catherine L. Backman, PhD, OT(C), FCAOT
Associate Professor, Department of Occupational Science and Occupational Therapy
The University of British Columbia
Vancouver, British Columbia, Canada

Robert K. Bing, EdD, OTR, FAOTA (Deceased)
Professor Emeritus
The University of Texas Medical Branch
Galveston, Texas, USA

Charles H. Christiansen, EdD, OTR, OT(C), FAOTA
Executive Director
The American Occupational Therapy Foundation
Bethesda, Maryland, USA

Jane A. Davis, PhD (candidate), MSc, OT(C), OT Reg (ONT), OTR,
Lecturer, Department of Occupational Science and Occupational Therapy
Faculty of Medicine,
University of Toronto
Toronto, Ontario, Canada

Toby Ballou Hamilton, PhD, MPH, OTR/L
Assistant Professor, Department of Rehabilitation Science
College of Allied Health
University of Oklahoma Health Sciences Center
Oklahoma City, Oklahoma, USA

Andrew S. Harvey, PhD
Professor Emeritus of Economics
Director, Time Use Research Program
Saint Mary's University
Halifax, Nova Scotia, Canada

Michael K. Iwama, PhD, OT(C), OT Reg (ONT)
Associate Professor, Department of Occupational Science and Occupational Therapy
University of Toronto
Toronto, Ontario, Canada

Jennifer Jarman, PhD
Assistant Professor, Department of Sociology
National University of Singapore
Singapore

Hans Jonsson, PhD, OT (reg)
Associate Professor
Director of Master Courses in Occupational Therapy
Division of Occupational Therapy
Department of Neurobiology, Care Sciences, and Society
Karolinska Institutet
Stockholm, Sweden

Annah R. Lesunyane, M Occ Ther
Lecturer, Department of Occupational Therapy
Faculty of Health Sciences
University of Limpopo
Medunsa, Pretoria, South Africa

Matthew Molineux, BOccThy, MSc, PhD, AccOT
Head of Occupational Science and Occupational Therapy
School of Allied Health Professions
Leeds Metropolitan University
Leeds, United Kingdom

Wendy Pentland, PhD, OT(C), OT Reg (ONT)
Associate Professor, Division of Occupational Therapy
School of Rehabilitation Therapy
Queen's University
Kingston, Ontario, Canada

Helene J. Polatajko, PhD, OT Reg (ONT), OT(C), OT Reg (ONT) FCAOT
Professor, Department of Occupational Science and Occupational Therapy and Graduate Department of Rehabilitation Science
University of Toronto
Toronto, Ontario, Canada

Alfred T. Ramukumba, B Occ Ther (Hons), M Phil Adult Education and Training
Senior Lecturer and Head of Department, Occupational Therapy Program
Faculty of Health Sciences
University of Limpopo
Medunsa, Pretoria, South Africa

Robin L. Stadnyk, PhD, OT(C) OT Reg. (NS)
Assistant Professor
School of Occupational Therapy
Halifax, Nova Scotia, Canada

Elizabeth A. Townsend, PhD, OT(C), OT, FCAOT
Professor and Director, School of Occupational Therapy
Dalhousie University
Halifax, Nova Scotia, Canada

Gail Whiteford, PhD
Professor and Head of Albury Wodonga Campus
Charles Sturt University
Albury, New South Wales, Australia

Ann A. Wilcock, PhD
Adjunct Professor
School of Occupational Therapy
Dalhousie University (Canada)
Normanville, South Australia, Australia

Simon Kam Man Wong, MAIS, MBA, PDOT
Manager, Occupational Therapy Department
Tai Po Hospital
Hong Kong

Jiri Zuzanek, PhD
Professor, Department of Recreation and Leisure Studies
Faculty of Applied Health Sciences
University of Waterloo
Waterloo, Ontario, Canada

CONSULTANTS

Kate Barrett, OTD, OTR/L
Assistant Professor, Department of Occupational Therapy and Occupational Science
The College of St. Catherine
St. Paul, Minnesota, USA

Linda Buxell, MA, OTR/L
Professor, Department of Occupational Therapy and Occupational Science
The College of St. Catherine
St. Paul, Minnesota, USA

Kristine L. Haertl, PhD, OTR/L
Associate Professor, Department of Occupational Therapy and Occupational Science
The College of St. Catherine
St. Paul, Minnesota, USA

Julie Bass Haugen, PhD, OTR/L, FAOTA
Professor, Department of Occupational Therapy and Occupational Science
The College of St. Catherine
St. Paul, Minnesota, USA

Reviewers

Second Edition Reviewers

Debbie Amini, MEd, OTR/L, CHT
Director, Occupational Therapy Assisting
Cape Fear Community College
Wilmington, North Carolina, USA

Melba Arnold, MS, OTR/L
Assistant Professor, Occupational Science/Occupational Therapy
Saint Louis University
St. Louis, Missouri, USA

Linda Duncombe, EdD, OTR/L, FAOTA
Clinical Associate Professor
Academic Fieldwork Coordinator
Occupational Therapy and Rehabilitation Counseling
Boston University
Boston, Massachusetts, USA

John Fleming, MOT, OTR/L
Assistant Professor, Occupational Therapy
College of St. Catherine
St. Paul, Minnesota, USA

Sue Gallagher, MA, OTR/L
Assistant Professor, Occupational Therapy
Quinnipiac University
Hamden, Connecticut, USA

Anita Hotchkiss, MS, OTR/L
Instructor, Occupational Therapy
Gannon University
Erie, Pennsylvania, USA

Lisa Hubbs, MS, OTR/L
Program Coordinator, Occupational Therapy Assisting
Suffolk County Community College
Brentwood, New York, USA

Janet Nagayda, OTD, MS, OTR
Associate Professor and Chair, Occupational Therapy
Saginaw Valley State University
University Center, Michigan, USA

Claudia Peyton, PhD, OTR/L, FAOTA
Coordinator, Occupational Therapy
California State University
Redondo Beach, California, USA

Janeene Sibla, MS, OTR/L
Associate Professor, Occupational Therapy
University of Mary
Bismarck, North Dakota, USA

Beth P. Velde, PhD, OTR/L
Professor, Occupational Therapy
East Carolina University
Greenville, North Carolina, USA

First Edition Reviewers

Kathy P. Bradley, EdD
Chair, Occupational Therapy Department
Medical College of Georgia
Augusta, Georgia, USA

Barbara Rom, OTR/L
Program Director, Occupational Therapy Assistant Program
Green River Community College
Auburn, Washington, USA

Amy Solomon, OTR
Denver Technical College
Denver, Colorado, USA

CHAPTER 1

An Introduction to Occupation

Charles H. Christiansen and Elizabeth A. Townsend

OBJECTIVES

1. Define key concepts related to occupations, including occupation, activity, task, habits, routines, automaticity, and embedded occupations.
2. Discuss the different ways in which occupations create meaning.
3. Describe several examples of occupational classifications/taxonomies discussed in this chapter.
4. Identify specific biological, psychological, and contextual factors that influence occupational choice and patterns.
5. Discuss current evidence of the relationships between occupations and health, well-being, and participation.
6. Summarize how understanding of occupation is enhanced after reading about the history of occupations, sleep, leisure, play, and paid work.

KEY WORDS

Automaticity
Embedded occupations
Everyday life
Folk taxonomy
Habit
Human occupations
Narrative
Occupation
Occupational classification/taxonomy
Occupational habits
Occupational routines
Occupational science
Occupations
Routine
Taxonomy

www.prenhall.com/christiansen

The Internet provides an exciting means for interacting with this textbook and for enhancing your understanding of humans' experiences with occupations and the organization of occupations in society. Use the address above to access the interactive Companion Website created specifically to accompany this book. Here you will find an array of self-study material designed to help you gain a richer understanding of the concepts presented in this chapter.

CHAPTER PROFILE

In this chapter, the term *occupation* is defined and examined broadly to provide a context for viewing the daily pursuits of humans. The chapter seeks to establish a beginning point for understanding the scope of ideas in the book and to introduce an *occupational perspective* of human life and society. Several key questions regarding occupation are posed. These questions enable the exploration of concepts regarding how occupations have been defined and classified in the past. Human time use reveals broad types of human endeavor, each having implications for behavior, development, social interaction, well-being, and participation in society. Factors influencing occupational engagement are explored, and a brief history of occupations through the ages is summarized from the work of Robert Bing. The chapter closes with a review of ideas related to the perceived beneficial effects of human occupation on individuals and our participation in societies. It is acknowledged that the chapter and the book overall are written largely from the perspective of Western cultures.

INTRODUCTION

The word *occupation* in English is derived from the Latin *occupatio*, meaning "to occupy or to seize." To be occupied is to use and even seize control of time and space (or place) as a person engages in a recognizable life endeavor. Daily human occupations are invested with form and a sense of purpose, meaning, cultural style, and social/economic significance or power (1, 2). Those who take an occupational perspective of life and society raise questions and seek answers about occupations. One looks at life and society using an occupational lens to understand what people are doing, or want and need to do to survive, be healthy, and live well as valued citizens. Conversely with such a lens, one can look at systems and society to understand how occupations are named, classified, and organized in different economies and sociocultural practices. Our reference to human occupation in this book includes more than engagement in work. Everyday lives reflect participation in a broad range of pursuits. Occupational engagement—the occupying of place and time in a rich tapestry of experience, purpose, and attached meaning—is how we broadly define human occupation (2).

UNDERSTANDING THE COMPLEXITY OF OCCUPATION

Humans have occupied their lives with the goal-directed pursuits necessary for existence and well-being since the dawning of time. As group-living animals, early humans used primitive or proto-occupations to ensure their survival. They cooperated in their pursuit of food, water, and shelter and in protecting and nurturing their offspring. Undoubtedly, these early group behaviors were genetically influenced as part of nature's adaptations for survival of the human species. The evolution of language enabled meanings to be attached to occupations and events, and as the human brain increased in size, greater intelligence led to new ways to adapt, survive, and contend with the challenges of nature. The division of labor within groups is an example of this. As humans evolved, so did occupations. Yet, even now within different cultural groups, we can still identify distinct types of occupational pursuits necessary for survival and maintenance. In considering these ideas, it is useful to think about the socioculturally diverse roles individuals play in serving the needs of groups. Social roles, such as mother, father, and leader are, at their core, defined by the occupations that are used to maintain families, groups, communities, and organizations. These differ in context, depending, for instance, on cultural rituals and social conditions. Box 1-1 provides a brief glimpse of how occupations have changed since early history.

BOX 1-1 A History of Occupation

An understanding of occupations today is better achieved if a person has an appreciation for what people did during previous eras. Archeologists and anthropologists agree that from the dawn of time, humans' primary purpose was to survive. As early humans developed language and intellect, adaptation to the forces of nature required a division of labor. In very early times men were the foragers and gatherers, and women, being child-bearers, were the preservers and fashioners of materials for eating and bartering. The basic occupations at this time included agriculture, the making of essential tools, and the creation of pottery, textiles, and basketry (59).

Although an in-depth exploration of the history of work and leisure could easily fill volumes, a review of everyday occupations through the ages and how these influenced (and were influenced by) the cultures and attitudes of the time provides a useful context in which to view the present. History illustrates how work and play coexisted and were jointly influenced by the cultures and environments of the times.

In later centuries, the Greeks were among the first advanced culture to appreciate the importance of work and leisure (60). Work was seen as the gods' curse on humankind. The Greek word for work was *ponos*, meaning a sense of a heavy burdensome task, downright drudgery. Within this culture, however, the division of labor was based on status within the culture. There was little dignity or value in work, other than as a means for avoiding hunger and death, or for reaching prosperity and the opportunity for leisure. Slaves, peasants, and craftsmen did the work of gathering and preserving raw materials and fashioning goods. A middle class was made up of merchants, who did the bartering. The nobility and priests became the upper class, whose work was to indulge in the pleasurable occupations of life, such as teaching, discovering, thinking, or composing music. At this time, leisure became one of the foundations of Western culture. The English word *school* is derived from the Greek word *skole,* for the place where education and teaching occurred (60).

(*continued*)

BOX 1-1 Continued

Three prominent Greek philosophers provided classic insights regarding work and the pursuit of the thoughtful life (61). Socrates was known to frequent the shops of Athens, observing artisans at work, doing what he thought were nonessential tasks. Aristotle, on the other hand, believed that well-being did not come from the pursuit of pleasure (hedonism); rather, it came from the meditative life (leisure). Plato, late in his writings, declared that life must be lived as play, playing certain games and making sacrifices. In this manner a person could gain favor with the gods and provide a defense against enemies (62).

The Roman philosophers also held views about occupation (63). Cicero, the great orator and philosopher, claimed there were but two worthy occupations: agriculture and business, especially if the latter led one to an honorable and stately retirement into the quiet of the countryside. The Hebrews also held an admiration for work and the meditative life. The Talmud states that labor is a holy occupation, and even if one does not need to work to survive, he or she must nevertheless labor, for idleness results in an early death (64).

Alfred the Great (849–899 AD), King of Wessex, established the right of freeborn Englishmen to the three-eights division of the day into work, rest, and leisure. During this same time various festivals emerged, particularly to recognize sacred or seasonal events. Consecrations, sacrifices, sacred dances and contests, and performances were all occupations for celebrating a festival. During the period from 350 to 800AD, people returned to a simpler life (65); yet, the class stratification remained as peasant, merchant, and nobleman. In the early 16th century, Martin Luther believed that work and serving God were synonymous, and one was expected to do the best job possible, thereby earning dignity. One was called to one's work because all daily occupations were divinely inspired (66).

In the 17th century, a Frenchman, John Calvin, whose writings have had a significant impact on Western cultures, added to the prevailing beliefs by declaring there was no room for idleness, luxury, or any activity that softened the soul (67). Meditation was not acceptable because Calvin believed that God was not in the habit of revealing himself to humans through thinking. A person was expected to extract the greatest good from work, including a profit. Successful work would result in wealth, which was to be used to care for those less fortunate. This link between work and wealth became known as the Protestant work ethic.

The Agrarian Age (c.1800–1880) brought the tools necessary to produce the goods required by the world. Because most occupations were seasonal, the worker could control periods of leisure and rest. This ended with the onset of the Industrial Revolution, beginning in the middle of the 18th century, and lasting for one hundred years. Time took over as the key to nearly all daily occupations. One no longer worked at home in what often had come to be thought of as "cottage industries." The worker left home to work in large buildings, with large numbers of individuals, often accomplishing the same occupations alongside one another.

Machinery replaced tools as the focus of labor. Compensation was determined by someone other than the worker and was based on the clock, usually displayed prominently in the workplace. This was the beginning of paid occupations in the industrialized world.

During the industrial revolution, leisure occupations departed from the home and became centered in the community. Many factory owners assumed responsibility for their workers' play time. An example was the community established by the Pullman Company, south of Chicago. The town was carefully laid out to include a wide variety of parks and structures for the pleasure of all members of the workers' families. Despite this, there was considerable unrest, and strikes often occurred over wages and the adequacy and control of leisure time.

During the Great Depression of the 1930s, the U.S. federal government assisted with numerous occupational programs, including the WPA, or Works Progress Administration (68). As one WPA enrollee said after just three weeks on the job: "Now I can look my children straight in the eyes. I've gained my self-respect. It's different now" (42, p. 812). Allied nations rallied behind the war effort. Yet, there was time for leisure occupations. Movie attendance set new records. Nightclubs, sporting events, vacations, and entertainment at home, such as listening to the radio, reading paperbacks, and various parlor games, became popular leisure occupations (69).

The present era, sometimes known as the Postindustrial or Information Age, was described by Ferguson as a social transformation resulting from personal transformation—change from the inside out (70). Naisbitt claimed that Western society was reluctantly leaving behind the Industrial Age and entering the Information Age, where the new wealth was in know-how (71). In the current era, with the universal two-income family, leisure occupations have undergone a drastic change. Cross says that there is now a stressed leisure class with great inequities between men and women. Women in the workplace return home to care for children and housework. They are frequently denied the after-work leisure time enjoyed by many men. Cross speculates that home-based entertainment, such as rented movies and high-quality sound systems, are used as convenient substitutes for other forms of leisure, but probably fall short of giving the satisfaction that other more-involved options might (72).

We can speculate about how attitudes toward work and leisure occupations are influenced by cultures. We can ask why many people are feeling less satisfied with their work and leisure than in the past. Or we can consider how the information age might influence the types and locations of occupations in the future. A better approach is to study occupations systematically, taking a broad look at the many dimensions that influence everyday human pursuits. Durant stated it well when he observed: "The present is the past rolled up for action, and the past is the present unrolled for understanding" (73, p. viii).

The History of Occupation was written by the late Dr. Robert K. Bing (1932–2004).

Histories are cultural accounts that may report the individual and/or collective occupations of humans over time in situations shaped by places and systems that influence what humans do there. The study of history is itself an occupational pursuit. Yet, occupation itself has only recently become a topic of deep interest and study. Human occupation is so embedded in human existence that it largely has been overlooked as a topic worthy of serious scholarly attention until recently. The emergence of occupational science, a field devoted to understanding human occupation, has addressed this oversight by focusing on what people do in their lives under different circumstances.

This chapter addresses five important questions that portray a Western perspective and serve as a framework for understanding human occupation in the 21st century. These include:

1. How do people occupy their time?
2. What influences what people do?
3. How do people describe their occupation?
4. How does context, i.e., place or environment determine what people do (and when they do it)?
5. How does occupation affect health, well-being, and just participation in society?

HOW DO PEOPLE OCCUPY THEIR TIME?

How do you occupy your time? is such a classic question that it is asked repeatedly in ordinary conversation to discover how people typically allocate their time, attention, and energy. The answer may include a description of someone's paid work, but the question invites a far more extensive exploration of occupation in relation to time, that elusive yet defining feature of human existence. Implied in the question is an interest in how time is used in particular places, through particular routines and habits, and in particular sociocultural conditions. To be fully answered, the simple question, *How do you occupy your time?* requires that we consider *what* people do in their daily routines and habits, *when* they do their occupations, *where* they do them and *why*, and *how* the context determines what they do (and conversely, how what people do influences their context).

Consider this scene: It is one o'clock in the afternoon on a pleasant Monday in May. Main Street is bustling with people enjoying nice weather. Some are moving quickly with a given destination in mind, perhaps in a hurry to get back to jobs after their lunch breaks. Others are watching children play, carrying shopping bags, walking dogs, or simply strolling two by two and enjoying conversation. Two male police officers eat sandwiches while talking with a street vendor who is selling lunch snacks. On a corner, a musician strums a guitar behind an open instrument case, hoping for the coins of a passersby. A delivery van speeds by to a destination in the country. It stops at an intersection where nearby, children are entering school buses for an afternoon outing. Further along the road, builders are completing roadwork. On the edge of town the van passes farmers who are selling local produce. Earlier in the

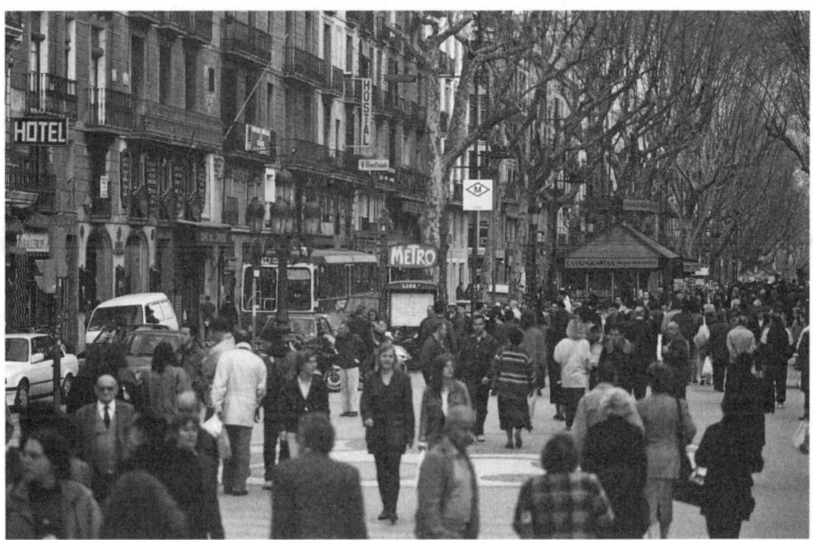

FIGURE 1-1 Occupations surround us.
(Photodisc/Getty Images)

day, the farmers have delivered produce to a local warehouse, where managers are preparing it for shipment to other communities.

This scene could occur in nearly any town or city in the world (see Figure 1-1 ■). It describes people living their lives, engaged in many occupations. Although it does not seem especially remarkable, the scene provides a way to begin addressing the question, *How do you occupy your time?* Observation of such a scene is a good way to raise awareness about the vast range of occupations that comprise daily life, as well as the ways in which occupation is related to time and space (or place) and the context in which people live. It is also useful to associate people and what they do with the necessary roles and activities that must be performed to maintain families, groups, communities, and organizations.

Now imagine an occupational science experiment in which a participant embeds a tiny digital camera with a transmitter into a pendant to be worn around the neck continuously during waking hours for 1 month. In reviewing the many hours of video that result, the occupational scientist might be interested in what the person did, where the person spent time, and how much time the person spent doing various occupations. A quantitative, statistical analysis of this information could answer the question, *How do you occupy yourself?*

During your quantitative analysis, you find that the 25-year-old participant, whose month long video you are analyzing, spent 73 hours on the telephone, either at home or at various locations, using a cell or mobile telephone. Being a university student, the participant also spent 80 hours reading and studying, again at various locations, 80 hours in class, and 80 hours at a part-time job in a clothing store. Another 78 hours were devoted to eating, 22 hours to shopping, 15 hours to housework, 63 hours to dressing and grooming, and 75 hours in socializing with friends during the

30-day experiment. Another 47 hours were devoted to driving from one location to another. Nearly 200 hours were spent sleeping.

Here, the occupational scientist would need to categorize what the participant did. To answer the question *How do you occupy your time?* the researcher would calculate how much time was spent in various *occupational categories.* A progressively detailed statistical analysis could correlate the use of time spent in particular places with specific occupations, or analyze the allocation of time devoted to particular routines and habits, or further yet, relate particular occupations to specific places or geographic locations. In other words, the simple question, *How do you occupy your time?* invites a wealth of exploration about occupation, time, space and the sociocultural structures of different communities and societies.

The term *occupational engagement* is sometimes used to describe people doing occupations in a manner that fully involves their effort, drive, and attention. Sometimes the description, "being engaged in an occupation," refers to vocational pursuits, or doing work necessary for daily existence. As demonstrated above in the street scene, some occupations produce goods and services necessary for people to live. However, being engaged in an occupation might suggest that one is captivated and fully attentive to the experience. A Swedish occupational scientist, Hans Jonsson, has described this phenomenon in his studies of what people do after retirement, suggesting that people are drawn to occupations, even in retirement, that fully engage their time and attention in a manner similar to that provided by satisfying work (3).

A simple starting place for understanding human occupation and developing an occupational perspective of life and society is to list the variety of occupations that comprise everyday life—for an individual, a family, a community, an organization, or a society. Discussion and analysis of the list might consider the complexity of occupation in relation to time and space and the categories of occupations because it is not actually easy to list or classify occupations based on what people are doing.

For example, the professional tennis player does not experience nor perceive tennis in the same way as the amateur athlete who plays for fun and fitness. For the professional, tennis is a form of paid work. For the amateur, it is considered active play or leisure. Similarly, some people sew or play the piano for relaxation, whereas for others, these same occupations constitute necessary paid work or employment.

Discussion could consider further the complexity associated with simultaneous participation in more than one occupation. It is usual for occupations to be "nested" or "embedded" within other occupations (4) so that it is difficult to determine precisely how time is divided among various occupations. Consider someone traveling on the train and at the same time talking on a cell telephone or working on a portable computer (see Figure 1-2 ■); or someone planning the building of a new shed while also monitoring children at play; or someone playing a musical instrument while also conducting a group of musicians.

Economists who study human time use address the simultaneous multitasking just described by attempting to distinguish primary occupations from secondary occupations. Primary occupations are often but not exclusively discerned by observing the location of the occupation. If you are responsible for watching that children play safely and your cell phone rings, your primary occupation would be observing and

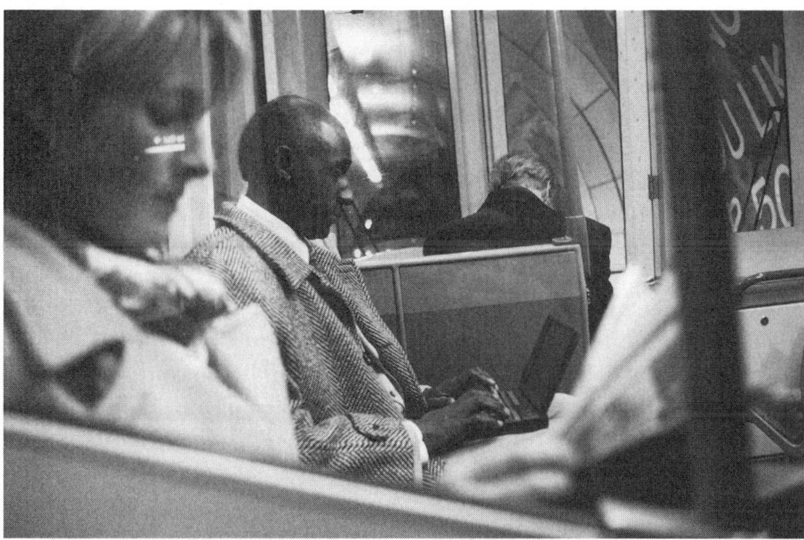

FIGURE 1-2 Nested or embedded occupations occur when people do more than one thing simultaneously.
(Photodisc/Getty Images)

interacting with the children, and your secondary occupation would be communicating by cell phone with the caller.

Let's return for a moment to the scene described earlier of the vibrant town at midday. Consider how the occupations observed represent habits or routines—the habituation associated with many occupations. Habits are relatively automatic, repetitive patterns of human behavior (5). Some, but not all habitual behaviors are occupations. For example, chewing a pencil or biting your nails may be habitual actions, but fail to qualify as occupations. On the other hand, driving a certain route to work, or getting coffee first thing in the morning, could be considered habitual occupations (6). Routines have been defined as "habitual, repeatable and predictable ways of acting" (7). Clark observes that routines provide a structure that serves to organize and maintain individual lives (6). Most people have routines that help them move efficiently through their regular daily occupations. For example, many people have a particular morning or bedtime routine. This may include first putting on a robe and getting breakfast, then getting the morning newspaper and showering and dressing for the day. The items and sequence of the day define the characteristics of the routine, which in the morning often includes the occupations of dining, hygiene, grooming and dressing, and reading or getting the news from television or radio. For those working at a location outside the home, the routine also involves using transportation from home to the workplace.

In contrast, a habit might involve a particular style or characteristic embedded within an occupation or occupational routine. For example, some people may have a habit of putting cream in their coffee and stirring it three times before taking a sip. Others may habitually comb their hair or brush their teeth in a particular manner.

Still others might feel the need to light a cigarette as soon as they pour themselves a cup of coffee, answer the phone, or begin to read the paper.

Many people, if asked, would identify habits and routines as an important influence in their individual pattern of time use. Despite their importance in accounting for how we spend time, until recently, most research on repetitive behaviors has focused on recurring patterns of behavior that are destructive, antisocial, or unhealthy. These include physical addictions (e.g., smoking, alcoholism, or drug use) as well as psychological addictions (e.g., gambling, eating, or excessive engagement), or preoccupation (e.g., with computer games).

A more recent approach has viewed habits from the standpoint of their neurological foundations, suggesting that habits, or patterns of time use, can range along a continuum (8). This view proposes that certain habits and routines may be necessary for well-being, whereas other states, such as not having life structure or being dominated by excessive repetitive behavior, are not adaptive and thus not conducive to health and well-being (8). It is clear that regular employment outside the home can provide a certain structure for daily routine. Whether a person owns a business or works for someone else, the necessary tasks associated with work-oriented occupations provide a regular routine that can be useful in helping to organize a person's life. When people lose or are constrained in developing the structures that support the organization of their lives, they may be at risk for physical or emotional consequences, such as depression, lowered self-esteem, or sleep disorders (9).

The idea that some occupational routines are useful may seem contrary to prevailing views that focus on their negative consequences. However, habits and routines can be useful when they support behavior or thought by enabling attention or energy to be conserved so they can be directed toward thoughts or actions where they best serve the interests of the individual. Inasmuch as routine and necessary behaviors do not require highly focused attention, they conserve energy and attention to enable quick responses to unexpected contingencies or pursuits that have a higher priority or importance (10).

John Bargh has devoted a career to studying *automaticity*, a term that refers to behaviors that represent automatic responses based on situational conditions that lead to behaviors and choices that are activated or triggered by subconscious mechanisms reacting to features of the environment (11, 12). Although automaticity leads to behavioral responses that are stereotypical, automatic behaviors are not the same thing as habits. They can perhaps best be considered habits of choice or fixed behavioral tendencies because when triggered, they can and do result in predictable goal choices in situations with similar characteristics. Bargh believes that these unconscious behavioral influences are more pervasive than we may think in influencing our choices and behaviors (13).

Both automatic responses (automaticity) and habits can be either problematic or helpful. For example, automaticity can lead to stereotypical responses based on another person's skin color or social status, thus causing people to avoid social interactions that could be helpful (14). Similarly, habits can also lead to errors, such as getting off an elevator on the wrong floor when the door opens or turning off the alarm and oversleeping (see Figure 1-3 ■). On the other hand, automatic choices that influence nurturing, altruistic, or ethical behaviors can be socially beneficial, just as the habit of fastening a seatbelt can lead to greater safety in driving. Much additional study on habits, routines, and automatic behaviors is necessary before definitive conclusions can be drawn about the role of repetitive patterns of occupation in everyday life.

Considered separately, habits, routines, and automatic behaviors constitute portions of daily lives, or building blocks of lifestyles. But, are there larger patterns or tendencies that describe lives? The answer to this question is yes. The word *lifestyle* is used to describe these larger patterns, often influenced by societal and cultural forces.

Conventional wisdom holds that some patterns of behavior may be more wholesome, sustainable, or balanced than others, leading to a longer life, less stress, or better health and happiness (15). Although much research remains to be done, emerging evidence shows that occupations that address certain basic and universal needs, or those with characteristics that buffer (or provide resilience) against the negative consequences of stressors, may help to promote health and prevent disease. Thus, lifestyles with patterns including habitual, buffering occupations could be construed as more conducive to wellness and participation in society. (2, 16–18).

Most people know inherently from personal experience that the whole of everyday life is comprised of occupations, and that time use, places for doing, and habitual routines constitute defining aspects of any lifestyle. There is implicit, general

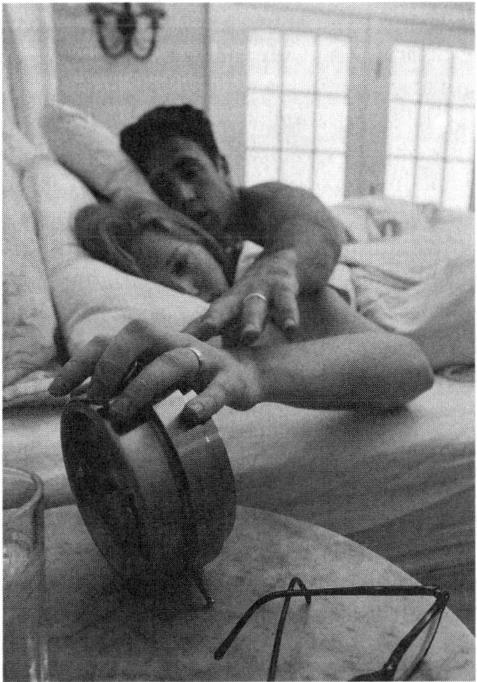

FIGURE 1-3 Much of daily life involves habits and routines. (Photodisc/Getty Images)

knowledge that doing is part of being, that humans are doers, and that places influence what we do. We also understand implicitly that there are societal influences on how, when, and where humans occupy themselves. So, what can be done to make this knowledge more explicit and to deepen understanding of how people occupy themselves? Is such knowledge just common sense? If so, how could this *common* sense be made more explicit to help people to recognize and organize the richness of human experience in different ways? What new insights would come to light by asking questions from an occupational perspective?

WHAT INFLUENCES WHAT PEOPLE DO?

The question *What occupies you?* sounds similar to the question, *How do you occupy yourself?* More carefully considered, the question, *What occupies you?* brings to mind the qualitative aspects of occupation—encouraging us to consider *why* people engage in occupations? Suppose for a moment that an occupational scientist invites a study participant both to wear a pendant to make a video record of occupations and also to keep a diary to explain *why* he or she is engaging in particular occupations in the times and places recorded.

The qualitative analysis of the diary of the day described earlier might reveal that during the 73 hours the participant spent on the telephone with a partner, a major topic of conversation concerned questions about the nature of their relationship. Moreover, the 15 hours of housework were undertaken because the participant valued spending only a half hour per day to keep the barest minimum of order at home. In contrast, approximately 2 hours per day were devoted to dressing and grooming and even more to socializing with friends, these being highly valued occupations to this young university student.

This brief suggestion for a qualitative study of occupations could address questions about the relationships between occupational choice and the identity humans generate by selecting and participating in particular occupations. There is a growing sentiment among social and developmental psychologists that a person's sense of self emerges largely as a result of what he or she experiences on a daily basis and over time (19–21). Some researchers suggest that goals are fashioned around imagined selves, to the extent that occupations are chosen with an aim toward becoming a particular kind of person (e.g., rich, popular, or skillful) or to avoid the unpleasant outcome of becoming impoverished, unpopular or clumsy, thus risking or encountering social rejection (22). Clearly, fashions and trends in modern society tend to support the idea that self-expression and identity-building are important factors in the selection of occupations and, by extension, how time is used.

Occupations Create Meaning

The diary described earlier could also be analyzed to consider the meaning or meanings of the occupations recorded. Occupations are complex also because they have diverse meanings with social as well as individual significance.

In everyday life, occupations frequently provide the context for interaction with others. As group-living animals, our lives are filled with social occupations and the abundant relationships that these interpersonal situations provide. Human interactions create social meaning. Rituals and ceremonies, such as weddings and funerals, are occupations that have widely understood shared meaning within cultures. Other experiences have shared meaning but are also likely to represent opportunities for creating individual or personal meaning.

Consider the meaning of a camping trip for pleasure. Planning such an outing invites certain expectations about the kind of clothing that one will wear and the kinds of occupations in which one will participate to collect, prepare and eat food, to find shelter, to enjoy the area, and to interact with others. The conveniences of modern times have made the camping experience symbolize self-reliance and an opportunity to get in touch with the natural surroundings so often absent in the built environment. But the experiences encountered during the camping trip often go beyond these shared meanings and may be intensely individual. A person may always remember the first fish caught, the first bear seen in the wild, or the stories told around the campfire that provided a rare opportunity to gain insight into life's problems or provided an occasion to share a special experience with a close friend or relative—to be part of a group or community.

One dimension of meaning-making in occupations can be described as spiritual (23). Some occupations, such as listening to music or appreciating art and design, can touch the human spirit and enrich the experience of living beyond the practical needs of survival and physical comfort. A related spiritual dimension of occupations pertains to making sense of the larger purpose of life. The very term *"contemplate"* derives from the Latin words referring to that which takes place within a temple. Thus, the sense of a larger purpose may for some be related to beliefs that one's occupations have a purpose or significance beyond the individual.

Typically, people understand the meaning of their lives by considering their occupations as part of their life story. It seems that occupations gain meaning over time by becoming part of an individual's unfolding autobiography, or personal narrative (24, 25). Contemplation of one's occupations over time may contribute to a sense of satisfaction about life and the emergence of a satisfactory identity.

The question, *What occupies you?* also sparks reflection and introspection about *why* people engage in particular occupations. To explore this question, one might also ask *Why do you choose to be occupied as you do? What motivates you to select some occupations and not others? Why are you interested in particular occupations?* or *What occupations give your life meaning?* If occupation is more than a job—if identity, development, meaning, and possibly other facets of human existence are intricately linked to occupation—what knowledge already exists and what else needs to be known? It is true that jobs and paid work may contribute to identity, development, and meaning for some people at some times in their lives. But how do humans use the multiplicity of daily occupations to create a life for themselves and to create the policies and other structures that determine what humans can and even want to do?

WHAT IS YOUR OCCUPATION?

When people are casually asked, *What is your occupation?* or the previous question, *How do you occupy yourself?*, they generally use what is known as a *folk taxonomy* to describe different types of occupations. Typical folk taxonomy descriptors are, *I work as a plumber, I am taking time off, I'm home with the children now, I'm retired, I don't do much of anything, I'm just a homemaker.* This folk system is used to describe occupations and to convey the ways in which certain occupations are valued. For instance, feminists such as Germaine Greer (26) and Betty Frieden (27) have pointed out how homemaking is such a socially devalued occupation that those for whom this is their primary occupation are not only unpaid but are viewed as lesser contributors to society, being *just* homemakers. The folk taxonomies of everyday language also lack the level of detail or precision that would be necessary for rigorous analysis. For example, someone may describe their day as including time to play, leisure, hanging out with friends, or resting. At any particular moment, they might say they are *eating junk food.* This folk category uses the value-laden term *junk,* which suggests that their food is less than healthy. A more careful analysis would possibly describe this as being occupied in *eating popularized food,* such as hamburgers and pizza. These are foods that have healthful aspects (inclusion of meat and cheese proteins, carbohydrates in bread or pizza dough, and vegetable products in the condiments) as well as unhealthful aspects (high salt and fat and unhealthy additives).

In contrast to this commonsense, folk manner of describing occupations, occupational scientists and others are developing taxonomies, sometimes referred to as occupational classifications or occupational categories, to group objects or events according to like characteristics. The development of taxonomies is complex and not without problems, but the grouping of occupations enables comparisons and other analyses of particular occupational categories, populations, cultures, or topics of interest (28, 29).

There are many ways to classify or group human occupations. One approach is to organize occupations according to their purpose or goal. In this approach, clusters of occupations can be identified based on their intended outcome. For example, grocery shopping, taking out the garbage, cleaning the house, and doing laundry are all considered chores. Their common purpose is to maintain the living environment. Similarly, dressing, bathing, and grooming are all directed toward personal care of the self. Notice that all occupations involve goal-directed behavior. A study by Graham and colleagues attempted to identify categories based on the goal-driven activities of a group of volunteer subjects (30). Their study led to the identification of 18 goal categories, many of which emphasized the social nature of occupations. These goals are (30)

- Be accepted by others.
- Convey information to others.
- Help look after other persons.
- Be in control of the situation.

- Have fun.
- Reduce own anxiety.
- Maintain self-respect or self-esteem.
- Identify financial prospects.
- Attain physical well-being.
- Meet hunger or thirst needs.
- Engage in sexual activity.
- Perform competently.
- Make a favorable impression.
- Seek help, advice, or reassurance.
- Persuade someone to do something.
- Obtain information, learn something new, or solve problems.
- Engage in pleasant social activity.
- Make new friends, develop relationships.

These goal situations were studied further and reduced to just three categories: *interpersonal goals, self-achievement goals,* and *pleasure-seeking goals.*

The classifications for everyday occupations include many categories and typically identify a range of daily pursuits not limited to paid work. Scientists who study time use within populations have developed classifications for use in describing how people occupy their time (31). Other taxonomies have evolved in psychology, leisure studies, and occupational therapy, using categories such as recreation, rest, sleep, relaxation, housework, sports, travel, retirement, labor, work, productivity, worship, celebration, and personal care. These occupational descriptors are general rather than specific and can be further defined with specific types or subcategories of occupational pursuit.

For example, the category of employment or work can be subdivided into literally hundreds of specific paid and unpaid, formally recognized occupations, ranging from airline pilot, to zoologist, to homemaker. Occupational classifications of paid work have developed for use by researchers and policy developers, including sociologists and government workers (see Box 1-2; see also Table 4-1 in Chapter 4)

Another approach to classifying what people do has evolved from scholars interested in places and locations. For example, social geographers and architects are interested in understanding the places or locations in which certain occupations are performed and how places or locations influence habits, routines, or particular kinds of behavior or feelings (32).

Another way of classifying occupations is to simply designate them as obligatory, necessary, or chosen (29). For example, eating and sleeping (and most occupations devoted to care of the self) are necessary for survival and health (see Box 1-3). They are classified as obligatory. On the other hand, free time gives us the opportunity to choose what we will do at our discretion—to select occupations that bring pleasure or satisfaction.

As noted earlier in relation to the question, *How do you occupy your time?* occupational classification is problematic. What is work for one may be leisure for another

BOX 1-2 Classifying Paid Work

Most of the effort in developing systematic classifications of occupations has been done in the area of paid work. Occupations that produce goods and services are necessary for economic strength. Nations, therefore, have had a strong economic incentive to study, understand, and support information about work-related occupations—that is, jobs.

An example of a frequent method for classifying jobs is known as the *behavioral requirements approach.* For example, Fine developed a classification that examines vocational occupations on the basis of the objects (things), information (data), and people required for the job. Using these three categories, jobs can be described according to the degree of complexity of skill required as the worker encounters things, data, or people in the job. This approach formed the basis for developing the classification system in the *Dictionary of Occupational Titles,* which for many years was used in the United States for classifying types of paid work or vocations (74, 75).

Most countries around the world have developed similar classifications of paid occupations (76), such as Canada's National Occupational Classification (77) and Britain's National Vocational Qualifications System (78). Jarman (Chapter 4) highlights the interests of sociology and governments in developing these economically oriented classifications of occupations.

A related approach to classification of occupations is known as the *ability requirements approach.* In this approach, tasks are described based on the abilities required of the performer, such as reasoning, strength, or vision. Early work by Fleishman (79) identified 52 abilities that could be used to describe and classify various worker roles. These abilities still serve as a basis for classifying jobs in the United States. The current system for organizing information about job categories in the United States is called O*NET. This online system, operated by the Department of Labor, relies on a combination of abilities, task requirements, and other factors to differentiate among jobs and provide easily accessible information to employers and workers (80).

(see Box 1-4 and Figures 1-4 ■ and 1-5 ■). Play may be unknown in some cultures; rather, work and play may be intermingled into the rhythm of everyday life. Occupations are not often discrete actions because multiple occupations are often enfolded or nested, occurring simultaneously in the same time and space. Folk taxonomies to describe what people do are often nonspecific but may also be far richer in portraying everyday experience.

Psychological, social, and economic forces may determine what people can or even want to do rather than what they would like to do with their time. The availability

BOX 1-3 Is Sleep an Occupation?

Despite the fact that humans spend nearly one third of their lives sleeping, scientists have known little about sleep until the past two decades. To name sleep as an occupation is itself controversial because occupations are usually equated with action. Nevertheless sleep requires actions to prepare for sleep (making beds, engaging in relaxation routines) or to create a sleep environment (closing curtains, shutting out noise, arranging for a suitable sleeping surface whether sleeping on a mattress indoors or camping on a mat outdoors). Most people, not only scientists, now understand that sleep is essential to good health, that all mammals, not only humans, require it, and that disturbed sleep leads to difficulties during wakefulness (81).

A full understanding of bodily processes during sleep is not yet known. It is known that sleep consists of five phases and that the body cycles through these phases several times each night. Each cycle includes a stage of deep (delta) sleep and culminates in a paradoxical condition in which the eyes move rapidly and the brain shows high electrical activity. This is known as REM, or rapid eye movement, sleep. During this REM stage, lasting 20 to 30 minutes, the body has no control over muscles of the posture and extremities, even though respiration and heart rate have increased substantially. It is during REM sleep that dreams occur.

Some evidence exists to suggest that stressors during the day can affect REM sleep (82, 83). It is known that certain compounds found in foods or pharmaceuticals can disrupt sleep patterns and diminish the restfulness of sleep (84). A number of sleep disorders (such as insomnia, narcolepsy, and sleep apnea) affect significant numbers of people. Because some of these disorders are quite disabling, the amount of scientific attention devoted to understanding sleep is increasing.

Because dreaming is associated with REM sleep, questions are also being asked about the relationship that dreams may have with wakened states (85). Some have speculated that dreaming reflects unconscious mental processes, whereas others speculate that sleep serves as a respite from the need to process environmental information. Sleep seems to be related to restoration of the body, immune function, energy conservation, memory function, temperature regulation, and general development (86).

of time for leisure pursuits has been viewed historically as an indication of social class (31). The political nature of occupations means that some occupations are officially recognized for pay whereas others are not, or some people are paid more for the same occupations than are others. Nevertheless, the question, What is your occupation? is so prevalent in daily life that it is important to consider common ways in which occupations are classified (see Table 1-1 ■).

BOX 1-4 Classifying Leisure

Leisure has been defined as an occupational classification, as discretionary time, and as a state of mind (87, 88). Freedom of choice in participation without a particular goal other than enjoyment seems to be the defining characteristic of leisure (89). This "state of mind philosophy" dates back to the Greek philosophers Aristotle and Plato, who viewed leisure in terms of its opportunity for expression and self-development.

Stebbins (90) has identified two broad categories of leisure, which he has termed casual leisure and serious leisure. Casual leisure seems to be derived from occupations that are pleasurable, are of short duration, are intrinsically rewarding, and require no special training for enjoyment. In contrast, serious leisure includes amateurism, hobbyist pursuits, self-development, and volunteering.

Serious leisure can be identified by six characteristics. These include significant personal effort (including acquisition of knowledge, training, or skill), perseverance, lasting benefit, strong feelings of identification, and a set of beliefs and subculture (90). Fandom and hobbies are two subsets of serious leisure. Fandom pertains to those serious leisure occupations surrounding media (radio, television, and movies) personalities, sports, science fiction, and musicians. Hobbies include engaging in various kinds of crafts (such as sewing or carpentry, collecting, model-making). Stebbins (91) has also identified liberal arts hobbies as a type of serious leisure, which he describes as a fervent pursuit of knowledge for its own sake during free time. Although other types of serious leisure may require study, the pursuit of knowledge in those cases is secondary to participation in the activity. In liberal arts hobbies, the acquisition of knowledge is the primary goal (92).

According to more recent theories, leisure participation fulfills important psychological needs. Recent attempts to classify specific leisure occupations have focused on the personality types attracted to them or the psychological needs they meet. For example, research (93) has matched leisure preferences to six personality types from John Holland's theory. More recently (94), a taxonomy of leisure based on need gratification has been proposed. This classification has eleven clusters of leisure pursuits that fulfill identified needs and was based on analysis of 82 leisure occupations that were ranked by nearly 4,000 subjects (94). These needs include agency, novelty, belongingness, service, sensual enjoyment, cognitive stimulation, self-expression, creativity, competition, vicarious competition, and relaxation.

Leisure participation has economic as well as personal and social implications. Historically, wealth and the time available for leisure were related (94). As industrialized nations developed, more leisure time became available for the working classes. In contemporary Western nations, the time available for leisure activities seems to be declining (46).

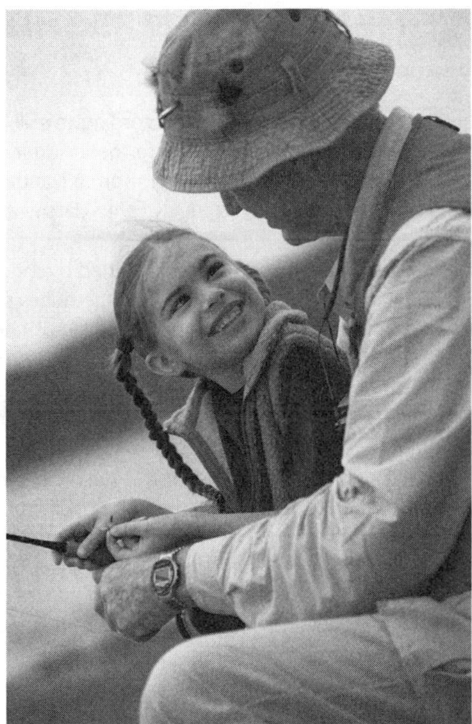

FIGURE 1-4 Fishing is a popular form of casual leisure for young and old alike.
(SW Productions/Getty Images, Inc.- Photodisc.)

What is your occupation? is such a commonplace question, but like the other questions raised in this chapter, there are many answers and many complexities. The question opens the floodgates of occupational classification and the categorization of occupations. General categories, such as paid work and leisure, seem straightforward, but there is much to be known about these and other occupations. Moreover, the categorization is itself controversial given that each category has cultural implications, and occupations are rarely easily and simply assigned to one category. Because occupations are more than activities and tasks, the answer to *What is your occupation?* requires more than the naming and listing of actions. Implied in the question is a request to distinguish the purpose of some occupations in relation to others, for instance, to reply with reference to paid or unpaid occupations. Cultural and social conditions will determine whether the answer raises issues of power, as in stating that your occupation is parenting, for which there is strong social value, but little economic value. There is a growing understanding, both in literature and in the general population, that people need to include more than paid work in everyday life. What else needs to be known so that responses to the question, *What is your occupation?* are more informed?

TABLE 1-1 *Selected Occupational Classification Systems*

Name	Brief Description
Australian Standard Classification of Occupations (ASCO)	Contains 1,079 occupations classified according to skill level (e.g., skilled vs. semiskilled) and the work performed. Administered by the Bureau of Statistics. Uses information from a standard set of descriptors called job content factors (JCFs) to classify and report data about occupations.
International Standard Classification of Occupations (ISCO)	This system is being developed and maintained by the European Union. Occupations are clustered based on the duties performed. Information reported includes a brief (one-paragraph) description of the duties and a listing of the education level generally required. These provide the basis for a hierarchical system that contains 10, 28, 116, and 390 titles at each respective level of the hierarchy.
National Occupational Classification (NOC) (Canada)	This system classifies occupations using two main criteria: skill type and skill level. There are 10 major categories of skill type ranging from management to manufacturing and processing. Under skill level, there are four categories, including university degree, college, technical school or apprenticeship training, high school completion and on-the-job training, and short demonstration training or no formal educational requirements. Using the skill type and level matrix, more than 900 profiles have been developed for 522 unit groups. Each is provided with ratings and descriptor scales in several areas using the updated 2001 classification.
National Vocational Qualifications System (Great Britain)	Based on the competencies required in particular occupations, NVQs are made up of a number of units which set out industry-defined standards of occupational competence. These describe the skills and knowledge people need to be able to perform effectively at work. Eleven major sectors of industry/commerce are identified, and each sector contains five levels of competencies, which range from general foundational skills to skills required in senior management positions.

HOW DOES CONTEXT DETERMINE WHAT PEOPLE DO (AND WHEN THEY DO IT)?

The occupations people choose influence their lifestyles, their comfort, their productivity, their social relationships, and indeed, their health, well-being, and participation in society.

That is, if you examine a person's typical week, there is likely to be a consistent pattern for what is done over time. Similarly if you examine the typical occupations of an organization, such as a government department or business, or of a community, there will be consistent patterns over time. These patterns are influenced by biological factors, by psychological factors including the interests and personalities of those involved, and by the contextual factors that may support or restrict what all or some people do. Typically, these factors interact to explain how time is used in different contexts by different groups or populations. Place or location, already considered earlier, is only one context influencing occupations over time. Consider some examples of other influences on daily occupation and time use.

Biological Factors

Biological influences on time use include age, physical status, and chronobiology, or bodily rhythms. Clearly, as people age their typical use of time changes over the life span. Most infants spend a great deal of time sleeping. In young adulthood, the amount of time spent in sleep often decreases.

Physical status may change time use because it imposes extra demands on the time required to perform different tasks. People with chronic diseases, for example, may have diminished strength or energy, which in turn influences their ability to engage in different occupations.

Our bodies also influence time use through natural rhythms of attention and activity that are influenced by hormones through the endocrine system. Chronobiology is a special field of biology that focuses on these influences. Daily patterns of activity may be influenced by circadian rhythms. The term *circadian* is from the Latin words *circa* (meaning around) and *dia* (meaning day). A 24-hour day constitutes a *round* of embedded or enfolded occupations. Scientists are just now beginning to understand the roles of hormones and how they influence our attention and engagement in occupations over time. This understanding helps us to find ways to cope with situations in which our required occupations are not aligned with our bodily rhythms. Most people know about jet lag, which occurs when travelers cross many time zones. The disruption that sometimes occurs following such travel is called circadian desynchronization. This disruption of internal biological clocks can also occur as a result of shift work and can be of limited duration or longer term. Common symptoms include sleep loss, fatigue, diminished performance, loss of appetite, nervous tension, and a feeling of malaise or ill health.

Biological clocks inside people depend on everyday events in the environment to "set themselves." Exposure to light, having meals, and other routines or patterns of social activity are now known to be important to daily occupational rhythms. The study of human occupation often shows the connection between internal and external influences (such as social factors) on occupational selection and time use (33).

Psychological Factors

As people mature, their preferences and beliefs begin to take shape within a unique personality, which influences their choices and everyday behavior. Personality type may influence the career choices of working adults, as well as preferences for how leisure time is spent (34). Values and beliefs, along with characteristic tendencies to view and interpret the world (sometimes called cognitive style), each strongly influence choices of occupations. These preferences include not only what people choose to do, but also where and with whom we choose to spend time. Current theories of occupational choice emphasize psychological factors, such as personality and self-identity, as important influences on occupational time use and lifestyle patterns.

Contextual Factors

There is no doubt that situational factors, or context, influence what people do. Physical factors include natural conditions, such as the weather, landscape and built environment, and availability of objects such as tools, furniture, and equipment necessary to undertake certain activities. To cite some obvious examples, ice-skating is a limited occupation near the equator, and water sports are impractical in the Sahara desert. Near the arctic, long durations of daylight or darkness can influence occupational as well as circadian cycles. Similarly, differences in the built environment can influence transportation occupations. Traveling by water taxis is common in Venice, whereas traveling by taxis and subways is more practical in London.

Sometimes, the physical characteristics of landscapes and objects invite occupational engagement. For example, the horizontal design of chairs and other smooth horizontal objects invites sitting. Substances and surfaces that can be shaped or manipulated invite touch. Handles invite grabbing. These characteristics of objects and designs were named *affordances* by Gibson, the father of ecological psychology (35). Affordances are environmental properties that both induce and support goal-directed behavior (36).

Another factor that influences engagement in occupations in industrialized societies is the availability of raw materials, finished goods, and services. The supply of objects and tools necessary for some occupations can influence the ability to engage in certain occupations. Thus, without the basketball, the schoolyard game cannot take place. Without parts, repair technicians cannot perform their work. Without building materials and tools, the construction business comes to a standstill, whereas restaurants and supermarkets depend on the regular delivery of fresh produce. Most types of work, play, and leisure depend on the availability of some type of products or services.

In the industrialized world, people are finding increasingly that a key contextual factor influencing occupation is the availability of energy. Without electricity, natural gas, or refined petroleum products, transportation services and some occupations are constrained. Clearly, the availability of objects, manufactured goods, and services is tied to everyday life. This connection between occupations and commerce helps to explain why economists are interested in studying human occupations to understand how people produce or consume goods and services. Thus, people are not only citizens of states or nations; they also constitute a valuable resource known as human capital. This capital has value, however, only because of human occupations—the occupations related to producing or consuming goods or services.

Because humans are social beings, we live in groups and are influenced by other people and by the policies, laws, media, and other conditions that determine what is possible or even thinkable. Social theorists (37, 38) have long recognized that groups of people, whether they are families, cultures, or societies, influence behavior through rules, customs, and traditions. Social expectations, whether they are formal (such as policies and laws) or informal (such as traditions or customs) greatly influence patterns of daily occupations. Social groups influence beliefs about the world, about right and wrong, and about life in general. This influence occurs through implicit or formal teaching and through our lived experience. Beliefs, in turn, greatly influence occupational choices and patterns of time use. When people choose lifestyles that are different from societal norms, their behavior may be classified as deviant (39). There are many categories of deviance that result in lifestyle patterns that are unique to certain groups, sometimes called subcultures.

Flowing from social norms and expectations are the regulations that societies put in place to coordinate and control what people can and, indeed, want to do in the everyday world (40). People know implicitly that what they do is determined by what is allowable and accepted. But people are often unaware of what forces determine daily occupations. Theories of social norms and deviance address this issue of what is allowable and accepted from the point of view of values and beliefs.

However, the more directly powerful, practical forces that define norms and deviance in society are policies, legislation, and market forces. For instance, employment policies, occupational classifications, and market forces determine what occupations receive financial rewards and what occupations are considered private and unpaid (41). Consider the regulation of occupations in hunting-and-gathering societies. Likely such communities have very few written policies, but the economy and understood policies are that all males participate in gathering food, while all females and children participate in preparing food. The national policies that govern what people in communities can do may define some people as unemployed because their gross annual income is minimal. As unemployed people, they may not be eligible for health insurance or national pensions for seniors, even though they have engaged in meaningful occupations and "worked" all their lives.

Contrast the regulation of hunting-and-gathering occupations with that of occupations in the global telecommunications industry. There is a huge, interconnected, written, but often taken-for-granted network of policies, laws, and financial regulation of these occupations. Anyone who has invested in telecommunications, or has worked in this field, will know that the occupations that use video display terminals (VDT's), for example, are highly regulated as a component of international telecommunications. Salaries are low, and repetitive motion injuries are high for workers in front of VDT's. These are often (but not exclusively) women in office occupations, such as secretarial work (42–44) or those serving as online customer service representatives. Hence, the often taken-for-granted control of occupations is not always direct, but rather has a filter-down impact that is invisible and connected with world events and powerful forces that shape everyday life.

Social factors, whether they are traditions, expectations, or regulating policies, interact with biological factors to influence patterns of time use across the life span. During childhood, greater periods are spent in exploration and play occupations that are vital for learning and physical maturation (see Box 1-5 and Figure 1-5).

BOX 1-5 Play: The Occupations of Children

The inclusion of play as an occupational category is of interest, particularly in studying child development (see Davis & Polatajko, Chapter 6), but also in considering the relationships between occupation and health, well-being, quality of life, and justice (see Whiteford, Chapter 12, and Stadnyk, Townsend, & Wilcock, Chapter 13). Play is one of the primary occupations of childhood. It is often described as self-motivated or chosen, pleasurable, and important from a developmental perspective because play offers abundant opportunities for learning. Because it is self-chosen and pleasurable, play is also a term often used to describe the nonwork occupations of adults. Parham (95) and Takata (96) have each observed that play can be described best as a behavioral style or attitude. For this reason, periods of work may be interspersed with playful moments.

Dutch historian Johan Huizinga (97) expressed the notion of play as an attitude and behavioral style, rather than a specific type of occupation. In his 1938 book, *Homo Ludens,* Huizinga traced the evolution of play from preindustrial times. Huizinga noted that play comes from an attitude of finding and sharing joy in the requirements of everyday life, so that even seemingly serious events can reveal playful elements. He lamented that, in the modern age, the fundamental nature of play was being commercialized into sport and entertainment that lacked community-based and cultural values of play viewed as important in earlier times.

Most approaches to describing play have emerged from theorists interested in how play influences social, physical, and cognitive developments during childhood. Influenced by Jean Piaget (98) and others, these approaches describe play as intrinsically motivated and active, noting that play focuses on process rather than outcome.

Behavioral scientists have proposed various play classifications. For younger children, play is classified according to its social dimensions, beginning with solitary play and progressing to types of cooperative play with others. Another approach to classifying play focuses on its processes, including functional play, which consists of simple repetitive movements, to more advanced types of play involving creativity, imagination, and the use of rules. Typically, types of play in children correspond to particular stages of development because they require different levels of cognitive, physical, and social skill (99).

Typical patterns exist for students, for working adults, and for retired people. Many retired people have greater periods of discretionary time available to them than they did when they were employed. Certainly, some people are different, but general patterns of time use can be found that characterize different stages of life. These vary somewhat across cultures, although occupational patterns across the world are remarkably similar (45).

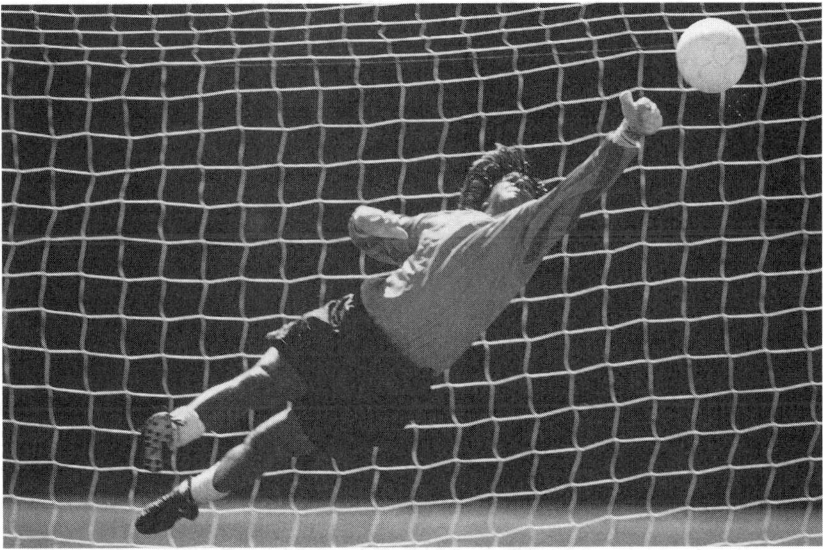

FIGURE 1-5 Play is a principal occupation of children.
(David Madison/Getty Images Inc.-Stone Allstock)

The availability of free time and how it is used is a topic of interest to social scientists from many fields. The amount of time apportioned toward leisure, paid work, and unpaid work has social, political, and economic implications. After several decades in which the amount of discretionary time for working-class individuals has steadily increased, there is evidence that these trends may have reversed so that the time available for relaxation and leisure now and in future may be diminishing (46).

HOW DOES OCCUPATION INFLUENCE HEALTH, WELL-BEING, AND JUST PARTICIPATION IN SOCIETY?

A growing body of literature is showing that lifestyle and occupational choices influence both physical and psychological well-being. The field of health promotion has for years recognized that most disease and injury is preventable, and that lifestyle choices such as regular exercise, nutrition, adequate sleep, and avoidance of stress, tobacco, and excessive alcohol use can improve health and increase the life span (47). What is important in modern health systems, critics argue, is attention to social, environmental, and behavioral issues that determine how, when and where people make responsible lifestyle choices (48).

Behavioral scientists interested in how individual differences, personality, and lifestyle factors influence well-being have shown that engagement in personally meaningful occupations can influence happiness and life satisfaction (49, 50). So-called

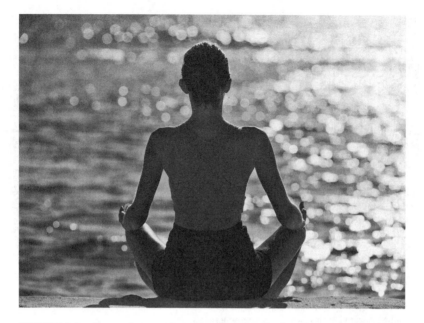

FIGURE 1-6 Occupations can have significant implications for personal health and happiness. Finding a balance in occupations is also important for reducing stress. (Photodisc/Getty Images)

person–environment or ecological models of adaptation suggest that people thrive when their personalities and needs are matched with environments or situations that enable them to remain engaged, interested, and challenged (51, 52). Humans participate, and they do so through occupation as a vital component of their overall well-being (53).

The relationship between lifestyles (which are largely defined by occupations) and health and well-being is now being considered from a more macroscopic viewpoint. Instead of focusing attention on isolated aspects of safety or health associated with particular occupations, social scientists are now concerning themselves with overall patterns of occupations and how they work to define optimal and equitable lifestyles (16). These concerns have arisen from the increasing pace of change and the time crunch experienced by people living in modern industrialized nations as they try to fit more productivity occupations within each day. The stress created by these circumstances has given rise to research on life balance, variously called work–life balance, role balance, or work–family balance, because employers are interested in avoiding the economic costs associated with absenteeism, turnover, or stress-related illnesses (15, 17) (see Figure 1-6 ■). In addition, increasing life expectancy in many societies has created a larger number of healthy, active people in retirement. This increasing period of life beyond the child-rearing and paid employment years has created interest in finding ways to promote active lifestyles to enrich the lives of older persons and prevent the psychological and biological consequences of lonely or inactive lifestyles (54).

Occupations are fundamental to participation in society, and participation, in turn is fundamental to social equity. The ideal of equitable personhood depends on all people participating in their communities as they are able and wish to be included in the central occupations of a society. For instance, persons with intellectual, physical, or psychiatric disabilities, single parents at home with children, refugees, retirees, and unskilled persons may be excluded from full participation in paid and other occupations by poverty, stigma, lack of transportation, or regulations that limit their participation (55). They become more fully participating citizens when they are included either by their engagement in paid work or by social recognition of their economic and social contributions (56). Participation in the cultural, economic, social, and political occupations of a society requires a respect for differences to transcend discriminatory and sometimes abusive forms of exclusion (57). Bourdieu, a French sociologist (58), expressed an occupational perspective, although not in such terms, in his recognition that participation in everyday life is a basic requirement for citizenship. Thus, values, beliefs, and social structures are contextual factors that influence and are influenced by participation in occupations. And occupations are directed related to health, well-being, and just or unjust participation in society.

CHAPTER SUMMARY

To rethink occupation is to recognize the richness and complexity of occupation. The task of defining occupation is not simply a matter of translating the Latin word *occupare.* Nor can occupation be fully understood by listing categories of paid occupations. When the Roman poet and philosopher Horace offered the admonition *Carpe Diem,* meaning seize the day, he was suggesting something far more than merely passing time or existing. In rethinking occupation, one can imagine that Horace was recommending that people live life to the fullest by learning about and making full use of occupation as the fabric for experiencing and structuring everyday life.

In the preceding pages, the complexity of human occupation has been introduced. It has been shown that occupations reflect time use according to both individual and cultural characteristics, and that biological (i.e., ecological) and psychological factors, as well as social conditions, influence occupational choices.

Approaches to identifying categories of occupational pursuit were described. It was noted that international time use studies provide useful information on human productivity and social trends. These studies are helping to provide a beginning taxonomy for describing and classifying human occupations. Some categories of occupations, including paid work, leisure, sleep, basic self-care, and household work were introduced. In each of these areas of human endeavor are implications for health, well-being and participation in society.

As an area of interest and study, human occupation cuts a broad swath across the biological, social, environmental design, and behavioral sciences, yet only recently has occupational science emerged as an interdisciplinary science. Occupation appears to be fundamental to human existence and to the organization of societies. An Introduction to Occupation is only a beginning.

STUDY GUIDE

Study Guide Author: Julie Bass Haugen

Summary of Main Points

This chapter emphasized the complexity of the seemingly simple concept of occupation. It was observed that occupations support peoples' very existence and overall sense of well-being. The chapter introduced five questions and several strategies that may serve as a foundation for learning about occupation. Observations of everyday scenarios, like a street scene, provide opportunities to expand our knowledge about the breadth of occupations. The meaning and importance of occupations may be studied through measures of time use, classification schemes, and individual narratives. The depth of knowledge about occupation may be appreciated by examining specific areas of inquiry, like paid work, play, and sleep. All of these approaches help us to appreciate the importance of occupations in the human experience.

Application to Occupational Therapy

In the practice of occupational therapy, it is important to remember that the occupations of a person are complex, unique to the person and even shape the sense of self. Thus, when a health or social condition or a disability changes a person's engagement in occupations, there are corresponding changes in identity, well-being and participation in society. The five questions discussed in this chapter are also evident in the occupational therapy evaluation process. The answers to these questions from the client's perspective provide client-centred occupational therapy practitioners with valuable information for intervention planning, and evaluation of the effectiveness of services. Occupational therapy services that address the client's priorities and needs for occupation will also influence overall health, well-being and just or unjust participation in society.

This introductory chapter on occupation provides an important foundation for addressing occupations within occupational therapy practice with individuals, families, groups, communities, organizations or populations. Occupational therapists use classifications/taxonomies to document occupations for interventions that introduce new or restored habits and routines that may improve occupational engagement.

Individual Learning Activities

1. Keep a detailed occupational journal for one weekday and one weekend day. Using the concepts from the chapter, write a summary of your journal for these two days to provide
   a. Two to three examples of occupations
      Meaningfulness
      Purpose or goals of occupations
      Context
      Approximate time involvement
   b. Two to three examples of
      Habits
      Routines
      Roles

Nested or embedded occupations
Primary and secondary occupations

c. A description of your lifestyle based on your occupations

2. Conduct an interview of a person who has had recent health or social issues and is willing to share an occupational story with you. Discuss the following:
   a. What were the primary roles and lifestyle prior to the health or social issues?
   b. Did the health or social issues change how time is used or the way in which occupations are done? If yes, how?
   c. Have habits or routines been modified as a result of the issues?
   d. What occupations have been particularly meaningful during this time and why?
   e. How has the "doing" of these occupations influenced the person's health status?
3. Identify two to three of your own questions related to occupations and health, well-being or participation in society.
4. Write a summary of your interview and your analysis of the relationship between health, well-being, participation in society and occupational engagement for this person.
5. Examine the website for the World Health Organization's International Classification of Functioning, Disability, and Health (ICF) (http://www.who.int/classifications/icf/en/).
   a. What are the occupational categories listed under Activities and Participation?
   b. What are the contexts for occupation listed under Environment?

Group Learning Activity

Select one vocation/job of interest for each member of your group. Examine the occupational characteristics for each vocation/job using two classification systems.

a. Explore the websites for O*Net Online (http://online.onetcenter.org/) and Canada's National Occupational Classification (http://www23.hrdc-drhc.gc.ca/2001/e/generic/welcome.shtml).
b. Identify the general factors included in occupational descriptions for the two systems. How are they similar and different? Summarize what you have learned about these two classification systems.
c. Compare and contrast the occupational descriptions of specific vocations or jobs in both systems.
d. Did one classification system provide you with more information (the what) about the vocation or job and the meaning it might have for an individual (the why)? Explain.

Study Questions

1. The word *occupation* comes from the Latin root word *occupatio*, meaning to
   a. Do
   b. Seize
   c. Participate
   d. Occur

2. Nested or embedded occupations may be defined as
   a. Simultaneous participation in more than one occupation
   b. A classification system for occupations
   c. Doing occupations in a manner that fully involves effort and attention
   d. The underlying meaning of an observable occupation
3. "Relatively automatic, repetitive patterns of human behavior" is a definition of a
   a. Lifestyle
   b. Occupation
   c. Routine
   d. Habit
4. Automaticity in behaviors can be both helpful and problematic.
   a. True
   b. False
5. Biological factors influencing occupation include all of the following EXCEPT
   a. Age
   b. Chronobiology
   c. Personality
   d. Physical status

REFERENCES

1. Nelson, D. L. (1988). Occupation: Form and performance. *American Journal of Occupational Therapy, 42*(10), 633–641.
2. Christiansen, C., Clark, F. A., Kielhofner, G., & Rogers, J. (1995). Position paper: Occupation. *American Journal of Occupational Therapy, 49*(10), 1015–1018.
3. Jonsson, H., Josephsson, S., & Kielhofner, G. (2001). Narratives and experience in an occupational transition: A longitudinal study of the retirement process. *American Journal of Occupational Therapy, 55*(4), 424–432.
4. Bateson, M. C. (1986). Enfolded activity and the concept of occupation. In R. Zemke & F. Clark (Eds.), *Occupational science: The evolving discipline* (pp. 5–12). Philadelphia: F.A. Davis.
5. Camic, C. (1986). The matter of habit. *American Journal of Sociology, 91*, 1039–1087.
6. Clark, F. A. (2000). The concepts of habit and routine: A preliminary theoretical synthesis. *The Occupational Therapy Journal of Research, 20*, 123S–138S.
7. Corbin, J. M. (1999). *The role of habits in everyday life. A Synthesis of Knowledge Regarding the Concept of Habit.* Pacific Grove, CA: American Occupational Therapy Foundation.
8. Dunn, W. W. (2000). Habit: What's the brain got to do with it? *The Occupational Therapy Journal of Research, 20*(Supplement 1), 2s–5s.
9. Christiansen, C. H. (2005). Time use and patterns of occupation. In C. Christiansen & M. C. Baum (Eds.), *Occupational therapy: Performance, participation and well-being* (3rd ed., pp. 70–91). Thorofare, NJ: Slack, Inc.
10. Young, M. (1988). *The metronomic society.* Cambridge, MA: Harvard University Press.
11. Bargh, J. A. (1997). The automaticity of everyday life. In R. S. Wyer (Ed.), *Advances in social cognition.* Mahwah, NJ: Erlbaum.

12. Ferguson, M. J., Bargh, J. A. (2004). Liking is for doing: The effects of goal pursuit on automatic evaluation. *Journal of Personality and Social Psychology, 87*, 557–572.
13. Bargh, J. A. & Chartrand, T. L. (1999). The unbearable automaticity of being. *American Psychologist, 54*, 462–479.
14. Bargh, J. A., Chen, M., & Burrows, L. (1996). Automaticity of social behavior: Direct effects of trait construct and stereotype priming on action. *Journal of Personality and Social Psychology, 71*, 230–244.
15. Backman, C. M. (2004). Muriel Driver Lectureship: Occupational balance: Exploring the relationships among daily occupations and their influence on well-being. *Canadian Journal of Occupational Therapy, 71*(4), 202–209.
16. Sheldon, K. M. (2004). *Optimal human being: An integrated, multilevel perspective.* Mahwah, NJ: Erlbaum.
17. Christiansen, C. H., & Matuska, K. M. (2006). Lifestyle balance: A review of concepts and research. *Journal of Occupational Science, 13*(1), 48–61.
18. Christiansen, C. (1993). Three perspectives on balance in occupation. In F. Clark & R. Zemke (Eds.), *Occupational science: Selections from the symposia* (pp. 431–451). Philadelphia: F. A. Davis.
19. Erikson, E. H. (1982). *The life cycle completed.* New York: Norton.
20. Christiansen, C. (1999). Occupation as identity. Competence, coherence and the creation of meaning. *American Journal of Occupational Therapy, 53*(6), 547–558.
21. Bateson, M. C. (1990). *Composing a life.* New York: Penguin.
22. Markus, H., & Nurius, P. (1986). Possible selves. *American Psychologist, 41*, 954–969.
23. Hammel, K. (2001). Intrinsicality: Reconsidering spirituality . . . Occupation as spiritual activity. *American Journal of Occupational Therapy, 51*, 181–185.
24. Bruner, J. (1990). *Acts of meaning.* Cambridge, MA: Harvard University Press.
25. McAdams, D. P. (1993). *The stories we live by: Personal myths and the making of the self.* New York: Guilford Press.
26. Greer, G. (2000). *The whole woman.* New York: Anchor Books.
27. Frieden, B. (1963). *The feminine mystique.* New York: W. W. Norton.
28. Christiansen, C. (1992). The study and classification of occupation. In N. Gillette (Ed.), *AOTF Research Colloquium.* Houston: American Occupational Therapy Foundation.
29. Christiansen, C. (1994). The study and classification of occupation: A review and discussion of taxonomies. *Journal of Occupational Science, 1*(1), 3–21.
30. Graham, J. A., Argyle, M., & Furnham, A. (1980). The goal structure of situations. *European Journal of Social Psychology, 10*, 345–366.
31. Harvey, A. S. (1993). Guidelines for time use data collection. *Social Indicators Research, 30*(2–3), 197–228.
32. Rowles, G. (1991). Beyond performance: Being in place as a component of occupational therapy. *American Journal of Occupational Therapy, 45*(3), 265–271.
33. Halberg, F. (1994). *Introduction to chronobiology.* Minneapolis, MN: Medtronic.
34. Furnham, A. (1981). Personality and activity preference. *British Journal of Social Psychology, 20*(1), 57–68.
35. Gibson, J. J. (1979). *The ecological approach to vision perception.* Boston: Houghton Mifflin.
36. Shaw, R. E., Kugler, P. N., & Kinsella-Shaw, M. M. (1990). Reciprocities of intentional systems. In R. Warren & A. H. Wertheim (Eds.). *Perception and control of self motion* (pp. 579–619). Hillsdale, NJ: Erlbaum.
37. Cooley, C. H. (1902). *Human nature and the social order.* New York: Charles Scribner's.
38. Mead, G. H. (1996). *Mind, self and society.* Chicago: University of Chicago Press.
39. Goode, E. (1996). *Social deviance.* Boston: Allyn & Bacon.

40. Smith, D. E., (2005). *Institutional ethnography: A sociology for people.* Walnut Creek, CA: Alta Mira Press.
41. Townsend, E. (1997). Occupation: Potential for personal and social transformation. *Journal of Occupational Science, 4*(1), 18–26.
42. Houtman, I. L. D, Bongers, P. M., Smulders, P. G. W., & Kompier, M. A. J. (1994). Psychosocial stressors at work and musculoskeletal problems. *Scandinavian Journal of Work, Environment and Health, 20,* 139–145.
43. Landisbergis, P., Schnall, P. L., Dietz, D. I., Warren, K., Pickering, T. G., & Schwartz, J. E. (1998). Job strain and health behaviors: Results of a prospective study. *American Journal of Health Promotion, 12,* 237–245.
44. Tittiranonda, P., Burastero, S., & Rempel, D. (1999). Risk factors for musculoskeletal disorders among computer users. *Occupational Medicine, 14,* 17–34.
45. Szalai, A. (Ed.). (1972). *The use of time.* The Hague, Netherlands: Mouton.
46. Sullivan, O. G. (2001). Cross national changes in time-use. *British Journal of Sociology, 52*(1), 331–348.
47. McKeown, T. (1976). *The role of medicine: Dream, mirage or nemesis?* London: Nuffield Provincial Hospital Trust.
48. Callahan, D. (1998). *False hope.* New York: Simon & Schuster.
49. Christiansen, C., Backman, C., Little, B. R., & Nguyen, A. Occupations and subjective well-being: A study of personal projects. *American Journal of Occupational Therapy, 53*(1), 91–100.
50. Diener, E. (2000). Subjective well-being: The science of happiness and a proposal for a national index. *American Psychologist, 55*(1), 34–43.
51. Csikszentmihalyi, M. (1990). *Flow—The psychology of optimal experience.* New York: Harper and Row.
52. Christiansen, C. H., Little, B. R., & Backman, C. (1998). Personal projects: A useful approach to the study of occupation. *American Journal of Occupational Therapy, 52*(6), 439–446.
53. Cantor, N., & Sanderson, C. (1999). Life task participation and well-being. The importance of taking part in daily life. In D. Kahneman & E. Diener (Eds.), *Well-being: The foundations of hedonic psychology* (pp. 230–243). New York New York: Sage Foundation.
54. Ryff, C. D. (1995). Psychological well-being in adult life. *Current Directions in Psychological Science, 4,* 99–104.
55. World Health Organization. (2001). *International classification of functioning, disability and health.* Geneva, Switzerland: World Health Organization.
56. Whiteford, G., & Wright-St. Clair, V. (Eds.). (2005). *Occupation and practice in context.* Merrickville, NSW: Elsevier Australia.
57. Thibeault, R. (2002). Occupation and the rebuilding of civil society: Notes from the war zone. *Journal of Occupational Science, 9*(1), 38–47.
58. Bordieu, P. (1999). Weight of the world. Social suffering in contemporary society. Polity press.
59. Stringer, C., & Gamble, C. (1993). *In search of Neanderthals: Solving the puzzle of modern human origins.* New York: Thames and Hudson Inc.
60. Pieper, J. (1963). *Leisure: The basis of culture.* New York: New American Library.
61. Warner, R. (1958). *The Greek philosophers.* New York: Mentor.
62. Brunschwig, J., & Lloyd, G. E. R. (Eds.). (2000). *Greek thought: A guide to classical knowledge.* Cambridge, MA: Harvard University Press.
63. Cicero, M. T. (1960). *Cicero: Selected works.* London: Viking Penguin-Putnam.

64. Rappaport, S. (1910). *Tales and maxims from the Talmud.* London: George Routledge's Sons.
65. Dark, K. (2000). *Britain and the end of the Roman Empire.* Stroud, United Kingdom: Tempus Publishing.
66. Lindberg, C. (Ed.). (1999). *The European reformations sourcebook.* Oxford: Blackwell.
67. McGrath, A. E. (1990). *A life of John Calvin: A study in shaping the Western culture.* Oxford: Blackwell.
68. Leuchtenburg, W. (1963). *Franklin D. Roosevelt and the New Deal.* New York: Harper & Row.
69. Jeffries, J. W. (1996). *Wartime America: The World War II home front.* Chicago: Ivan R. Dee.
70. Ferguson, M. (1980). *The aquarian conspiracy: Personal and social transformation in the 1980s.* Los Angeles: J. P. Tarcher.
71. Naisbitt, J. (1982). *Megatrends: Ten new directions transforming our lives.* New York: Warner Books.
72. Cross, G. (1990). *A social history of leisure since 1600.* State College, PA: Venture Publishing, Inc.
73. Durant, W. (1957). *The story of civilization: Part VI: The Reformation.* New York: Simon & Schuster.
74. Fine, S. A. (1988). Functional job analysis. In S. Gael S (Ed.), *The job analysis handbook for business, industry, government* (pp. 1019–1035). New York: Wiley.
75. Fine, S. A. (1955, October). A structure of worker functions. *Personnel and Guidance Journal, 34,* 66–73.
76. Hoffman, E. (1991). *Mapping the world of work: An international review of the use and gathering of occupational information.* Washington, DC: Bureau of Labor Statistics.
77. *National occupational classification.* (2001). Ottawa, Canada: Human Resources Development Canada.
78. Elias, P. (1996). *A review of the standard occupational classification.* Coventry: Institute for Employment Research, University of Warwick.
79. Fleishman, E. A., & Quaintance, M. K. (1984). *Taxonomies of human performance: The description of human tasks.* Orlando: Academic Press.
80. Peterson, N., Mumford, M., Borman, W., Jeanneret, P., Fleishman, E., & Levin, K. (1997). *O*NET final technical report* (Vols. 1–3). Salt Lake City, UT: National Center for O*NET Development, U.S. Department of Labor.
81. Aronoff, M. S. (1991). *Sleep and its secrets: The river of crystal light.* Los Angeles: Insight Books.
82. Horne, J. A., & Minard, A. S. (1985). Sleep and sleepiness following a behaviorally "active" day. *Ergonomics, 28,* 567–575.
83. Meguro, K., Ueda, M., Yamaguchi, T., Sekita, Y., Yamazaki, H., Oikawa, Y., et al. (1990). Disturbance in daily sleep/wake patterns in patients with cognitive impairment and decreased daily activity. *Journal of the American Geriatrics Society, 38*(11), 1176–1182.
84. Minors, D. S., Rabbitt, P. M. A., Worthington, & H., Waterhouse, J. M. (1989). Variation in meals and sleep-activity patterns in aged subjects; its relevance to circadian rhythm studies. In *Chronobiology International* (pp. 139–146). Oxford: Pergamon Press Inc.
85. Siegel, J. M. (1994). Brainstem mechanisms generating REM sleep. In M. K. Kryger & W. C. Dement (Eds.), *Principles and practice of sleep medicine* (2nd ed., pp. 125–144). New York: W. B. Saunders.
86. Hobson, J. (1995). *Sleep.* New York: Scientific American Library.
87. Gunter, B. G., Stanley, J., & St. Clair, R. (1985). Theoretical issues in leisure study. In B.G. Gunter, J. Stanley, & R. St. Clair (Eds.), *Transitions to leisure: Conceptual and human issues* (pp. 35–51). Lanham, MD: University Press of America.

88. Witt, P. A., & Goodale, T. (1982). Stress, leisure and the family. *Recreation Research Review, 9*(3), 28–32.
89. Iso-Ahola, S. E. (1979). Basic dimensions of definitions of leisure. *Journal of Leisure Research, 11*, 28–39.
90. Stebbins, R. A. (1997). Casual leisure: A conceptual statement. *Leisure Studies, 16*, 17–25.
91. Stebbins, R. A. (1998). The liberal arts hobbies: A neglected subtype of serious leisure. *Leisure and Society, 17*(1), 173–186.
92. Holmberg, K., Rosen, D., & Holland, J. L. (1990). *The leisure activities finder.* Odessa, FL: Psychological Assessment Resources.
93. Tinsley, H. E., & Eldridge, B. D. (1995). Psychological benefits of leisure participation: A taxonomy of leisure activities based on their need gratifying properties. *Journal of Counseling Psychology, 42*(2), 123–132.
94. Veblen, T. (1899). *A theory of the leisure class: An economic study of institutions.* New York: The Macmillan Co.
95. Parham, L. D. (1996). Perspectives on play. In R. Zemke & F. Clark (Eds.), *Occupational science: The emerging discipline* (pp. 71–88). Philadelphia: F. A. Davis.
96. Takata, N. (1971). The play milieu—a preliminary proposal. *American Journal of Occupational Therapy, 23*, 314–318.
97. Huizinga, J. (1964). *Homo ludens: A study of the play element in culture* (4th ed.). Boston: Beacon.
98. Piaget, J. (1969). *The psychology of the child.* New York: Basic Books.
99. Bergen, D. (1988). *Play as a medium for learning.* Portsmouth, NH: Heinemann.

CHAPTER 2

Cultural Perspectives on Occupation

Michael K. Iwama

OBJECTIVES

1. Present an historical view of the concept of culture and its influence on worldviews.
2. Discuss culture from a social lens to understand the meanings of occupation.
3. Compare and contrast cultural influences on ways of knowing and concepts of truth.
4. Compare Western individualistic ideas of occupation with the Eastern (Japanese) collectivist view.

KEY WORDS

Amae
Culture
Epistemology
Occupation
Ontology
Postmodernism
Relativism
Social constructionism
Soto
Uchi
Universalism

CHAPTER PROFILE

In this chapter, a particular view of culture is considered as a variable social lens or medium through which the concept of occupation is understood. So much of what is "normal" and commonplace in our daily lives remains hidden from view, blended into the familiar routines, habits, and patterns of activity that fill the day. Much of the evolving study of occupation is based on meanings common to the industrialized world and in the familiar Western ways of knowing. The empirical method—or

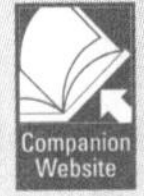

www.prenhall.com/christiansen

The Internet provides an exciting means for interacting with this textbook and for enhancing your understanding of humans' experiences with occupations and the organization of occupations in society. Use the address above to access the interactive Companion Website created specifically to accompany this book. Here you will find an array of self-study material designed to help you gain a richer understanding of the concepts presented in this chapter.

science—is one familiar way of knowing. When a competing view or explanation of phenomena is presented, the mundane and normal become transformed into something remarkable, interesting, and worthy of consideration. In the same way that a vacation takes on greater importance in the context of having to endure a particularly stressful job, or a cup of drinkable water rises in value in the wake of a terribly long drought; this chapter presents a competing view of occupation based on East Asian society and culture. It provides a dramatic point of comparison to an empirical, Western view to shed new insights into the complexity and breadth of human occupation. Numerous worldviews of occupation could have served as points of comparison to the empirical view, such as views of occupation that take into account sexual orientation, gender, socioeconomic status, class, age group, or any constructed category of shared experiences. However, an East Asian comparative context is chosen as a social lens on occupation because of its familiarity and interest to the chapter's author.

The chapter begins with an exercise of considering fundamental differences in how people perceive and make sense of themselves and the world in which they exist. This individual viewpoint is called a worldview. Differences in worldviews can explain cultural variations in understanding aspects of the world, such as human occupation. The chapter then questions the universality of social concepts like culture and occupation. Culture's variability in meaning according to place and time is offered as a point to consider how the concept of occupation can also vary according to unique, individual situations. In particular, descriptions of Japanese social structure and cultural patterns are used to illustrate how assumptions can differ about the nature of occupation. The purpose of this chapter is to broaden the growing discussion about occupation by exposing readers to an alternative (cultural) view of the meaning of human actions in the world, thereby stimulating some reflections regarding how the study and discussion of human occupation might proceed.

INTRODUCTION

Does truth exist outside the self—out there—universally and waiting to be discovered and understood through some valid method? Or does truth exist within the self, varying and changing according to the broader contexts in which the self is inextricably imbedded? This fundamental issue, and variations of it, debated among great philosophers throughout the ages, remains current today and holds significant implications for the study and understanding of occupation. Where one's own worldviews reside along the continuum spanning the poles of this great debate could influence to a large extent how human occupation is comprehended and appreciated.

If one's worldview is found at one end of the continuum, where reality and truth are perceived to exist external to the self, there may be a tendency to place one's self, or one's point of reference, in a central location. The tendency may be to comprehend the environment to exist outside the self—both the self and the environment separated as distinct entities or objects. Such a view of reality and truth often accompanies an understanding of occupation as an individual matter. This view supports an intepretation of occupation as a bridge or connection between a distinct self and a separate and distinct environment.

When such a rational view of reality persists, a convincing case can be made about the relationship between what one does and what one comprehends about personal fulfillment, satisfaction, and well-being. This view of a separate self and environment enables an emphasis on self, agency, and personal well-being, as well as on the ability of the individual to exploit the surrounding environment. The emerging interest in a science of humans as occupational beings (occupational science), when directed toward studying the forms, functions, and meanings (1) of what people do, is largely consistent to date with this particular worldview.

A worldview that regards truth as existing universally "out there" may prefer rational explanations of how the world and its phenomena are connected in some ultimate logical way. The preference for "grand" or overarching theory as valid explanations of phenomena, knowable through the human senses (objectivism/empiricism), is a hallmark of this particular perspective. This is the same perspective that has given rise to the prevalent, Western, positivist scientific tradition of the modern era, representing empiricism as the dominant standard of truth in the industrialized world. Proponents of empirical science may treat matters of culture as a feature found within people—an embodiment or categorical marker of distinction. Definitions of culture expressed along matters of race and ethnicity are common artifacts of this particular view, for these concepts lend themselves well to definition and measurement.

An alternative perspective for considering human occupation is one in which the individual is not the central focus. Rather than considering the individual self as a central point of reference from which to make sense of the universe and truth, this alternative worldview regards humans as just another part of the an environment that includes the totality of the universe. People who follow traditional East Asian religious or philosophical forms, such as Buddhism, will be familiar with this type of worldview. In this worldview, humans are not necessarily given a place of privilege vis-à-vis the world, but "no less than the trees and the sky, (humans) have a right to be here" (2). The self is de-centered, and truth is interpreted in relation to other elements that share the surrounding context. Truth, from this regard, is not singular and universal, but rather is viewed as being multiple and changing according to nuances in the situation. The meanings of things and phenomena are not necessarily seen to be universally stable and "out there" waiting to be discovered, but rather they are viewed to be socially constructed (3, 4, 5) and varied. Subsequently, such pluralistic and particular worldviews shun or dismiss the authority of a grand and overarching theory. This perspective is often opposed to Western, empirical scientific views of being because it regards this type of science as merely one of many ways of knowing.

This latter worldview is congruent with postmodernism (6), taking a typical relativistic view, preferring to explain phenomena and meaning in relation to other embedded phenomena and objects found in a common context. Here, there is no gap between self and environment (7). This view challenges objectivist and pragmatic assumptions about the forms, functions and meanings of occupation. A key point with such a worldview is that the forms, functions and meanings of human occupation are not necessarily universal but rather understood to be socially constructed and varying according to the underlying context as viewed by persons within a particular situation.

RELATIVISM AND THE CONSEQUENCES OF CULTURE

Relativism provides an alternate way of viewing culture to the empirical view. As much as culture represents the categories and distinctive markers of human activities, objects and phenomena (for example, the construct of race and the stereotypical behavioral patterns and practices associated with a particular identified group of people), culture is also a process. Distinctive markers are created, maintained, and translated by people who share a common sphere of experience, situated in a particular place and time (context) (8). For example, taxonomists within the field of biology may point out the various categories and subcategories of the flora and fauna in a certain geographical region during a specific era, and articulate the inclusion criteria used in the nomenclature process. Although these categories and rules of inclusion can be taken for granted among those who share a similar outlook, they may conflict with another group's view and organizing schema of the same phenomena. Rather than accept taken for granted categories as a description of reality—of what is universally "out there," relativists may argue that particular categories and inclusion criteria are arbitrarily determined—or constructed (9). The relativist argument is that the organization, structure, and content of categories may differ when viewed from different cultural spheres of experience or situation.

From one side of the continuum of worldviews, the views of the other can appear incredible and be judged simply as "wrong." Depending on what is at stake, alternate views can be interpreted as misguided and, at times, even threatening. Using the authority that has been given to empiricism or "objective science" in the industrialized world, the views of the relativist can be discredited as irrational, being particularly "unscientific." However, from the other's vantage point, empiricism may appear to be similarly misguided with its restricted, positivistic explanations of the meaning of it all. The constellation of shared values, beliefs, and views of what is normal and what is viewed as truth by one group can render other groups' values and beliefs to be invalid. This is the challenge and paradox of forms, functions and meanings of occupation when framed in terms of culture. Are our worldviews, our meanings of truth(s), and our patterns regarding human activities and their meanings in the larger scheme (context) of things acquired through our biological ancestry—through our DNA? Or are they acquired through a social process of mutual or different experiences of phenomena and shared or diverse understandings (or meanings) bound in time and place?

The lack of consensus or universal agreement on what is worth knowing and what is worth doing between these two cultural views of reality—empirical and relativist—raises important issues over just how the study of human occupation ought to proceed. By remaining partial to an empirical view of human occupation, the study of occupation runs the risk of remaining relatively narrow in its scope, catering to a particular dominant worldview and interpretation of the meaning of human agency. The science of occupation may privilege certain (Western) cultural interpretations of occupation and, in turn, limit or devalue the worldviews of cultures that hold a different view of truth and the meaning of human existence and action. Will the relevance and study of occupation be confined to the culture of modern, empirical science and the rational leanings of the Western industrialized world, or will it proceed to also include the diverse cultural comprehensions of human activity beyond empiricism and current familiar cultural boundaries?

In this chapter, the concept of culture, interpreted in its most current and progressive way, is used to consider how varying worldviews and shared experiences of the social world might affect one's understanding of the forms, functions, and meanings (1) of occupation in the contexts of daily life. The same view of culture is also used to gain some insight into humans as occupational beings. Subsequent chapters provide convincing views and explanations of what human occupation is understood to be. Intentionally, the relativists' position, situated at the "other" extreme of the ontological continuum presented at the beginning of this chapter, is taken, and some brief but compelling examples of Japanese social structure and cultural patterns are used to challenge the relatively uncontested, empirical, objectified assumptions about the nature of occupation. The purpose of this chapter is to broaden understandings of occupation by exposing readers to an alternative, relativist (cultural) view of the meaning of human actions in the world and thereby to stimulate some reflections regarding how the study of human occupation might evolve in a more globally encompassing and equitable manner in the future.

Culture in Time and Place

Culture can mean something different to different groups of people, depending on where, when, and with whom it was experienced and comprehended. Historical narratives of culture since the period of time in history known as the Enlightenment have followed a series of transformations. John Stuart Mill, by the mid 19th century, spoke about culture as cultivation of the human mind. "The cultivated mind is one to which the fountains of knowledge have been opened and which has been taught, in any tolerable degree, to exercise its faculties" (10). Matthew Arnold, a contemporary of Mill, added that culture could be properly described as "the study of perfection" (11), and that the evidence of having culture is to "know the best that has been said and thought in the world" (12). Culture was, before the end of the 19th century, taken largely to be expressed in human actions and something valuable to pursue in developing individual potential. Culture was a marker of distinction that involved the cultivation of one's mind to transcend to a higher plane and status in society. Perhaps it was not yet apparent that what constituted "good," "beautiful," "ideal," and "proper" might vary according to time and place. Remnants of such a view of culture still persist today, observed in its association with the fine and performing arts. A person may be seen as "cultured" if he or she frequents the ballet and knows the difference between, for example, a Dom Perignon Enothique 1990 and a La Grande Dame 1996.

By the mid 20th century in Western societies, the meaning of culture had undergone a transformation from its connotations with high culture and the process of cultivation of human potential to also include considerations of ordinary culture. "Culture is everything; culture is the way we dress, the way we carry our heads, the way we walk, the way we tie our ties—it is not only the fact of writing books or building houses" (13). This particular transformation of the meaning or definition of culture in the mainstream of Western life, from high culture to ordinary culture (14), is a significant one, because current ways of comprehending culture, both in the popular public realm and in the realm of social science discussion, appear to uphold this perspective. The theme of cultivating individual potential remains prominent, but the definition is less restrictive and reflects to a large extent how people in the Western world talk about and experience culture. Music, dance, visual and performing arts, food, literature, and forms of human activity now also qualify as culture. In these definitions, culture is connoted with the naming and representations of the forms of everyday life and not so much with its functions and meanings. Yet culture is not always connoted with the contexts and processes in which people find meaning of those particular phenomena and objects.

Culture as Shared Experience and Meanings

Along with the previous view of how the concept of culture has changed historically are two important observations concerning the evolving definitions of culture. Like most social concepts, the meanings of culture have evolved and been influenced by the same social contexts they are meant to describe and explain. This would suggest that even culture, itself, is also cultural (8)—that its definitions, meanings, and uses will vary according to the specific and varying contexts in which it is being examined.

Franz Boaz, an American anthropologist of Prussian descent, is often credited with developing the field of "historical particularism" which had a significant bearing on the study of culture in the first half of the 20th century. The importance of his ideas was based on the notion that every society or distinct social grouping carries its own unique historical development and ought to be understood in its own context—in particular its historical process (15). Boaz's work, along with that of his successors, would influence social science in a direction leading to its present concern with "meaning." Decades later, symbolic anthropologists, like Clifford Geertz, would advance the understanding of culture in a direction closer to how it is currently viewed.

Clifford Geertz, the well-known champion of symbolic anthropology, most recently argued that culture is "a system of inherited conceptions expressed in symbolic forms by means of which people communicate, perpetuate, and develop their knowledge about and attitudes toward life" (16). In other words, the purpose and function of culture, from this regard, was also to ascribe meaning on the world and make it understandable. Geertz used the phrase "thick description" (17) to describe his own specific mode of practice to gather the rich contextual characteristics and factors that more fully explained the meaning of identified human behavior and practices. For example, Shinobu, a Japanese exchange student is observed as he sits in a Western university classroom. He appears to be gazing out the window throughout the lecture being given by the professor. He rarely speaks or asks questions in the class and only responds when asked a specific question by the professor. Shinobu's behavior, compared to his non-Japanese peers, may lead the professor to believe that his student was uninterested or lacking adequate intellect to follow the material presented in the lectures. The student on the other hand may think to the contrary and feel surprised to have invited such an interpretation of his behavior by his professor. After all, he felt he was respecting the professor by not speaking, and turning his gaze away from the professor was helping him to meditate on the professor's words. Certainly, in a Japanese classroom, this student's behavior would not necessarily invite the same interpretation. The behavior taken out of original cultural context becomes miscast, causing a conflict of meaning. As the context changes, the meaning of familiar patterns of behavior phenomena change. A more profound, thick description of the behavior of interest would better reveal the contextual conditions and value patterns that plausibly support a more accurate interpretation of Shinobu's behavior.

Limited selections of Boaz and Geertz's substantial contributions to the social scientific discourse on culture over the last century have been presented here. Many others, including, but not limited to, George Herbert Mead (symbolic interactionism), Harold Garfinkle (ethnomethodology and the study of the commonplace), Kenneth Gergen (social constructionism), Jean Francois Lyotard (the postmodern condition), and the "postmodernists" were not elaborated, but have collectively shaped the current state of social scientific views on culture and the meanings of human being and action.

Science as Culture and Context for Occupational Knowledge

Accepted knowledge systems of any era are developed and validated within the particular circumstances and conditions of the greater societies in which they are used. These circumstances and conditions include cultural shifts. Parallels in this development of understanding of the meaning of human activities, objects and phenomena in the world can be seen in changes in the scientific method, both within the physical and biomedical fields.

Traditional forms of empirical scientific inquiry are based on a deductive approach in which the phenomena of interest are reduced to postulates or plausible explanations to be tested and verified. Concepts, and the principles that connect them are described by coinciding or causative postulates, and are set with an expectation of testing and validation. The notion of understanding something in greater detail, according to this empirical tradition of knowledge, often means taking wholes and reducing them to smaller parts. The movement of inquiry goes from the external toward the internal; from distal to proximal layers of complexity, down to the simple, naked truth or essence of the matter.

More recently, the scientific world has begun to yield some interest in inductive methods to understand phenomena and its meanings in a more profound way. There is growing awareness that concepts and their unifying principles are not always known ahead of time. An inductive approach is taken to dig deeper into phenomena to derive a richer or thicker description (17). Rather than moving deeper into the center for answers, the focus of inquiry moves from the center outward, and from the inside to the outside and uncontrolled surrounding context. Qualitative inquiry is a research paradigm that coincides with this inductive worldview. From the empirical side of the great ontological debate, empirical scientists may feel that qualitative research lacks the necessary methodological rigor to be valid. Seen from the other "cultural" extreme, qualitative researchers may feel that empirical science is much too rigid, simplistic, and hopelessly lost when trying to appreciate and understand (the complexities of) social and cultural phenomena.

SITUATED VIEWS OF OCCUPATION: A CULTURAL EXAMPLE

In the preceding section, the concept of culture was examined with respect to how meanings of social concepts can change, transform, and subsequently differ significantly according to time and place. Now we will view the concept of occupation in particular contexts. We will use the example of Japanese social structure, worldviews, and expressed value patterns to examine how the concept of occupation and its meanings might vary according to the Japanese cultural situation. Many descriptions of Japanese society and its usual cultural patterns and practices have been written, yet they still fall short of adequately explaining or defining the breadth of Japan's complexity. Nevertheless, several aspects and descriptions of the Japanese social structure, as reported by Japanese social scientists, have been selected and presented here as a limited backdrop for a broader understanding of occupation.

When considering the descriptive comments about Japanese society's structure and cultural features in this chapter, readers may imagine how to make sense of and to classify their own actions when transplanted into a very different surrounding context. One might ask oneself: To what extent does the surrounding social context play a role in ascribing meaning and importance to human activities? The process of classifying human activities, objects and phenomena in one's own familiar world, according to importance or value, is a process we all seem to understand, and in which we tacitly participate. Classification is a process of creating or adopting criteria that separate the human activities, objects and phenomena we perceive in our worldviews, then putting them into categories. Criteria for classification, which are constructed rules of inclusion and exclusion, determine to a significant extent the meanings of human activities, objects and phenomena in our own shared spheres of experience.

Classification is a process that displays values and priorities. For example, when you think about what you want to spend time doing on your holidays, you might create a list of activities or tasks in your mind based on a particular system of values. Why have you chosen to spend time with your children; to see a movie; to go for a long drive; or to help paint the church's new building addition? The factors (some internal and some external) that underlie our priorities (the ranking or classification of things set in categories in some order of status) are inferred here to be cultural; they are formed through a dynamic interaction between the self and the environment. The degree of influence of these factors on our actions is referred to in this context as cultural agency.

What is being suggested here is that you, the reader, consider cultural agency toward "doing" from the perspective of your own cultural context and from the limited description of Japanese social context presented earlier. After considering cultural agency toward "doing," we will revisit whether postulates about human "doing" constructed from one particular dominant (Western Empirical) worldview can be considered universal. We will consider whether universal postulates about human "doing" resonate with people situated in varying social contexts. Then we will examine the implications of different worldviews for the study of occupation.

PARTICULAR WORLDVIEWS: EAST ASIAN VIEWS OF THE COSMOS

When you think about the universe and your place within it, what do you imagine? Do you imagine a supreme being—a singular, omnipotent ruler of the universe who also represents a single moral code of life? Where do you place your own status in relation to deities, to other human beings, and to the elements of the environment, including living organisms and inanimate objects such as rocks and wood? These imaginations about the grand schema of the universe are sometimes referred to as "cosmological myths" (18). As trivial as this may appear, it is suggested here that these worldviews have a certain amount of relevance in determining one's own interpretation of the structure and content of truth and the meaning of it all. The myths or imaginations we hold to make sense of it all have parallels with the philosophical debate around empirical science and relativism presented at the beginning of the chapter: whether truth lies universally "out there"—stable, unchanging, waiting to be discovered—or "within" each of us—varied and changing according to context.

An Examination of the East Asian Version of the Cosmological Myth

Descriptions of a model Japanese worldview, as evidenced in Japanese folklore, religious rituals, philosophical literature, and artistic products, suggest the possibility of significant, if not dramatically differing, worldviews existing according to varying situations of time and space. The Japanese worldview, similar to many aboriginal and indigenous people's worldviews, appears to place nature, self, and society typically in a "closed," tightly integrated whole. Nature, with all its animate and inanimate objects, deities and spirits, so-called complex and simple organisms, are all part of one inseparable whole. There are no social-structural aftereffects of a radical transcendence of a single God, single truth, or single moral code from this primordial milieu. Rather than linear ties of loyalty and trust extending vertically toward a single deity or universal ideal, lines of trust settle into a complex, flexible constellation of horizontal relations. With regard to human behavior, in the absence of an omnipotent deity, the complex social situation or context becomes the variable entity by which all things are evaluated and judged. Persistence of the cosmological myth in Eastern understandings of nature, self, and society, compared to the Western transcendent, rationally separated version, can be correlated to certain observable social-structural patterns. The empirical Western worldview, for example, may limit the notion of the centrality of "self" in the universe and attribute accomplishment to a solitary, centrally situated self.

When one's basic worldview is such that self, others, animate and inanimate objects, and deities, which would usually be viewed empirically in Western societies as rationally separated entities, are inseparably unified, the value of human agency or doing becomes less clear. If occupation is seen as a bridge or transaction between self and the distinct, separated environment, what value, form, function and meaning does occupation hold when there is no gap between self and environment to be bridged? In other words, an Eastern relativist worldview would not interpret an act of doing by a person within an environment as having a particular purpose or outcome sought by the doer, but rather view it as an action that is part of a changing set of circumstances. From this perspective, things that happen in life are not necessarily earned or achieved. Things happen due to "karma," or a constellation of other factors—interrelated yet outside the realm of one's own control. The meanings of human activities, objects and phenomena are not necessarily determined or judged from a singular point of reference, within a centrally placed self, through an acquired singular code of ethics, but as occurrences that are part of an unfolding whole that consists of other equally important occurrences.

Vertical and Horizontal Social Indexing

From what has been popularly observed and written about Japanese society across various academic disciplines in the postmodern era, a strong tendency has been to describe the Japanese social system as collectivistic, or group oriented, and arranged in a rigid hierarchical structure. This is to be expected to a certain degree, as these distinctions are made remarkable when ascribed from a referent context of individualistic, egalitarian ideals. This is often apparent in common caricatures of Japanese tour groups to Western countries and their "amusing" group-behavior patterns comprehended through Western cultural norms. What seems remarkable to non-Japanese observers are the tour members' seemingly uniform behavior patterns, whereby they move in groups and seem to follow a tacit chain of command. When common Japanese social patterns are observed through the analytical lens of language and communication, it is hard to deny that collective social tendencies and hierarchies profoundly affect interaction between Japanese people in their everyday lives. So normal is this tendency toward social hierarchy that it is challenging for a socially adjusted, mature Japanese adult to comprehend the sensation of equal relations between two people or to view their acts in isolation from the larger group with which they identify themselves.

Vertical Social Indexing

Social scientists like Hendry (19), Nakane (20), Lebra (21), and Doi (22), contend that most Japanese would experience some difficulty in knowing how to behave in social interactions without being able to definitively place the other surrounding people in a hierarchical order in relation to themselves. This process of indexing one's self in relation to others differs remarkably between Western and Japanese social contexts. Whereas in the West, one might evaluate self and the other in terms of personal attributes (skills) and accomplishments (performance outcomes), the Japanese will often examine age, seniority in the group, and each individual's affiliation with other prominent people or institutions to index self to social environment (20).

The ritual of exchanging business cards between individuals on first meeting is another common example of Japanese collectivistic social tendencies. By examining the business card of another, one can place the other in some (situated) frame of reference; the kind of (reputable) organization each belongs to, and their rank within their respective frames. The evaluation made in that instance will immediately take effect in each person's behavior toward the other and will affect the nature and characteristics of their relationship for as long as they maintain that particular context of relation. How low one should bow and what level of speech and register to use to reflect the level of respect accorded to each other, among numerous other tacitly assumed factors, are determined by this situational ritual. The act of exchanging business cards is a common occurrence among Japanese businessmen, but the same type of social ritual and consequences can be observed among most other instances of social interaction in Japan.

Housewives, university students, and children in primary school interacting within their own groups and across groups all participate in these Japanese patterns of hierarchical social indexing. Perhaps part of the awkwardness that many Japanese people feel about conversing with complete strangers is the lack of clear social indexing between parties. Without knowing whether the other is higher or lower in hierarchical status, and without being able to place the other in some sort of common context, the choice of correct vocabulary, use of register, and fixing of attitude relative to the other persons is left uncomfortably open. When one's own view of truth is tied to the social, as opposed to a stable, unchanging single code or deity, such an unfixed situation can be awkward, if not downright paralyzing.

The meanings with which occupation have been imbued and appreciated thus far have been constructed largely within the cultural contexts of Western societies and within the institutional social norms of the world of modern, empirical science and its system of knowledge. *The concept of occupation, with all of its ascribed meanings, has no parallel concept in Japanese (and many other) lexicons.* The meaning of human agency and acts on the world differ when the understandings and meanings that make up the concept of occupation are construed differently. If the self is not central (and therefore does not assume such a privileged situation of reference) and the environment is not viewed to exist separately to the self, but rather as part and parcel of the self, the comprehension of occupation—occupation's purposes, forms, functions, and meanings—will differ. Therefore, the idea of occupation looks remarkably different in a context whereby truth is believed to exist within and around the person as opposed to existing separate to the self and "out there" waiting to be discovered.

The meanings of occupation also differ when understood from the perspective of hierarchical collectivism. If one has never acquired a sense of right to social equality based on the value of individual ability, the meanings and values tied to one's own acts (in the world) would also likely differ from the present individualistic and egalitarian referenced interpretations of occupation based on Western worldviews. In social hierarchies like those of Japan, the meaning of doing is determined or negotiated through the social situation, more than through some universal, individual-centered ethic. When the ethic of belonging is valued over one's perceived right and desire to freely act or "do," the ascription of meaning to one's doing becomes more the domain of the group or social situation than of the self. It is very difficult for the well-acculturated Japanese person to comprehend how one's identity is attained through what one chooses to do. Identity and self-value are seen to be bestowed by the social group to which one has been given membership, and not determined unilaterally through one's solitary effort and drive. Within the Western worldview, one creates identity through individual action, and within the Japanese worldview, one receives identity through association and involvement with the group.

Horizontal Social Indexing

In addition to collectivist tendencies and a vertical, hierarchical structure, another pattern peculiar to Japanese social structure holds implications for how occupation can be understood differently. Japanese social structure is organized as well by horizontal social indexing. Horizontal indexing is discussed in a variety of widely used terms with paired opposites in Japanese language, such as uchi and soto, omote and ura, and tatemae and honne. These and other dyadic terms have been frequently observed and commented on in the social scientific literature on Japan; for example, in situational relativism (21), in political hierarchy (23), in business enterprises (24, 25), in health and illness (26), in constructions of "self" (27), and in religion (28).

These commonly used Japanese terms, which can be roughly translated into English as inside and outside, in front and in the rear, and outer display and inner truth, respectively, imply that such dichotomies may be part of Japanese people's construction of reality and, subsequently, how their social worlds are structured, perceived, and navigated.

For many Japanese people, the purposes of occupation (interpreted here as "purposeful doing") and its expression have to be understood within the tension between "inside" and "outside." This tension, which pervades all social conventions, separates people's actions into those which can be classified as basic, personal intent (inside) and deliberate, outer, or public intent (outside) (21). Situations vary in time and space, and the well-socialized Japanese person is partial to differentiating others' words and actions on the world according to whether those expressions are meant to communicate the inside or outside meaning. The boundaries between inside and outside are situation specific and, therefore, vary according to situation.

This contrasts with the Western tendency to interpret social conventions universally (i.e., "a lie is a lie and is wrong no matter what the circumstance"), which can cause some difficulties when these universals become the standards by which the actions of other people, set in different sociocultural contexts, are interpreted.

Inside and outside may refer to a distinction within an individual, one's family, a group of friends, an institution, a community, or a nation. For example, an individual will carefully separate his private inner feelings from his outer public expression. On a larger level, one might be concerned about not allowing an embarrassing incident of national proportion to be known to other nations. Administrators of a college or university may conscientiously limit any information that might taint its reputation—either interdepartmentally or to the outside. The inside-outside conscientiousness, which also can be similarly observed in Western societies, is especially prominent in the Japanese social context, giving the common observation about "face" particular credence. In a collectively oriented society, where one's "face" and position are strongly determined by the surrounding social context, proper attention is paid to presentation or outer expression. Failure to do so may result in profound negative consequences to one's daily life and future circumstances.

Though the opposites of inside and outside are comprehended best within social contexts, these values are manifested in practically all dimensions of Japanese daily life. Anyone who has been to a Japanese home will note that one's physical environment is also structured similarly. Shoes are removed and kept at the "genkan" situated just inside the door to the outer world. The genkan serves as the threshold between the outside world and the inner, private world. The pattern and meaning of, motivation toward, participation in, and functional value of activity are profoundly modified by this bisecting treatment of the world and daily life context.

It is interesting to know that in normal Japanese uses of these social-structural pairings, the terms that denote outside, or the public domain, almost always supersede the term denoting the commonly hidden inner or private realm. In social dynamics that privilege the collective over the individual, the social group's aspirations are frequently placed ahead of individual aspirations. The group's interests are often seen as public knowledge, whereas individual concerns are often relegated to the hidden private realm. They are hidden because one's own interests and aspirations run the risk of being inconsistent with or contrary to those of the group. The Japanese worldview values harmony and belonging above everything.

Occupation has been discussed by Westerners as being important in shaping identity (29), enabling meaning in life, and influencing one's sense of well-being. The reader may get a sense of how such individual-centered values associated with human activity are complicated when examined in a different sociocultural context. The meaning of human doings needs to be reconsidered when passed through the filters of hierarchical and horizontal social structure and collective-oriented worldviews, such as those situated in Japan. Once again, we are afforded glimpses below of the special sociocultural contexts in which individual behavior, and perhaps *occupation* must be defined and expressed.

Interdependence and "Amae"

Although dependence in social relationships can be observed and described in most societies, social scientists and Asian studies researchers have come to accept the concept of "amae" into their interpretations and descriptions of dependent behavior patterns in Japanese society. Some contend that amae is a unique form of dependence that sets Japanese society apart from other modern industrial societies (19). Takeo Doi (22) articulated this behavior pattern over 30 years ago in his publication titled "Amae no Kouzou" (the structure of dependence). Since then, amae as a concept has found its way into the lexicon of social scientific research in Japan, and it seems that no comprehensive work on the Japanese social structure can avoid mention of this common term.

Amae is defined as "the need of an individual to be loved and cherished; the prerogative to presume and depend upon the benevolence of another" (22, p. 165). In this way, amae is seen to be both a noun (a concept to describe a pattern of behavior) and a verb (an action word to symbolize a behavior; seeking the indulgence of another). Doi states that "... amae is, first and foremost, an emotion, an *emotion* (italics added) which partakes of the nature of a drive and something instinctive as its base" (22, p. 166), and that "in its most characteristic form, (amae) represents an attempt to draw close to the other person" (22, p. 167). Doi likens amae to "the craving of a new born child for close contact with its mother, and in the broader sense, the desire to deny the fact of separation that is an inevitable part of human existence, and to obliterate the pain that this separation involves" (22, p. 169). It takes some effort for Western adults (especially men, perhaps because of the lack of experience of maternity and the maternal instinct) to recall emotions that were associated with childhood and the intimacy of the infant–parent relationship. This may be due to most Westerners having been socialized strongly toward developing independence and an identity that is distinctly separate from others. It may seem, for many situated in the Western world, that most Japanese, as Doi would have us believe, do not frustrate the "drive to dependence" (22, p. 169) but, rather, prolong it throughout their lives.

Most people living in the Western world would be able to relate to the basic emotion underlying amae, as this emotion to draw close to another human being is not only plausible but can be experienced normally even in Western social situations. However, to impose the quality of intimacy, which Westerners reserve for the sanctity of mother–child relations, onto adult interpersonal relations is to impose a negative value to the behavior. What is positively regarded in one sphere of shared experiences can be negatively regarded in another. Such variations in value patterns speak to the issue of culture. For societies that celebrate individuality, independence, and self-efficacy, dependent behaviors (especially those that emulate the infant–parent relationship into adulthood) are discouraged.

The existing value pattern that supports vertically structured collectivism in Japanese society affords much leeway for amae (interdependent) behavior. Life in present-day Japan would be extremely difficult to navigate without demonstrating some aspect of amae behavior or its associated language. Amae, or "Japanese interdependency," holds profound consequences for how Japanese people construct meaning in social interactions and participation in community or societal life. Not only are states of dependence tolerated, but they are actually expected, as part of a pattern of normal adaptive, behavior in Japanese social contexts of meaning. Amae is the glue that supports the social hierarchy that is characteristic of Japanese social structure and, likewise, plays into matters of meaning of human doing—or occupation (as people in the West are apt to say).

CULTURAL PERSPECTIVES OF OCCUPATION

The beginning of this chapter included an examination of the evolving definitions of the concept of culture. Like most concepts that purport a connection to the social, the definition of culture can be explained to be bound and affected by time and place. Culture has moved from the extraordinary (such as "high culture") to the ordinary in daily life and from individual embodiment (as witnessed in matters of race and ethnicity) to its location in the social realm as shared spheres of experience and as social processes of ascribing meaning to the human activities, objects and phenomena we encounter. Culture represents all these constructs and will likely continue to vary and change according to the beholder's situation and its contexts of interpretation.

The implications of this chapter for the study of occupation are found in how we construct the point of reference from which the forms, functions, and meanings of occupation are comprehended and evaluated. As introduced earlier in the chapter, key assumptions influencing understanding, including views of the universe, the self and meanings of occupation will differ depending on whether the self is believed to be independent of and acting on the environment, or the self is inextricably integrated within the environment.

In the Western objective, rational context, occupation is readily understood as a viable and universally meaningful concept because it, like other phenomena, is viewed as existing "out there" and can be understood more accurately by direct observation and rigorous measurement. From an individualistic, empirical perspective, humans are tacitly understood to be occupational beings. The explanatory power of this particular view often goes unchallenged, for it is understood according to modern empirical-scientific ways of knowing—which probably represents the most powerful validation of truth in the industrialized world.

Contrasted against this dominant view is an alternative position regarding the meaning of occupation as seen from a social constructionist's relativist view. From this viewpoint, the self is removed from a privileged central location of reference, becoming instead a self embedded in the environment rather than being separate and distinct from it. Meaning is not reflected back to a solitary self, but rather is dependent more on the self in relation to the proximal social. Therefore, in this regard, truth is context specific and varies according to place and time. Like the evolution and changes witnessed in the meaning or definitions of culture when reflected back to varying contexts of shared experiences, truth is not necessarily universal, residing out there in a separately situated environment. Rather than taking certain facts for granted as true (like the widely held idea of humans as occupational beings and the assumption of a direct causative effect of occupation on human health and well-being), the constructionist view concedes no such assumptions.

What is occupation? What forms do occupations take in a given culture/context? And is it really important to humans' senses of well-being? Do people in other cultures (like the Japanese) see themselves as occupational beings, or is this a quality put on them by people abiding in a different cultural reality and acquired value pattern? What are the boundaries of the contexts that give such meaning to these phenomena and objects? These would represent the kind of questions arising from this comparative perspective.

These two empirical and relativist interpretations or views of truth represent the breadth of the possibilities of cultural perspectives on occupation. Varying spheres of shared meanings, as contexts, matter significantly in understanding the meanings of occupation and may present a formidable dilemma concerning how occupation is conceptualized and researched in the future. In any credible research, how the concept of study (occupation) is defined will influence the design and methods used for its study.

In conventional, empirical inquiry, concepts and their connecting principles (theory, models, hypotheses and postulates, etc.) are tested and verified (some would say reified) through the arbitrative authority of mathematical laws. Here, subjective data are often of secondary interest and regarded to be less preferred over "hard," rational, evidence.

In research within the tradition of relativism or social construction, concepts are seen to be dependent on context, and truths to be socially situated. Concepts become discovered through inductive processes and are assumed to be limited to the contexts from which they arise. Consequently, from this perspective, the empirical method and its supporting worldview are stripped of their universality and relegated to a status of being merely one (albeit currently the most powerful) of many alternative views and interpretations of truth.

The dilemma facing the science of occupation is not so different from the larger debates that are currently occurring in the wider (Western) intellectual community. Thomas F. Gieryn refers to this great debate as "the science wars" (30). On one side of the line of tension stand reason, empiricism, and the objective truth of positivistic science. On the other side stand social constructionism, relativism, and postmodernism. The ideas of the great natural scientists that have progressed all the way from the age of reason (enlightenment), including Paul Gross (31), Norman Levitt (32), and Noretta Koertge (33), have had their ideas and ways of knowing aggressively challenged by the academy of postmodern social scientists, like Stanley Fish (34), Stanley Aronowitz (35), and Ruth Hubbard (36).

In this chapter, examples of the Japanese social context, albeit translated into the language and vocabulary of Western social science, were presented for the purpose of provoking some fresh perspectives into the cultural construction of the concept of occupation. This was attempted through the exercise of contrasting two distinctly different spheres of experience: of the (Western) reader's, and of the Japanese writer's, representing two remarkably varying cultural contexts from which to make sense of occupation.

So, how is the meaning of human activities affected and shaped by the social and cultural context in which they are considered? Human performance of activity takes on a certain constellation of meanings when regarded from the cultural norms of individualism, egalitarianism, and independence, as it would when regarded from the cultural norms of collectivism, hierarchy, and dependent social relations.

The comparisons of worldviews and social contexts here were meant to also mirror or represent the two contrasting worldviews presented at the beginning of the chapter. Cultural researchers, proponents of postmodernist perspectives, and the majority of Japanese people would probably support and legitimize the existence of multiple views of being. If multiple views of being exist, then those dedicated to the study of occupation have much to consider in their pursuit of knowledge and truth. In regard to the scientific debate, one side is prone to view occupation as nature—out there, universal in meaning, and knowable through methodical, impirical inquiry, whereas the other side is prone to view occupation as culture—internally comprehended and varying in meaning, being bound by contexts that include time and place. This chapter has taken, admittedly, the viewpoint of the latter with the hope of presenting a provocative discussion regarding the implications of culture on the understanding of occupation. How will you make sense of occupation and comprehend explanations of its qualities in this and other parts of this book? The body of knowledge around this compelling concept, though in a relatively fledgling stage, continues to evolve and capture the attention and imaginations of people from different walks of life or different "spheres of shared experience." How occupational scientists and people who acquire an interest in occupation consider and wrestle with the issue of culture in the coming years will greatly influence the manner in which occupation is comprehended and used in a globally inclusive manner. This inclusive approach will become increasingly important as the world becomes more of a global community.

CHAPTER SUMMARY

Although understanding the cultural dimensions that influence what people do may seem like a straightforward exercise, it is clear that the task has great complexity. In this chapter, it has been shown that with some cultures, or social groups, considering culture it is not simply a matter of understanding customs and traditions and using those to make broad generalizations about what different acts mean. Where occupation is concerned, what is required is reconsidering the perspectives that people in a culture have about life in general.

The chapter has intended to draw sharp contrasts between different views of life or experience, called worldviews, which characterize different social groups. In particular, Japanese and Western perspectives have been compared. Western worldviews often understand occupation from the perspective of discrete, objectively viewed activities that fulfill prescribed purposes for a central doer, who engages and views experiences from the standpoint of the self. In contrast, in the Japanese worldview, the doer, or self, is not central but rather one element in an overall context. Context is described here as the situation in which a given occupation is embedded. In some cultures, particularly in the West, the person, or self, is at the center of that context, whereas other factors, such as place, other people, objects, and circumstances, are viewed as peripheral or external. In Japan, however, a collectivist worldview is more typical. This view considers all elements as vital and necessary pieces of a dynamic and integrated whole.

A key difference in the two worldviews is thus how context is viewed and whether or not occupation ought to be viewed as a natural phenomenon that can be studied and understood externally and objectively, or in a more inclusive way that accepts that it can be viewed as an internal phenomenon that must be understood from the perspective of multiple internal meanings that vary by time and place.

STUDY GUIDE

Study Guide Author: Kristine Haertl

Summary of Main Points

Personal worldview is influenced by culture and context. Often, one's understanding of occupation is heavily influenced by Western scientific methods and belief systems. This chapter compares and contrasts the understanding of occupation from a Western individualistic, societal viewpoint where the self is considered the center and environment external to the self, to an Eastern Japanese collectivist worldview, which places nature, the self, and society in an integrated whole. In order to advance our knowledge within occupational science, multiple worldviews in diverse cultural contexts must be studied to expand our awareness and comprehension of occupation.

Application to Occupational Therapy

Therapists often guide practice in familiar conceptualizations, theoretical frameworks, and worldviews. As the emphasis on evidence-based practice has grown in the past decade, the field must acknowledge multiple ways of knowing, develop an appreciation for quantitative and qualitative methods of inquiry, and strive to increase awareness of multiple perspectives and diverse cultural worldviews.

Occupational therapy practice should not only focus on the micro (individualistic, occupation-based) perspective, but also on the macro (collective, societal) viewpoint. In order to affect global health at a systems level, readers should expand their cultural lenses and acknowledge societal variations within occupational therapy practice.

Occupational therapy upholds the importance of context in relation to practice with individuals, families, and communities. A comprehensive understanding of multicultural views that do not always uphold an individualistic approach is integral to expanding practice to include theoretical frameworks that extend beyond the Western world. The concept of occupation is not universally understood, and consideration of ways of living and doing within multicontextual situations and worldviews will serve to expand views and methods of scientific inquiry to serve the needs of persons from diverse cultural backgrounds.

Individual Learning Activities

1. Review the occupational science literature and identify three to four articles of authors from at least two distinct different cultures. Write a two- to three-page paper on the similarities and differences the articles reveal in worldview and perception of occupation.

2. Select a culture distinctly different from your own. Write a reflection paper on how your life would have been influenced growing up in this culture. Consider the following questions:

   a. What would your occupations entail and how would they differ from your current occupational patterns?
   b. How would your worldview differ?
   c. What differences do you envision in your relationships, daily routines, and career choice?
   d. As an occupational therapist, how would your focus differ in working with individuals from this culture?

Group Learning Activity

Form groups of three individuals. On your campus or within your community, identify three individuals each from different cultures (e.g., the international student organization on your campus may be a good resource). As a group, design a common questionnaire that addresses (a) distinguishable features of the culture; (b) cultural conceptualizations of meaning through religion, worldview, and the aesthetics (forms of art within the culture); (c) the daily occupational patterns of individuals within the culture; and (d) any additional questions you'd like to know about the culture.

Each group member will conduct one interview with an individual from another culture. Have each individual within your group write down preconceived ideas about the culture of the individual to be interviewed. Following the interview, as a group, prepare a 30-minute presentation comparing and contrasting responses from individuals from each culture. Discuss the implications of findings for the field of occupational science.

Study Questions

1. The empirical method, often associated with quantitative inquiry, is aligned best with:
   a. Eastern worldview
   b. Western worldview
   c. Both
   d. Neither

2. Which of the following is most closely aligned with relativism?
   a. A philosophical viewpoint that adheres to the idea that truth and criteria of judgment are relative to the circumstances, people, and contexts involved
   b. A philosophical viewpoint that purports an overarching theory or truism that is universal
   c. The idea that cultures are created and maintained by a supreme God
   d. The philosophical viewpoint that empirical scientific study is the best way to seek knowledge

3. Along with a collectivist viewpoint of society, Japanese culture emphasizes the heterarchy, or equal structure and place of individuals in society.
   a. True
   b. False

4. The meaning of occupation and "doing" in Japanese society:
   a. Emphasizes the individual, the occupation, and the environment as separate but equally weighted entities
   b. Is considered in reference to a collectivist society, whereby the environment is considered a part of the self and society
   c. Both of the above
   d. Neither of the above

5. Postmodernism takes:
   a. An empirical view
   b. An objective view
   c. A relativist view
   d. None of the above

REFERENCES

1. Yerxa, E., Clark, F., Frank, G., Jackson, J., Parham, D., Pierce, D., et. al. (1989). An introduction to occupational science, a foundation for occupational therapy in the 21st century. *Occupational Therapy in Health Care, 6,* 1–15.
2. Ehrmann, M. (1972). *Desiderata.* Brooke House, Los Angeles.
3. Berger, P., & Luckmann, T. (1967). *The social construction of reality; a treatise on the sociology of knowledge.* London: Allen Lane.
4. Burr, V. (1995). *An introduction to social constructionism.* London, Routledge.
5. Gergen K. J. (1985). The social constructionist movement in modern psychology, *American Psychologist 40,* 266–275.
6. Lyotard, J.-F. (1984). *The postmodern condition: A report on knowledge.* Minneapolis: University of Minnesota Press.
7. Iwama, M. (2003). The issue is: Toward culturally relevant epistemologies in occupational therapy. *American Journal of Occupational Therapy, 57,* 582–588.
8. Smith, M. J. (2000). *Culture; reinventing the social sciences.* Buckingham: Open University Press.
9. Gergen, K. J. (1999). *An invitation to social construction.* Thousand Oaks, CA: Sage.
10. Mill, J. S. (1863). *Utilitarianism.* London: Parker, Son, & Bourn.
11. Arnold, M. (1993). *Culture and anarchy.* Cambridge: Cambridge University Press. (Original work published in 1869)
12. Arnold, M. (1879). *Mixed essays.* London: Smith, Elder, & Co.
13. Cesaire A. (1972). "From Discourse on Colonialism." In P. Williams & L. Chrisman (Eds.), *Colonial discourse and post-colonial theory: A reader* (pp. 172–180). New York: Columbia University Press.

14. Williams, R (1958). Moving from high culture to ordinary culture. In N. McKenzie (Ed.), *Convictions.* London: MacGibbon and Kee.
15. McGee, R. J., & Warms, R. L. (2004). *Anthropological theory: An introductory history.* New York: McGraw-Hill.
16. Geertz, C. (1973). *The interpretation of cultures: Selected essays.* New York: Basic Books.
17. Geertz, C. (1973). Thick description: Toward an interpretative theory of culture. In *The interpretation of cultures* (pp. 3–30). New York: Basic Books.
18. Bellah, R. N. (1991). *Beyond belief: Essays on religion in a post traditional world.* New York: Harper & Row.
19. Hendry, J. (1995). *Understanding Japanese society* (2nd ed.). London: Routledge.
20. Nakane, C. (1970). *Tate shakai no ningen kankei* [Human relations in a vertical society]. Tokyo: Kodansha.
21. Lebra T. S. (1976). *Japanese patterns of behavior.* Honolulu: University of Hawaii Press.
22. Doi, T. (1971). *Amae no kozo* (The anatomy of dependence). Tokyo: Kobundo (in Japanese).
23. Ishida, T. (1984). Conflict and its accommodation: Omote-ura and uchi-soto relations. In E. Krauss, T. Rohlen, & P. G. Steinhoff (Eds.), *Conflict in Japan* (pp. 16–38) Honolulu: University of Hawaii Press.
24. Kondo, D. (1990). *Crafting selves: Power, gender, and discourses of identity in a Japanese workplace.* Chicago: University of Chicago Press.
25. Hamabata, M. M. (1990). *Crested kimono: Power and love in the Japanese business family.* Ithaca, NY: Cornell University Press.
26. Ohnuki-Tierney, E. (1984). *Illness and culture in contemporary Japan: An anthropological view.* Cambridge: Cambridge University Press.
27. Doi, T. (1985). *The anatomy of self: The individual versus society.* Tokyo, Japan: Kodansha International.
28. Hardacre, H. (1986). *Kurozumikyo and the new religions of Japan.* Princeton, NJ: Princeton University Press.
29. Christiansen C. H. (1999). Defining lives; occupation as identity: An essay on competence, coherence, and the creation of meaning. 1999 Eleanor Clarke Slagle Lectureship. *American Journal of Occupational Therapy. 53*(6), 547–558.
30. Gieryn, T. F. (1999). *Cultural boundaries of science; credibility on the line.* Chicago; University of Chicago Press.
31. Gross P. L. (1998). Evidence-free forensics and enemies of objectivity. In N. Koertge (Ed.), *A house built on sand: Exposing postmodernist myths about science* (pp. 99–118). New York: Oxford University Press.
32. Gross P. R., & Levitt N. (1994). *Higher superstition: The academic left and its quarrels with science.* Baltimore; The Johns Hopkins University Press.
33. Koertge, N. (1998). Scrutinizing science studies. In N. Koertge (Ed.), *A house built on sand: Exposing postmodernist myths about science* (pp. 3–6). New York: Oxford University Press.
34. Fish, S. (1996, May 21). Professor Sokal's Bad Joke. *New York Times* Op-Ed, p. A23.
35. Aronowitz, S. (1988). *Science as power, discourse and ideology in modern society.* Minneapolis: University of Minnesota Press.
36. Hubbard, R. (1990). *The politics of women's biology.* New Brunswick, NJ: Rutgers University Press.

CHAPTER 3

The Study of Occupation

Helene J. Polatajko

It is neither wealth nor splendour, but tranquility and occupation which give happiness.

Thomas Jefferson

OBJECTIVES

1. Define four modes of understanding or epistemologies based on the work of Perry and Belenky.
2. Compare and contrast naturalistic and positivistic paradigms.
3. Describe study designs used in naturalistic and positivistic paradigms.
4. Give examples of subquestions for each of the six questions of basic inquiry related to human occupation.

KEY WORDS

Epistemology
Metacognition
Methods of inquiry
Multivariate
Naturalistic paradigm
Occupationology
Occupations
Occupational science
Paradigm
Positivistic paradigm
Qualitative research
Reductionistic

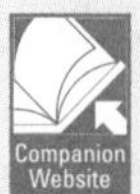

www.prenhall.com/christiansen

The Internet provides an exciting means for interacting with this textbook and for enhancing your understanding of humans' experiences with occupations and the organization of occupations in society. Use the address above to access the interactive Companion Website created specifically to accompany this book. Here you will find an array of self-study material designed to help you gain a richer understanding of the concepts presented in this chapter.

CHAPTER PROFILE

This is a "how-to" chapter. The reader will learn how to learn about occupation, that is, how to become a student of occupation. Some would describe this as learning how to be an occupationologist, a scientist who specializes in studying occupation, sometimes also described as an occupational scientist. In this chapter, a range of formal and informal methods for studying occupation are introduced. The chapter offers a point of entry to the world of scholarly inquiry into occupation. First, the chapter will discuss what it means *to understand* occupation. Six questions form a template to unravel the mysteries of occupation and current methods of inquiry.

INTRODUCTION

We each engage in numerous **occupations** every day. As well, we see people around us engage in occupations and see occupations portrayed in print, on television, and at the movies. As a result, each of us has a great deal of familiarity and personal experience with occupation. So, it would be easy to assume that we all understand occupation, that we are all occupational experts. But are we? Do we know, for example, whether children in Papua, New Guinea, are occupied in playing the same games as children in Atlanta, Georgia? Would Michael Jordan have been as successful if he had chosen the occupation of hockey rather than basketball? Or, can we be certain if Wayne Gretzky, the Canadian hockey player, did, in fact, *choose* the occupation of hockey? Do we know what makes a person a gifted musician or a great surgeon? Can we predict which child will grow up to be the prime minister of Canada, president of the United States of America, or a leader in the United Nations? Do we know which occupations a community will determine are worth developing when that community's primary occupations of livelihood—for example, a steel mill—become obsolete?

Our personal experiences are very important in helping us develop an understanding of occupation, but they are not sufficient! An understanding of occupation, as that of any phenomenon, cannot be gained from direct experience alone. Constructing an understanding of occupation requires careful examination of the doing, the doer, the context or situation in which the occupation is found, and the relationships among these elements. The process of examination always starts with a question. Six basic questions about occupation are asked in this chapter to help bring about an understanding of this phenomenon. These same questions guide journalists in their investigative reporting: *Who? What? When? Where? How?* and *Why?*

Each of the six questions leads us to various **methods of inquiry.** The methods of investigative journalism, like personal experience and observation, can be applied to the study of occupation and can tell us a fair amount about it. However, no *single* method of inquiry is sufficient. Occupation is a complicated, **multivariate** phenomenon. Consequently, its understanding requires a multifaceted approach. Methods, ranging from stories to statistics, drawn from both qualitative and quantitative paradigms of inquiry, are needed. The chapters in this book illustrate many methods of inquiry associated with the six basic questions. These questions provide a template for inquiry (1) that can be used to understand occupation. To explain and demonstrate the process, an overview of possible methods of inquiry will be presented along with at least one example for each of the six questions.

WAYS OF KNOWING

Understanding the Who, What, When, Where, How, and Why of Occupation

> *To understand: To perceive the meaning or explanation of, grasp the idea of, or comprehend: to be thoroughly acquainted with or familiar with. (2)*

How people go about understanding something depends on what it is they want to know and how well they want to know it. If we want to know someone's name, we might ask that person. If we want to know how we can hear the answer, we can read a book on the human auditory system. If we want to know more than a person's name, that is, if we want to get to know the person, we might share time with that person to observe and learn about their everyday routines and interests. If we want to truly understand our best friend, we might do all of the above and more.

Researchers tell us that how we go about understanding something depends not only on what we want to understand, but also on who we are: our age, gender, and education (3, 4); our social and economic advantage; and our perspective on the nature of the world and its reality (5).

Shared learning and deeper understanding require representational thought, built on reflection, abstraction, and an exchange of ideas. Once an exchange of ideas occurs, any number of ways of knowing can be adopted. William Perry, in his classic work, *Forms of Intellectual and Ethical Development in the College Years* (6), described a scheme for representing the various ways of understanding. He called these ways of knowing *epistemological positions.* Later, Belenky and her colleagues (4), among others, argued that women and men, although similar, approached understanding in different ways (see Table 3-1). The simplest way of knowing involves personal experience and direct observation of the actual, the concrete, and the specific in the present. Belenky and her colleagues (4) noted that personal experience and observation were the ways of knowing used by the youngest and most disadvantaged women in their study. They referred to this way of knowing, this epistemological perspective, as *Silence* to denote the total submissiveness of disadvantaged women to authority. This approach provides for a very rudimentary understanding of the here and now but does not allow for any understanding of the past or the future, for any reflection, or for any shared learning (see Table 3-1■).

Taken together, the work of Perry and Belenky's research teams provides a comprehensive description of four modes of understanding, four **epistemologies.** In the first mode, knowledge may be accepted from authorities at face value and without question; truth is viewed as essentially dichotomous—black or white. In the second approach, authority is not considered absolute because a variety of perspectives or opinions are recognized. Truth is viewed as subjective, personal, and intuitive. This

TABLE 3-1 *Female versus Male Ways of Knowing*

Female Epistemological Perspectives	Male Epistemological Perspectives
Silence—The self is experienced as mindless and voiceless, subject to external authority. **Received knowledge**—The self is conceived of as capable of receiving, even reproducing, knowledge from the all-knowing external authority. **Subjective knowledge**—Truth and knowledge are conceived of as personal, private, and subjectively known or intuited. **Procedural knowledge**—The processes of learning and applying objective procedures for obtaining and communicating knowledge are values and actively cultivated. **Constructed knowledge**—All knowledge is viewed as contextual; The self is seen as a creator of knowledge and both subjective and objective strategies for knowing are valued.	**Basic duality**—The world is viewed in polarities: right/wrong, black/white, we/they, good/bad; everything is knowable; the learner is dependent on external authority to hand down truth. **Multiplicity**—It is realized that there is diversity of opinion and a multiplicity of perspectives in some areas; faith in absolute authority is shaken. **Relativism subordinate**—Opinion alone is recognized as inadequate; evidence and support that can stand up to scrutiny are required; an analytical, evaluative approach is actively cultivated. **Relativism**—Truth is understood to be relative; the meaning of an event is understood to depend on the context of the event and the framework of the knower; relativism is seen to pervade all aspects of life.

Source: As described by Belenky and colleagues (4)

second way of knowing is similar to the prevalent reliance on intuition that preceded scientific thought and is considered central to many Eastern philosophies. A third way of knowing concedes that knowledge from authority and intuitive knowledge are inadequate ways of knowing. Instead, only knowledge that is gained from reasoned reflection or is based on support and evidence, and subject to formal analysis and evaluation, is viewed as dependable. In this third mode of understanding, truth is viewed critically—that is, it is subject to verification. The fourth way of knowing is to recognize knowledge as constructed and changing, subject to the situation and the perspective of the knower. In this fourth approach, truth is recognized as relative and, thus, is viewed critically. Included in these perspectives of knowledge is the full range of methods for understanding, extending from the informal methods of the individual knower to the formal methods of disciplined inquiry used by recognized researchers.

Disciplinary Ways of Knowing

Disciplines, formed by groups of like-minded individuals concerned with understanding particular phenomena, are similar to individuals in that they have particular ways of knowing (7, 8). The modes of inquiry used by a specific discipline have to do with the nature of the phenomena of interest, as well as the epistemological perspectives of the members of the discipline (9). Put more simply, each discipline adopts a way of understanding, a mode of inquiry, that is appropriate to the people who make up the discipline and the nature of what is to be understood (3, 5, 7, 8).

Disciplinary ways of knowing, referred to as disciplinary **paradigms,** although specific to a discipline, are not necessarily unique to that discipline. A number of disciplines have adopted similar ways of knowing; for example, chemistry, physics, engineering, and psychology have all adopted the experimental method as a primary mode of inquiry. In addition, disciplines may adopt several ways of knowing. For example, sociology uses experimentation, survey, field study, and nonreactive study (10) as its preferred ways of understanding phenomena.

Disciplinary paradigms are not static or fixed. Rather, they change as the understanding of phenomena evolves (8, 11). Change may be prompted also by a need to gain deeper understanding, as has happened in psychology (12–14). Because of the changing nature of inquiry among disciplines, a large and ever-growing range exists of "how-to" literature on inquiry—a literature that covers a broad and varied range of methods in a number of disciplines.

Paradigms for Inquiry

Disciplinary paradigms have tended to emanate from one of two broad epistemological perspectives. The first perspective, called the **naturalistic paradigm,** is also referred to as **qualitative research.** The second perspective is the **positivistic paradigm,** which is also referred to as the quantitative, experimental-type, or **reductionistic** approach (7, 8, 10, 15, 16, 17, 18).

The **naturalistic paradigm** is based on the assumption that the world is made up of multiple, overlapping realities that are subjectively experienced, socially constructed, complex, and constantly changing. The role of the qualitative researcher is to come to an in-depth understanding of these realities and how they are constructed. Qualitative researchers immerse themselves, often over a long period, into the natural settings and lives of groups or individuals being studied to gain an understanding of and to interpret their experiences and perspectives. The **qualitative research** process is understood to be a subjective one, with the researcher as the main instrument of data collection.

The positivistic paradigm is based on the assumption that the world is made up of observable, measurable facts. In this approach, the role of the quantitative researcher is to uncover these facts and to discern laws that govern the relationship between cause and effect by conducting carefully planned studies that control as many variables as necessary. The ultimate goal of positivistic research is to explain and predict, and to this end, research is expected to be objective, unbiased, and logical (5, 12, 15–18).

With the advent of modern science in the Western world, the predominant Western perspective on understanding became firmly based in positivism. Until relatively recently, naturalistic perspectives were viewed as suspect or inadequate and thus were devalued (5, 7, 14). The growth of modern science produced a literature on methods of inquiry that was almost exclusively quantitative. However, this is changing rapidly. A number of disciplines are beginning to realize the limitations of reductionistic methods of inquiry and the potential contributions of naturalistic methods to a complete understanding of their phenomena of interest. More and more the merits of using these two paradigms for understanding the same phenomenon, used simultaneously or in stages, are being recognized (5, 7, 12, 14–16, 19). As a result, an excellent literature on methods for both paradigms of inquiry has emerged. Let us look at the different ways in which these two paradigms can help us to understand occupation.

Paradigms for the Study of Occupation

Interest in human occupation, as a phenomenon worthy of study in its own right, is relatively new. Although many excellent studies can be found that inform us about occupation, for example, *Working,* the documentary masterpiece by Terkel (20), or *The Historical Meanings of Work,* a collection of scholarly essays edited by Joyce (21), these emanate from a variety of disciplines. No one discipline has claimed the study of occupation as a central domain of concern, and hence, no paradigm of inquiry has been identified for the study of occupation.

It has been suggested that a new discipline, dedicated to the study of occupation, is needed (22), and indeed, some scholars, most notably Elizabeth Yerxa and her colleagues (23), have advocated for the development of a new **occupational science.** They have argued that this new science[1] ought to be a basic science, one that could support such professions as architecture, career counseling, environmental engineering, industrial psychology, kinesiology, leisure studies, and occupational therapy. Yerxa and her colleagues (23) have proposed that occupational science needs to define appropriate paradigms of inquiry. They have suggested disciplinary paradigms and research methods of inquiry that hold particular promise for the study of occupation, in particular, methods based in naturalistic inquiry. Notwithstanding the efforts of these and other scholars, the study of occupation is still in its infancy, and no single disciplinary tradition yet exists. Consequently, there is no well-established disciplinary paradigm of inquiry and relatively little accumulated literature detailing methods for the study of occupation.

Because the study of occupation remains in its infancy, understanding is still rudimentary. Further, there has been little open discussion of the methods of inquiry that are most appropriate to the study of occupation. Indeed, in the absence of a well-established discipline, no obvious forum exists for such a discussion. It is the opinion of this author that it is still far too early to adopt a particular epistemological perspective or a paradigm of inquiry for the study of occupation. It is proposed, therefore, that all basic questions of inquiry be asked. That is, who, what, when, where, how, and why seem to be appropriate questions to begin our study; and all methods of inquiry, particularly naturalistic and positivistic, should be considered potentially useful.

METHODS OF INQUIRY FOR THE STUDY OF OCCUPATION

An understanding of occupation can come from three primary sources: personal experience, existing data sources, and new investigations. Direct experience of engaging in occupations is very important in helping to understand occupation, but experience is insufficient. Constructing an understanding of occupation requires careful examination of the phenomenon in its entirety, including the doing itself, the context of the doing, the perspective of the doer, relationships among these elements, and the framework of the knower. This examination must be built not only on personal experiences but also on formal methods of systematic inquiry.

What follows is an attempt at explaining the formal methods of inquiry for the study of occupation, referred to here as occupationology,[2] and in other places in this volume as occupational science. The methods selected are those that are consistent with meeting the aims of any program of disciplinary inquiry, that is, to *describe* and *explain,* with a view toward predicting and controlling.[3] The methods identified are by no means novel. They have been drawn from the literature of a number of disciplines concerned with the study of humans and societies. Richard's (24) observations about his own work apply aptly to these methods: "Few of the separate items are original. One does not expect novel cards when playing so traditional a game; it is the hand which matters" (p. 1).

The scale of the literature on methods of inquiry is such that it is far beyond the scope of a single chapter to present all available methods, let alone describe them in any detail. The intent here is to be illustrative rather than exhaustive. Illustrations of various types of studies can be found throughout this book. Thus, an overview of the more common methods of inquiry is provided here. The purpose is to supply sufficient information on methods to afford the reader a point of entry into this vast literature. The reader is directed to the cited sources for in-depth explanations of the methods and for a broader, more comprehensive listing of available methods. These sources should be considered a starting point for identifying all methods of inquiry that may be useful in understanding occupation.

Methods of inquiry into occupation should have the same basic structure as any other inquiry: question, design, data collection, data analysis, data interpretation, and conclusion. Questions, designs, and data collection methods will be discussed here because these steps set an inquiry into motion. In the sections that follow, care has been taken to identify common methods from both the naturalistic and the positivistic paradigms. This has been achieved by surveying recent texts addressing both perspectives in related disciplines, in particular: education, social and behavioral sciences (5, 7, 10, 16, 18, 19, 25), health sciences (8, 9, 17), and psychology (12–15, 26).

The Question

The first step of any process of inquiry is the formulation of a question. Our understanding of occupation is so rudimentary that all the questions of basic inquiry are appropriate to ask. We can ask both the descriptive questions (who, what, when, and where) and the explanatory questions (how and why). The specific question will depend on the aspect of occupation that is of interest to the knower and the paradigm of inquiry. Table 3-2 ■ gives some examples of specific questions that could—and should—be asked about occupation.

TABLE 3-2 *Six Questions of Basic Inquiry and Possible Subquestions Applied to Human Occupation*

Purpose	Question	Subquestions
Describe	**Who** engages in occupations?	Do all people engage in occupations? Does age, gender, race, religion, ethnicity, ability, health, or socioeconomic status affect occupational engagement? Did early humans engage in occupations?
	What are occupations?	What are the patterns of occupations, i.e., are there occupational profiles?
	What occupations are there?	What are the occupational profiles of different individuals, groups, etc.? Does age, gender, race, religion, ethnicity, ability, health, or socioeconomic status affect what occupations people choose? What are the differences in occupational profiles?
	When do people engage in occupations?	Are occupations engaged in at any time of day, week, year, or life? Are there daily, weekly, seasonally, yearly or life patterns of occupational engagement? Are there particular times when people engage in occupations more; less? How does the cultural, economic, political, and social context determine when people engage in occupations?
	Where do people engage in occupations?	Are occupations specific to a specific context or can they occur anywhere? Are some occupations universal; are some environmentally specific? Are some environments more conducive to some forms of occupational engagement than others?
Explain	**How** are occupations performed?	How are occupations created/learned? How does the process of occupational engagement happen? How does ability affect occupational performance? How is occupational engagement supported? How is it hindered?
	Why do people engage in occupations?	Does occupation have meanings? Do all? Do all people ascribe the same purpose to all occupations? Why do people engage in some occupations and not others?

Design and Data Collection Methods

The design and data collection methods[4] reviewed here emanate from the two major paradigms of formal inquiry addressed. Once a question has been formulated, the next step is to carry out a literature search to determine if the question has already been answered. Knowing what is already recorded also helps to refine a research question. One then chooses a design that is consistent with the question and the paradigm of inquiry. Once the design is set, the actual data collection methods are chosen.

Many designs and data collection methods are available to answer questions about occupation. The more common ones are summarized in Table 3-3 ■. The classification appearing in Table 3-3 is an amalgam, or combination, of a number of different classifications,[5] not that of any particular author: The classification for quantitative designs is essentially that presented in Pedhazur and Schmelkin (19) and Portney and Watkins (9); the classification for qualitative designs is that presented in Creswell (16). The particular design elements that appear in Table 3-3 were chosen not only because they are commonly used but also because: (1) they fit well with the constructs of description and explanation, (2) they eliminate similar terms having different meanings, or (3) their meaning is logically intuitive.

Table 3-3 also provides a listing of the more common methods of data collection for both paradigms. Design and methods of data collection have been distinguished

TABLE 3-3 ***Common Research Methods in the Quantitative and Qualitative Paradigms***

Quantitative	Qualitative
Study Designs	**Study Designs**
Descriptive studies (aka, correlational, observational, survey)	Ethnography (observational)
Experimental studies (including quasi-experimental, true experimental)	Case study
	Phenomenology
	Grounded theory
Methods of Data Collection	**Methods of Data Collection**
(Passive) observation	(Participant) observation
Interview	Interview
Questionnaire	Document and record collection
Measurement	Audiovisual materials
Instrumentation	
Document and record collection	
Audiovisual materials	

Source: This classification is an amalgam of classifications presented by Banister and colleagues (12), Breakwell, and colleagues (26), Clark-Carter (15), Creswell (16), DePoy and Gitlin (17), Glaser and Strauss (25), Glesne (5), Lincoln and Guba (18), and Pedhazur and Shmelkin (19).

for two reasons: (1) *clarity;* frequently there is no distinction made between design and methods of data collection, resulting in confusion in the meaning of terms (e.g., an observational study versus observation as a means of data collection); and (2) *Commonalities/distinctions;* to make it obvious that some methods of data collection (i.e., observation and interview) span the quantitative/qualitative divide (15).

The more common designs for the quantitative paradigm are descriptive and experimental (9, 19). In *descriptive studies,* information is gathered for the purpose of documenting the nature and meaning of the phenomenon at a specific point in time, describing how it changes over time, and exploring relationships among phenomena. In *descriptive studies,* no assignment of subjects or control of variables occurs. In *experimental studies,* hypotheses regarding cause and effect are tested by the manipulation of certain variables and the control of others. In true experimental studies, assignment of subjects is random; in quasi-experimental studies, it is not.

The more common designs for the qualitative paradigm are *ethnography, case study, phenomenology,* and *grounded theory* (5, 16). Historical research may also draw on the qualitative paradigm, for instance, to trace the history of ideas or to interpret archival and archeological evidence using literature and folk stories passed down over time. In *ethnographic studies,* through a process of long-term immersion, a researcher gathers information, primarily by participant observation and interview, about the attitudes, beliefs, and behaviors of a group of people or a culture for the purpose of understanding the forces that shape those behaviors and feelings. In *case studies,* the researcher uses a variety of data collection methods, over a sustained period of time, for the purposes of understanding a particular activity or phenomenon. In *phenomenological studies,* through a process of extensive and prolonged engagement, using observations and interviews, the experience and meaning of individuals' lived realities are examined. In *grounded theory studies,* the researcher, using multiple stages of data collection, collects, codes, and analyzes observational and interview data until the data being collected become redundant. Through a process of constant comparison of data, relevant categories and their relationship are identified and theoretical constructs are formulated. In *historical research,* the researcher would design a study to critically appraise literature, statistics, archival documents, artifacts and other archeological evidence (data) to trace evolving ideas about occupation or about the choices people made about particular occupations in different contexts over time. The weight of evidence for historical truth depends on the completeness and accuracy of information and on gathering multiple forms of evidence from various sources, for instance, to compare literature, songs, and folk stories that reveal the occupations of women and men with statistics on the earnings, parenting, leisure time, social patterns and life span of women and men at particular points in history.

Several designs can be used to answer any particular question. In addition, the same design can be used to answer a number of questions. The designs corresponding to basic questions about occupation are discussed next and examples are given.

UNDERSTANDING WHO

It hardly seems necessary to ask the question, *Who engages in occupations?* Experience tells us that everyone we know, everyone we see around us, everyone we see in the media, everyone we hear about, and everyone we read about—whether in the present or past—engages in occupations. Further, the answer to this question seems to be well established in the historical, anthropological, social, and psychological literature; that is, all people, regardless of the variables that typically distinguish groups, engage in occupations because occupations are what people do. Although there are people whose engagement in occupations may be limited, either temporarily or consistently, it is self-evident that most humans engage in occupations most of the time and under most circumstances.

What warrants investigation, then, is the exception; that is, who does *not* engage in occupation? Generally, qualitative methods of inquiry, such as ethnographies, are more likely to lend themselves to finding the exception. Quantitative inquiry, if used to study both the rule and the exceptions, may also be useful. Examination of existing data can also be informative, for example, documents or records describing individuals or groups of individuals, biographies, and autobiographies.

A good example of an autobiographical account detailing an individual's nonengagement in occupation is *Terry Waite Taken on Trust* (27). Terry Waite was held in solitary confinement in Beirut by terrorists for 1,763 days. During most of that time, he was left with nothing to do because his environment did not allow it. This remarkable man created his own, albeit unorthodox, occupations. That is to say, he wrote his autobiography entirely in his head throughout the duration of his captivity. What becomes blatantly evident from this book is that nonengagement in occupation is difficult to induce. The mind seeks to occupy itself if external occupational stimulation is absent. Further, severely limited engagement is so difficult to bear that individuals create whatever activities or occupations the environment can support, and they resume more occupations or more meaningful occupations as environmental support increases. In other words, when one is considering a person doing an occupation (the who), what they are doing, along with when and where they are doing it, must also be considered. Because we know that context shapes our choices and opportunities to engage in occupations, one would consider how ability/disability, age, culture, gender, ethnicity, race, sexual orientation, social class, or other forms of diversity in humans and their living conditions affect who engages in particular occupations, These issues constitute the *what, when,* and *where* questions of occupation that must be addressed to establish a contextual story line.

UNDERSTANDING WHAT

Trying to answer the question *what,* with respect to occupations, seems a daunting endeavor. Personal experience tells us that there are many occupations—possibly too many to count. One merely needs to look in the do-it-yourself sections of bookstores, or in the hobbies or careers sections, to grasp the vastness of occupational possibilities. There are endless accounts of the occupations of people, regardless of where one looks, be it in the media, the popular literature, the arts, or the historical, anthropological, social, and psychological literature.

Moreover, the naming of occupations is such a culturally laden act that a set of occupations in one cultural context would surely be named differently by another. Understanding the *what* of occupation, then, requires a sensitivity to the context of the occupation; requires that we listen to and observe what people are doing in the context of their lives. As noted in discussing who engages in occupations, consideration of context raises questions about how ability/disability, age, culture, gender, ethnicity, race, sexual orientation, social class or other forms of diversity in humans and their living conditions affect what different people do and why human diversity is displayed strongly in what people need, want, are expected or choose to do.

First, however, it requires examination of what constitutes an occupation, that is, what is and what is not an occupation. This investigation requires the specification of a language and inclusion/exclusion criteria for the use of that language; in other words, it requires taxonomic work. Recently, Polatajko and colleagues (28), arguing that there was insufficient agreement on the language of occupation to guide scholarly development, introduced the *Taxonomic Code for Occupational Performance* (TCOP) as a method of bringing uniformity to the discussion of occupation. TCOP makes a clear distinction between what constitutes an occupation and what are merely subsets of occupation (e.g., turning the key vs. driving the car). TCOP may be a useful tool for advancing our understanding of occupation. However, it requires further examination and validation. An important step in understanding the *what* of occupation will be to continue the development of a taxonomic code.

Given the early state of our taxonomic development, understanding *what* humans do requires a careful descriptive approach to the study of occupational repertoires and profiles. This can be dealt with in a number of ways, including case studies or descriptive studies. Ethnographies provide detailed profiles of individuals or communities, and surveys generate profiles of large groups.

National census databases are excellent sources of survey data on large groups. Most countries have a national agency that routinely collects demographic, socioeconomic, and social information about the paid occupations of its population. The U.S. Census Bureau provides statistics on a large variety of topics that include information on what people do. In the area of labor and employment alone, the Census Bureau provides information on the demographics of the labor force, commuting to work, occupation, industry, and class of worker. It also provides links to statistics from more than 100 U.S. federal agencies. Under the Canadian Statistics Act, Statistics Canada is required to collect and publish statistical information on nearly every aspect of the nation's society and economy. Originally the census was just a simple population count, but today Statistics Canada collects and distributes information from a variety of surveys, offering a rich source of information on the occupations of Canadians. Two types of surveys are used routinely. The first involves population surveys (census) in which every possible respondent is approached. The second features sample surveys that gather data from representative groups of the population. Both types use various survey designs. For instance, a repeated survey design consists of a series of separate cross-sectional surveys. Longitudinal or panel surveys collect information on the same individuals at different points in time. A national census is a repeated survey that uses both census taking and sampling techniques.

Although a census provides a good overview of a nation's occupations, it does not provide a detailed breakdown on occupational patterns. However, a number of other population surveys are available that provide detailed information about occupational or activity patterns. The American (29) and the Canadian (30, 31) General Social Surveys (GSS) monitor changes in the health and activity of Americans and Canadians. The International Social Survey Programme (ISSP) (32), with 40 member countries, provides an archive for data from cross-national collaboration on social science surveys covering a wide variety of topics including work orientation, leisure, and sports. These surveys provide rich data on a huge range of occupations.

To use the Canadian population survey as an example, a repeated telephone survey is conducted approximately every 5 years and includes questions on education, paid work, unpaid work, personal care, physical activities, socializing, passive leisure such as watching television and reading, sports, and other entertainment. This survey also asks about activity limitations. The Canadian GSS is collected from a representative sample of residents 15 years of age and over who reside in Canada. It is noteworthy that the GSS survey refers to *activities,* which this book would define as either occupations or components of occupations, such as tasks or activities, depending on the specifics of the GSS *activities.* Consider what can be learned about a broad range of occupations from a GSS survey. Findings indicate that, aside from personal care, the most common occupations encompass activities and tasks around the home, with 90% of the people participating in household work and related home occupations for an average of 3.6 hours a day. Women spend an average of 1.5 hours more each day on housework than do men. Seventy-seven percent of the population over the age of 15 watches television for an average of 3 hours a day, ranging from a low of 2.3 hours per day for females age 25 to 34 to a high of 4.3 hours per day for males over age 65 (30). In Chapter 5, Pentland and Harvey illustrate how the GSS can be used to understand what people do with their time. One can surmise that future national surveys eventually may collect data on a wider range of occupations, posing questions focusing beyond the activity and task components of occupations, in order to understand how Canadians organize their occupations into routines, meaningful vocations, community building, or paid work.

What becomes evident from existing sources documenting human occupation is that humans have always engaged in a tremendous variety of occupations and that occupations differ among individuals, groups, cultures, and nations, as well as across time. Yet, patterns of occupations are commonly experienced, to which humans' occupational repertoires and profiles attest. Furthermore, it seems clear that understanding the *what* of occupation also requires an understanding of the *who, when,* and *where* of occupation.

UNDERSTANDING WHEN

Our personal experience clearly suggests an answer to the question, *When do people engage in occupations?* The answer is *Always*. Some might answer that occupations occur only during humans' waking hours, depending on whether or not they consider sleep an occupation. Yet sleep is planned, is goal directed, and is more active (both physically and mentally) than most people think. Indeed, those who have traveled with children in the back seat of a long car ride know that people always want to be doing something. Interesting questions about *when* include: *When do people not engage in occupations? Which people engage in which occupations at what times, and for how long?* Understanding *when* is a matter of understanding how occupations and time are related. Occupations occur in the context of time. By asking when, we will understand how humans create occupational patterns across the day, week, month, year, life, and indeed, across history.

We can understand when occupations occur by looking at the arts, popular stories, and literature in history, anthropology, sociology, health, and psychology. The work on circadian rhythms offers fascinating insights into the daily patterns of human occupation. The expression of the circadian rhythm through activity (33) reveals typical patterns of daily occupations (Figure 3-1 ■). The literature on human development also offers notable insights into the patterns of human occupation across the life span. Moreover, historical analyses of occupational patterns provide glimpses into how people's occupational possibilities and expectations have changed throughout history (34, 35).

A number of methods of inquiry can be used to study when occupations occur through patterns of occupational engagement. Virtually all qualitative designs can be used to record and reflect on occupational patterns. Within the quantitative methods of inquiry, time and motion studies, based either on self-report data or observational data, are commonly used.

A good example of a self-report time log is illustrated in the study conducted by Herrmann, who collected data from a group of 20 single adolescent mothers (36). Herrmann described the mothers' daily activities to learn about role conflicts between their maternal and adolescent roles. She asked the young women to keep a time log on which they chronicled all their activities over a period of 4 days, ascribing them to either the mothering or adolescent role and noting their level of satisfaction with the particular activity. The data from the time log showed that these young women spent the majority of their time (78%) doing adolescent activities, leaving much of the child care to others. Herrmann points out that, unexpectedly, this pattern did not differ between weekdays, when the women were in school, and on weekends.

Herrmann's findings (36) show that the individual alone does not determine occupational patterns, but rather they are determined in concert with the environment. With little change in occupational patterns from weekday to weekend, it seems that occupational patterns are affected not only by time but also by the environment in which these patterns occur. Once again, occupation cannot be fully understood by asking a single question, such as, *When do occupations occur?* The challenge of understanding *when* occupations occur is linked with questions about *who, what,* and *where.*

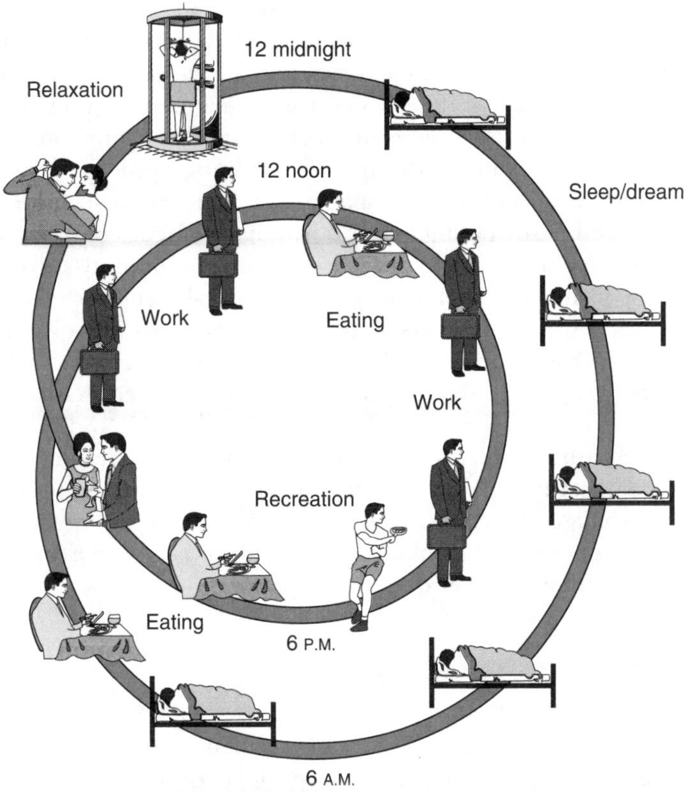

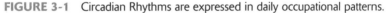

FIGURE 3-1 Circadian Rhythms are expressed in daily occupational patterns.

UNDERSTANDING WHERE

Personal experience, popular literature, and the arts all tell us that occupations happen everywhere—even in those environments where there are attempts to prevent occupational engagement, as Terry Waite experienced in captivity. A more interesting question to ask, therefore, is, *What impact does place, location, or geography have on occupational engagement?*

There are several ways of understanding the influence of place, location, or geography on occupations. All qualitative and quantitative methods are appropriate for studying these types of inquiries. Fields as diverse as human geography, industrial psychology, architecture, sociology of community, urban planning, and community development provide information on the interaction between occupations and environments. A rich and colorful source of data on the effects of place, location, and geography on occupations, now and in the past, is the magazine *National Geographic,* published in the United States. A browse through issues of *National Geographic* shows that occupations occur everywhere, including under the ocean and on the moon. Some occupations occur all around the world, such as infant care, but are done differently in different places, whereas others occur only in specific places, such as surfing, when the surf is up, or on the moon during a manned lunar expedition.

Schisler, who was interested in examining the impact of environmental change on occupational engagement, carried out an ethnographic study of Burundian refugees in Southwestern Ontario, Canada (37). Schisler spent more than a year interacting with and participating in the Burundian refugee community. She spent 17 months as an informal participant observer in this community and one academic term conducting formal participant observations. She also conducted in-depth interviews with 8 of the 18 adult members of this community and did individualized member checks with 6 of these individuals. Using the constant comparison method of data analysis, Schisler found that all participants experienced dramatic changes in their occupations as a result of the physical, social, cultural, and economic differences between Burundi in Africa and Southwestern Ontario in Canada. Of particular interest was the finding that the changes in occupation resulting from the environmental changes affected the people themselves, and they, too, changed. In other words, *where* people engage in occupations affects *when* and *what* they do, which in turn affects *who* they are. How does this happen?

UNDERSTANDING HOW

Whereas the who, what, when, and where of occupation are beginning to be better understood, less is known about *how* people perform occupations. Personal experience can only inform us, very superficially, about the *how* of occupations. Much of the process of occupational performance is not readily observable or knowable; that is, only relatively gross movements involved in the performance of a particular occupation can be observed and only processes that reach **metacognition, or personal awareness,** can be reported. A more in-depth understanding of how occupations are performed requires careful examination of the relevant components of persons and elements of the environment. Quantitative methods of inquiry, often involving specialized instrumentation in an experimental design, are useful for an in-depth understanding of many of the processes involved in occupational performance. Many examples of such studies exist, especially in the ergonomic, medical, movement science, occupational therapy, psychology, and social science literature.

Smyth and Mason (38) carried out an experimental study to investigate differences in the role of vision and proprioception in a positional, aiming task between normal children and children with a developmental coordination disorder (DCD). The two groups of right-handed children (73 with DCD and 73 control without DCD matched on age, sex, and verbal ability) were asked to move their hand under a tabletop into alignment with a target on top of the table. The position of the target was made known to the children by vision, proprioception (their body's sense of where their arms and hands were), or both. Accuracy of performance over 24 trials was measured in millimeters along the horizontal (x) and vertical (y) axes. Results indicated that, with proprioception alone, errors were made to the outside of the targets; the control children tended to favor proprioceptive input, whereas children with DCD tended to favor visual input—but only with their left hand. The authors concluded that detailed error analysis in aiming tasks provided information about target representation that cannot be gleaned from less-specific measurement strategies. This study provides experimental evidence of the impact of person and occupational factors on performance and demonstrates the usefulness of controlled studies in understanding how occupations are performed. Many more studies of this type, investigating all aspects of performance, are necessary before we can truly understand how occupations are performed.

UNDERSTANDING WHY

The final, and perhaps most difficult question to answer in this chapter about occupations, is *Why*? There is a general belief, supported by the media, that the basic reason for occupational engagement is survival. In other words, people work because they have to, because, directly or indirectly, occupations are necessary for subsistence, or enabling acquisition of food and shelter. The implicit notion is that other occupations, such as eating, sleeping, resting, or bathing and grooming, support the main task of work for survival.

Personal experience tells us that there are endless examples of occupational engagement that negate, or at least bring into serious question, this basic survival premise. For example, the survival premise does not explain why people who do not have to work do so, why very young children engage in occupations, or why some people do what they do even without pay. In particular, the basic survival premise does not explain why people do things that put them at serious risk of survival.

All available methods of inquiry need to be used to uncover the *why* of occupation, and new methods need to be developed. The American GSS (29) provides an example of how surveys can be used to look at work values and the meaning of work. Specifically, in the 1973 to 1996 GSS, this question was asked: "If you were to get enough money to live as comfortably as you would like for the rest of your life, would you continue to work or would you stop working?"[6] The examples referred to earlier by Terkel (20) and Joyce (21) provide evidence that a phenomenological study—designed specifically to uncover the meanings people ascribe to their work experiences—is useful, particularly, in learning to understand why people perform the work-related occupations they undertake.

In a smaller scale study, similar to that reported by Terkel, Rudman and colleagues (39) set out to discover the perspectives of community-dwelling, well-elderly persons on the role and importance of occupations in their lives. In-depth interviews were carried out with 12 informants chosen to allow for maximum variation. After an initial analysis of the interview transcripts using a constant comparative method, two-member checking group sessions were held. The results of these discussions were incorporated into the analyses, again using the constant comparative method. The emergent themes indicated that occupations were a means of: expressing and managing personal identity; staying connected to people, their past, and their future; and organizing time. More important, occupational engagement contributed to a sense of well-being for the seniors, to their continued existence, and to the quality of that existence. As one informant put it:

"Most people have a job and that's the only thing, one job all their lives. And the trouble with them is that when they retire, they don't know what the hell to do with themselves. In 2 years, they usually get sick and die." (39, p. 643)

CHAPTER SUMMARY

Understanding occupation, that is, *truly* understanding the who, what, when, where, how, and why of occupation, is a complex task, requiring many diverse methods of inquiry. This chapter illustrates how to learn about occupation. A range of formal and informal methods of inquiry was discussed to open points of entry into the world of scholarly inquiry in occupation. The six questions used to frame this chapter provide guideposts on the road to greater understanding of occupation. Readers are encouraged to participate now in unraveling the mysteries of occupation.

STUDY GUIDE

Study Guide Author: Julie Bass Haugen

Summary of Main Points

Although people have a lot of familiarity and personal experience with human occupations, the formal study of occupation is still in its infancy. This chapter introduced a framework for the study of human occupation and provided specific examples to illustrate how questions about occupation are answered through naturalistic and positivistic paradigms. The journalistic tradition of asking who, what, when, where, why, and how to understand a phenomenon was described as a useful approach to begin identifying questions of importance in occupational science.

Application to Occupational Therapy

Two major modes of understanding or epistemologies may help us to appreciate the different ways of knowing adopted by practitioners. The naturalistic (qualitative) and positivistic (quantitative) paradigms or modes may also be considered part of reflective practice or professional development plans. Three primary sources of information for understanding occupation are useful in gathering information for assessment/evaluation of individuals or communities: personal experience, existing data sources, and new investigations. The fourth primary source of information is to recognize knowledge as constructed, changing, and relative to the subject and situation. Practitioners are encouraged to critically analyze how systems and other environmental forces influence occupation in order to expand their understanding of the complex nature of human occupation.

The *who, what, when, where, why,* and *how* questions used as a basis for studying occupation also are relevant in a framework for assessment of occupation in occupational therapy practice. To fully understand an individual's occupational profile, the answers to these questions need to be obtained. The design and data collections methods associated with the naturalistic (qualitative) and positivistic (quantitative) paradigms provide us with two approaches to assessment. Each approach provides valuable insights that will guide intervention planning.

Qualitative and quantitative evidence from studies of human occupation strengthens support for the practice of occupational therapy. The two paradigms discussed in this chapter have direct parallels to approaches for assessment and intervention in occupational therapy practice. Our understanding of the who, what, when, where, why, and how of occupation is integral to providing client-centered, occupation-based, evidence-based practice.

Individual Learning Activities

1. Analyze a published study related to human occupation.
   a. Identify the who, what, when, where, why, and how questions that were addressed in this study.
   b. Identify the paradigm and specific design and data collection methods that were used to answer the questions in this study.
   c. Describe how you would apply the findings from this study in occupational therapy practice.
2. Discuss your current mode of understanding or epistemology for the following topics:
   - Treatment options for breast cancer or prostate cancer
   - The alignment of a political party's philosophy with one' personal values and beliefs
   - Comparison of the sleep patterns for you and a friend
   - The outcomes of a specific occupational therapy intervention

     a. Identify your current mode of understanding for each topic and provide a rationale for this status.
     b. How would further study of each topic change your mode of understanding?

Group Learning Activity

Form groups of three to four members and select a topic of interest related to human occupation.

a. Obtain two published articles on the topic for each group member and discuss your learning about the *who, what, when, where, why,* and *how* of this aspect of human occupation.
b. Based on your learning about this topic, develop a *who, what, when, where, why,* or *how* question that would further your understanding about this aspect of human occupation.
c. Select a paradigm and describe the design and data collection methods that you would use to answer the question.
d. Summarize your learning from the published articles and your study proposal in a group paper. Document your references.

Study Questions

1. Epistemological positions were defined as
   a. Multivariate statistics
   b. Research questions
   c. Ways of understanding
   d. Intellectual development
2. All of the following are true of disciplinary paradigms EXCEPT
   a. Ways of knowing are always unique to the discipline.
   b. Disciplines may adopt one or more preferred ways of knowing.
   c. Ways of knowing are not static or fixed.
   d. Similar disciplines may share similar ways of knowing.
3. The naturalistic paradigm is also referred to as
   a. Positivistic research
   b. Qualitative research
   c. Reductionistic research
   d. More than one of the above
4. The designs that are common for the positivistic paradigm include all of the following EXCEPT
   a. Descriptive studies
   b. Experimental studies
   c. Grounded theory studies
   d. All of the above
5. The relationship of occupations to time may be investigated through this question:
   a. What
   b. How
   c. Why
   d. When

REFERENCES

1. Ferguson, D. L., & Patten, J. (1979). *Journalism today: An introduction.* Skokie, IL: National Textbook.
2. *International Webster New Encyclopedic Dictionary of the English Language & Library of Useful Knowledge.* (1972). New York: Tabor House.
3. Kolb, D. A. (1981). Learning styles and disciplinary differences. In A. W. Chickering & associates (Eds.), *The modern American college: Responding to the new realities of diverse students and a changing society* (pp. 232–255). Washington, DC: Jossey-Bass.
4. Belenky, M. F., Clinchy, B. M., Goldberger, N. R., & Tarule, J. M. (1997). *Women's ways of knowing: The development of self, voice, and mind* (10th Anniversary ed.). New York: Basic Books.
5. Glesne, C. (2006). *Becoming qualitative researchers: An introduction* (3rd ed.). Boston: Allyn & Bacon.

6. Perry, W. G., Jr. (1970). *Forms of intellectual and ethical development in the college years: A scheme.* Toronto, ON: Holt, Rinehart and Winston.
7. Drew, C. J., Hardman, M. L., & Weaver Hart, A. (1996). *Designing and conducting research: Inquiry in education and social science* (2nd ed.). Toronto, ON: Allyn & Bacon.
8. Neutens, J. J., & Rubinson, L. (2002). *Research techniques for the health sciences* (3rd ed.). San Francisco: Benjamin Cummings.
9. Portney, L. G., & Watkins, M. P. (2000). *Foundations of clinical research: Applications to practice* (2nd ed.). Upper Saddle River, NJ: Prentice Hall.
10. Jackson, W. (2003). *Methods: Doing social research* (3rd ed.). Toronto, ON: Prentice Hall.
11. Kuhn, T. S. (1996). *The structure of scientific revolutions* (3rd ed.). Chicago: University of Chicago Press.
12. Banister, P., Burman, E., Parker, I., Taylor, M., & Tindall, C. (1994). *Qualitative methods in psychology: A research guide.* Philadelphia: Open University Press.
13. Haworth, J. (1996). Introduction: Contemporary psychological research: Vision from positional standpoints. In J. Haworth (Ed.), *Psychological research: Innovative methods and strategies* (pp. 1–14). New York: Routledge.
14. Hayes, N. (1997). Introduction: Qualitative research and research in psychology. In N. Hayes (Ed.), *Doing qualitative analysis in psychology* (pp. 1–8). Hove, England: Psychology Press.
15. Clark-Carter, D. (1997). *Doing quantitative psychological research: From design to report.* Hove, England: Psychology Press.
16. Creswell, J. W. (2003). *Research design: Qualitative, quantitative and mixed methods approaches* (2nd ed.). Thousand Oaks, CA: Sage.
17. DePoy, E., & Gitlin, L. N. (2005). *Introduction to research: Understanding and applying multiple strategies* (3rd ed.). St. Louis, MO: Mosby.
18. Lincoln, Y. S., & Guba, E. G. (1985). *Naturalistic inquiry.* Thousand Oaks, CA: Sage.
19. Pedhazur, E. J., & Schmelkin, L. P. (1991). *Measurement, design, and analysis: An integrated approach.* Hillsdale, NJ: Lawrence Erlbaum.
20. Terkel, S. (1975). *Working.* New York: Avon Books.
21. Joyce, P. (Ed.). (1989). *The historical meanings of work.* New York: Cambridge University Press.
22. Csikszentmihalyi, M. (1990). Foreword. In J. A. Johnson & E. J. Yerxa (Eds.), *Occupational science: The foundation for new models of practice* (pp. xv–xvii). New York: The Haworth Press.
23. Yerxa, E. J., Clark, F., Frank, G., Jackson, J., Parham, D., Pierce, D., et al. (1990). An introduction to occupational science: A foundation for occupational therapy in the 21st century. In J. A. Johnson & E. J. Yerxa (Eds.), *Occupational science: The foundation for new models of practice* (pp. 2–17). New York: The Haworth Press.
24. Richards, I. A. (1965). *Principles of literary criticism.* New York: Harcourt, Brace & World, Inc. (Originally published 1925)
25. Glaser, B. G., & Strauss, A. L. (1968). *The discovery of grounded theory: Strategies for qualitative research.* Chicago: Aline.
26. Breakwell, G. M., Hammond, S., Fife-Schaw, C., & Smith, J. A. (Eds.). (2006). *Research methods in psychology* (3rd ed.). Thousand Oaks, CA: Sage.
27. Waite, T. (1993). *Terry Waite taken on trust.* Toronto: Doubleday Canada.
28. Polatajko, H. J., Davis, J. A., Hobson, S., Landry, J., Mandich, A., Street, S. et al. (2004). National perspective: Meeting the responsibility that comes with the privilege: Introducing a taxonomic code for understanding occupation. *Canadian Journal of Occupational Therapy, 71*(5), 261–268.
29. National Research Council. (1999). *The changing nature of work: Implications for occupational analysis.* Washington, DC: National Academy Press.

30. Statistics Canada. (1999). *General social survey: Overview of the time use of Canadians in 1998* (Catalogue No. 12F0080XIE). Ottawa, ON: Minister of Industry.
31. Statistics Canada. (2004). General social survey: An overview. (Catalogue No. 89F0115XIE). Ottawa, ON: Ministry of Industry. Retrieved April 9, 2006, from, http://www.statcan.ca/cgi-bin/downpub/listpub.cgi?catno=89F0115XIE2004001
32. International Social Survey Programme. (n.d.). Retrieved April 9, 2006, from http://www.issp.org/homepage.htm
33. Fincher, J. (1984). *The brain: Mystery of mind and matter.* Toronto, ON: Torstar Books.
34. Davis, J. A., Polatajko, H. J., & Ruud, C. A. (2002). Children's occupations in context: The influence of history. *Journal of Occupational Science, 9*(2), 54–64.
35. Wilcock, A. A. (2006). *An occupational perspective of health.* Thorofare, NJ: Slack Inc.
36. Herrmann, C. (1990). A descriptive study of daily activities and role conflict in single adolescent mothers. In J. A. Johnson & E. J. Yerxa (Eds.), *Occupational science: The foundation for new models of practice* (pp. 53–68). New York: The Haworth Press.
37. Schisler, A. M. C., & Polatajko, H. J. (2002). The individual as mediator of the person-occupation-environment interaction: Learning from the experiences of refugees. *Journal of Occupational Science, 9*(2), 82–92.
38. Smyth, M. M., & Mason, U. C. (1998). Direction of response in aiming to visual and proprioceptive targets in children with and without developmental coordination disorder. *Human Movement Science, 17,* 515–539.
39. Rudman, D. L., Cook, J. V., & Polatajko, H. (1997). Understanding the potential of occupation: A qualitative exploration of seniors' perspective on activity. *American Journal of Occupational Therapy, 51*(8), 640–650.
40. Johnson, J. A., & Yerxa, E. J. (Eds.). (1990). *Occupational science: The foundation for new models of practice.* New York: The Haworth Press.
41. Polatajko, H. J. (1992). Muriel Driver lecture. Naming and framing occupational therapy: A lecture dedicated to the life of Nancy B. *Canadian Journal of Occupational Therapy, 59*(4), 189–200.

Endnotes

[1]Johnson, Yerxa, and her colleagues (40) have called the new science *occupational science.* Polatajko (41) has suggested that the study of occupation ought to be referred to as *occupationology.*

[2]Polatajko (41) uses the term *occupationology* to preclude the a priori presumptions inherent in the term *science.* The classic view of science is of inquiries that are conducted in a number of set stages starting with a hypothesis (15), thereby excluding qualitative inquiries.

[3]Clark-Carter (15) suggests that, for psychology, *control* is understood to mean intervene for the purposes of improving human life. In the case of occupational therapy, control is understood in the collaborative sense to mean "enable" for the purposes of prompting, facilitating, or otherwise enabling people to generate insights or opportunities to choose their occupations.

[4]Note, some confusion exists in the literature about the use of the terms *method* and *design.* Here the term *method* is used in conjunction with the phrase *of inquiry* (i.e., *method of inquiry,*) and refers to all aspects of a study including the paradigm to be used, the design, and the specific data collection methods and procedures, analysis, and interpretation. The term *design* refers to the overall structure and plan of a study that emanates from the paradigm of inquiry and the question and determines the specific procedures and data collection

methods to be adhered to in conducting the study. The term *method,* used either alone or in conjunction with the phrases *of data collection, analysis,* and *interpretation,* refers to the specifics of data collection, analysis, and interpretation, respectively.

[5]A number of ways can be used to classify designs. Some are based on purpose; others are based on data collection strategies or analytical strategies; many are based on a mixed model of naming (15, 26). There is no agreement on the best classification, nor is there any agreement on the terminology used to name what are essentially the same designs, for example, the terms *nonexperimental, correlational, survey,* and (passive) *observational* have all been used to refer to the same designs (19).

[6]Most Americans indicated that they would continue to work. The numbers range from a low of 65% in 1974 and a high of 77% in 1980. The most recent results from 1996 indicate that 68% would continue to work.

CHAPTER 4

What Is Occupation? Interdisciplinary Perspectives on Defining and Classifying Human Activity

Jennifer Jarman

OBJECTIVES

1. Challenge ideas about occupation.
2. Examine three perspectives on occupation: (1) occupational therapy and occupational science, (2) social science, and (3) official statistical agencies that collect and classify data associated with the formal workforce.
3. Explore how the different meanings of occupation affect our understanding of the social world.
4. Establish an understanding of perspectives to communicate effectively across disciplinary and professional boundaries and to learn from each other.

KEY WORDS

Division of labor
Gender
International Standard Classification of Occupations (ISCO)
Occupation
Occupational structure
Social class
Suboccupation

www.prenhall.com/christiansen

The Internet provides an exciting means for interacting with this textbook and for enhancing your understanding of humans' experiences with occupations and the organization of occupations in society. Use the address above to access the interactive Companion Website created specifically to accompany this book. Here you will find an array of self-study material designed to help you gain a richer understanding of the concepts presented in this chapter.

I would like to thank Elizabeth Townsend for her enthusiasm for this topic as well as for her help with locating relevant occupational therapy and occupational science literature. I would also like to thank Tracey Pye for her careful library research.

CHAPTER PROFILE

The purpose of this chapter is to examine three different ways in which human activities or *occupations* have been described or defined. Presented here are the perspectives of three communities with interests in occupation: (1) occupational therapy and occupational science, (2) social science, and (3) official statistical agencies that collect and classify data associated with the formal workforce. All three communities have arrived at working definitions of the concept of "occupation." Each community has somewhat different goals in relation to "occupation"; these variations are reflected in the definitions they create.

Additionally, the chapter explores what consequences the different meanings have for our understanding of the social world and important issues pertaining to it. Let us be clear that any one definition or classification of occupation is not better than any other, but that different criteria are used in order to define and classify occupation for different purposes. Most readers may come across the term *occupation* in several different contexts, so it is important to understand the reasons for these different definitions to communicate effectively and clearly across disciplinary and professional boundaries.

INTRODUCTION

People's occupations are such a basic part of their social world and culture that even very young children are well acquainted with their existence. Children's rhymes are full of references to a variety of occupations:

Rub-a-dub dub, three men in a tub,
The butcher, the baker, the candle-stick maker,
They all jumped out of a rotten potato.

Mother Goose Nursery Rhymes

Cobbler, cobbler, mend my shoe
Get it done by half past two.
Half past two is much too late!
Get it done by half past eight.

Mother Goose Nursery Rhymes

Children's songs are similarly full of references:

Oh, who are the people in your neighborhood?
In your neighborhood?
In your neighborhood?
Say, who are the people in your neighborhood?
The people that you meet each day?
Oh, the postman always brings the mail
Through rain or snow or sleet or hail
I'll work and work the whole day through

To get your letters safe to you
'Cause a postman is a person in your neighborhood
In your neighborhood
He's in your neighborhood
A postman is a person in your neighborhood
A person that you meet each day

(and so on through verses involving the fireman, the baker, the teacher, the barber, the bus driver, the dentist, the doctor [female Muppet], the grocer, the shoemaker, the cleaner and the trash collector).[1]

These rhymes and songs tell children a little about people in common work occupations. All these rhymes and songs suggest that occupation is most often viewed intrinsically as work; however, this book will challenge readers to consider the many ways in which humans are occupied, including ways that go beyond the endeavors we commonly view as work.

If a 5-year-old knows about occupations through nursery rhymes, you may be asking yourselves, why do we need an entire chapter devoted to the question of *What is occupation?* The answer is that the 5-year-old may have a straightforward answer to the question on a simple level. As a social scientist, I would argue that occupations are actually complex concepts that have different usages in different contexts. Defining the concept *occupation* is a complex task in all these contexts. It is even complex and controversial to define occupation as a "concept" versus a "phenomenon" or maybe a "process" or an "interaction" involving humans in their environments.

OCCUPATION IN OCCUPATIONAL THERAPY AND OCCUPATIONAL SCIENCE

It has been commonly believed that being occupied in a variety of ways makes people actually experience educational, health, social, and other benefits. In fact, occupational therapy became a profession in the early part of the 20th century and took its name both from its interest in occupation and its use of occupations to advance health and well-being in everyday life (1). Occupational therapists drew on an idea that is fairly old—the idea that people maintain or regain their health more quickly if they are involved in some kind of meaningful activity (i.e., occupation). In his Messenter Lectures, noted medical historian H. E. Sigerist noted that "our brain slips into chaos and confusion unless we constantly use it for work that seems worthwhile to us" (2). In 1922, Adolf Meyer, the father of American psychiatry, wrote: "Occupational therapy contends that what people do with their time, their occupation, is crucially important for their well-being. It is a person's occupation that makes life ultimately meaningful" (3). Much of current occupational therapy has developed around the notion of engagement between a therapist and a patient. Occupational therapists attempt to identify occupations that are meaningful and that assist people of all ages to develop their skills to deal with everyday life more successfully despite an illness, disability, or limitations faced by those who are aging.

Occupational therapists work toward a very finely nuanced understanding of what an occupation means with respect to any individual, family, group, or community, or to any category of health impairment, disability, or limitation on daily participation. This work can involve complex testing of motor skills, communication/interaction skills, and social, psychological, and organizational aspects of human existence in the natural or built environment. In scientific writings, the detail of the analysis of human occupation often used by occupational therapists is striking. The following excerpt is drawn by Nelson (4) from an analysis of the interaction between an occupational therapist and a woman trying to regain her driving skills after she incurred a brain injury in a car accident. In the excerpt, the woman is driving the car, and the occupational therapist is analyzing her actions.

> Fifteen minutes into the occupation, the patient's car is stationary for 40 seconds at a stop sign marking a major road. The route called for a right turn, but steady traffic moved by at approximately 50 miles per hour. The driver in the car behind her throws up his hands in apparent frustration.
>
> The traffic on the major road confused the patient. She misperceived the speed of oncoming cars, and the glare of the sun on the windshield compounded the problem. The apparent frustration of the man in the car behind her made her feel anxious. When it finally appeared that there was a break in the traffic flow, she overestimated the force necessary to depress the accelerator and underestimated the interval between accelerating and turning.
>
> Initially at the intersection, the patient simply wanted to make a right turn and be on her way. However, the longer she waited at the stop sign, the more she felt torn between wanting to be safe and wanting to escape the discomfort. When she almost lost control of the car, she had a powerful desire to right its course. Then she consciously wanted to learn from her mistake.
>
> At the busy intersection, the patient's occupational performance [driving] was marked by 40 seconds of repeated trunk and neck rotation with alternating glances at the rear-view mirror. Suddenly, she made an uncommonly quick move of the right foot from the brake to the accelerator and then plantar flexed her foot with power. Next, she forcefully rotated the steering wheel to the right. Immediately after, she frowned and declared forcefully "I've got to take my time and concentrate on the right thing." A few moments later in a calmer voice, she stated, "That guy behind us has his own problems . . . I had enough to concentrate on." She said further, "You know, I used to avoid situations like this and go only where there are stop lights. That's been the story of my life—avoiding things." (4, pp. 776–777)

In this case, "driving a car" is defined as an occupation. This is further divided into the **suboccupation** of "turning right in a stressful situation." Nelson also breaks the occupation down into "occupational performances,"[2] which include looking at the street map, adjusting posture in the driver's seat, pushing with the foot on the foot pedal and accelerator, turning the steering wheel, and speaking. What is noteworthy about the analysis is that the occupational therapist goes beyond observing the physical performances involved in the act of driving (pushing one's foot down, turning one's head a number of times in a particular way) and assesses much of the emotional and decision-making work that is also part of the occupation of driving.

The minute detail in which this occupation of everyday life is considered enhances an understanding of the complexity of human social life. Skills and acts that are taken for granted by most of us are revealed to be complex interplays of many different physical and social skills and processes when seen from the perspective of an ill or injured person by an occupational therapist. Occupation is not just something that is done, nor is it just a category of work. Instead, occupation involves a series of thoughts, actions, and interactions in particular places and times. To understand this, the observer must analyze the components of daily human engagement.

Although the example just given involved a daily occupation in the life of a person struggling with medical impairment, this is not the only area of interest expressed by occupational therapists. Loree Primeau is both an occupational therapist and an occupational scientist (the difference will be explained shortly). Her work examines how parents shape the balance between work and play in their interactions with their children to understand how these occupations may influence the health and life satisfaction of family members. She analyzes a number of "household" occupations. Let us look at one illustration of her use of the term *occupation.* In this illustration, Brent is the father, Riley is a young son, and Laura is a young daughter (5).

> Brent picked up a lawn edger, a long-handled, mechanical tool that trims the edge of the lawn. He took it and ran it along the grass at the edge of the driveway. Riley immediately asked, "Can I do it, Daddy? Can I do it?" When Brent was finished with it, he gave the lawn edger to Riley who began to edge the lawn along the curb of the street. Brent got the hedge clippers out and began to clip the hedges. After a couple of minutes, Laura got off of her tricycle and went over to Riley. She wanted to try the lawn edger too. Riley reluctantly gave Laura the edger. She tried to imitate Riley, but was having difficulty. When Riley asked for the lawn edger back, Laura gave it to him and then ran over to Brent, asking him to let her do what he was doing. Brent said, "Okay, but I'll have to help you." He put his hands over hers on the hedge clippers and helped her to cut off parts of the hedge. He would point out to her what part they were going to trim, then he would direct her hands over to that spot, and help her clip it. Riley, after watching this, asked for a chance to trim the hedge too. He told his dad that he didn't need help; he knew how to do it. Brent just pointed out the parts for him to trim, and Riley cut them off. (5, pp. 192–193)

This is an example of what Primeau calls *scaffolded play,* meaning that the parents structure an adult occupation so that it involves their children in as independent a manner as possible. Here the elements of the occupation can be seen to be different, depending on whose perspective is chosen. Looking at the actions of the parent, the occupation involves both child care and yard work, whereas a focus on the child makes us realize that the occupation involves both play and yard work. Primeau's conclusion is that families organize work and play as patterns of segregation and inclusion. This is an example of children being included in a parent's work occupation. A pattern of segregation would be one in which children were separated when a parent was engaged in a work occupation. For our purposes, we must note that an occupation may contain bundles of activities, and deciding where one occupation leaves off and another begins is a decision for the analyst. We should also note that there might be different levels of analysis, which in this case has been handled by the introduction of the idea of a suboccupation.

The second observation that we can make about the way occupational therapists view occupation is that the profession proceeds with a fairly broad and nonjudgmental way of thinking about what kinds of occupations are meaningful to individuals, families, groups, communities, or others. Occupational therapists work with people to identify "occupations" that are meaningful to them and to devise strategies that enable individuals, groups or communities to resume or relearn occupations, or indeed to learn new occupations to live a meaningful life. In so doing, occupational therapists are compelled to understand the complexity of the social aspects of what it means to be human—to come to terms with how complicated our everyday lives are, based on the ways in which we interact in social, physical, and policy environments. Occupational therapists also consider a wide range of ways in which people occupy their time and space. In assessing the occupations of children, for example, an occupational therapist goes beyond the commonsense notion that occupation innately has something to do with work. The occupations of children may revolve much more heavily around playing and learning in particular times and places; similarly, the occupations of elderly people may revolve around maintaining active, involved, and independent lifestyles, the options available being determined by where they live and when they decide to become engaged.

Not surprisingly, occupational therapists consider fundamental questions about the nature of modern society because they must consider what type of world they are helping people to actively negotiate. Indeed, they consider how that world has produced some of the dysfunctions associated with the occupations that they analyze. This takes them beyond the individual concerns to communal and societal considerations. Some occupational therapy writers are developing critiques of mainstream culture as a result. Not surprisingly, questions concerning the pace and nature of modern life—its speed, spiritual values, or lack thereof, and a concern for ritual and meaning arise frequently (6, 7).

Such is the importance of occupation in everyday life that an interdisciplinary research field, *occupational science*, was established in the 1980s with the goal of exploring and understanding the nature, meaning, and sociocultural structure of occupation. If occupations help to maintain health, then it is certainly important to have a good understanding of how they are constituted. Although occupational therapists have taken a strong lead in formulating occupational science, researchers from anthropology, economics, geography, political science, psychology, sociology, and other fields with concerns for everyday life have also been drawn to its study. Let's look at a few ways in which occupational scientists have defined occupation:

> Occupations are the ordinary and familiar things that people do every day. This simple description reflects, but understates, the multidimensional and complex nature of daily occupation. (8, p. 1015)

> Occupation, that is, purposeful activity. Occupation is the mechanism by which individuals demonstrate the use of their capacities by achievements of value and worth to their society and the world. (3, pp. 17–18)

> [O]ccupation is the active process of everyday living. Occupation comprises all the ways in which we occupy ourselves individually and as societies. Everyday life proceeds through a myriad of occupations, embedded in time and place, and in the cultural and other patterns that organize what we do. Moreover, occupations are named, organized, and given value and meaning by each culture. Occupation is highly gendered, with household work and parenting typically allocated to women. The active process of occupation is a basic human need since it enables humans to develop as individuals and members of society. To live is to enfold multiple occupations which provide enjoyment, payment, personal identity and more. (9, p. 19)

What do these definitions have in common? They all suggest that occupations emerge from the routine and everyday aspects of daily living, and they all contain the same assumption—that everyday living is actually a very complex process. Several of the definitions relate occupation to demonstrations of worth and value in society. Furthermore, Townsend informs us that "occupations are not random acts," but rather represent "purposes, goals, meaning and even express personal and cultural ideas of spirituality" (9, pp. 20–21). So occupations are not just any kinds of activities, they have a sense of purpose to them and give meaning. Daily life may comprise "myriads of occupations," but all these occupations are not necessarily viewed equally. Whereas it was mentioned earlier that occupational therapists tend to be fairly open minded about what constitutes a significant occupation viewed from the perspective of any particular individual, Townsend recognizes that some occupations are more highly valued within a society than others. Finally, she suggests that some occupations are **gendered** in the sense that they tend to be undertaken by one gender or the other.

So far, we have examined the concept of occupation as used by occupational therapists and occupational scientists. We have learned that occupations are finely nuanced and are assessed in great detail. Furthermore, we have learned that they may be drawn from activities usually considered to be "work," but that they may also go beyond these boundaries to include "play" occupations, "leisure" occupations, "therapeutic" occupations, or indeed any kind of occupation that is meaningful to the individual, the society, and the analyst. Sometimes it is difficult to decide precisely what constitutes the boundary between one occupation and another, so some writers have introduced terminology such as *suboccupation* or *occupational scaffolding* to describe the way in which occupations have components nested within them.

In defining occupations, occupational therapists and occupational scientists are led into a direct assessment of the commonsense notions that we typically have learned through our socialization. It also appears that occupations have a purposeful character and are meaningful to those engaged within them. Although they may be meaningful in different ways to various individuals, there are broad social understandings that certain occupations are more valued than others. These understandings are derived from the structures of social inequality present in most societies. In contemporary societies, "work" occupations have been more highly valued for a variety of historical, religious, and ideological reasons, notably based on sociocultural ideas about gender (10, 11). Many occupational therapists and scientists are currently seeking to challenge their primacy and assert the importance of occupations in other spheres of life.

OCCUPATION IN THE SOCIAL SCIENCES

"Occupation" has also been a concept of central concern to social scientists interested in understanding the nature of our contemporary world. One of the most significant early attempts to understand the role of occupations in society was outlined in what has become a classic sociological book, *The Division of Labor in Society* (12). It was written by the French sociologist Emile Durkheim (1859–1917), who is commonly regarded as one of the most important founding figures of the discipline of sociology. Durkheim made a distinction between traditional (preindustrial) societies and modern societies, and he based this distinction on the nature of the **division of labor** in society. In his view, earlier societies had a simple division of labor with a limited specialization of functions. Modern societies with modern industrial production systems developed with a fine division of labor. It looked to many 19th-century social observers that the old world that they had known was falling apart, and that a major amount of social conflict (revolutions, uprisings, class warfare) was a feature of industrial society. It was an essential part of Durkheim's argument, however, that the finer and finer divisions of labor that were emerging in modern societies created greater and greater *interdependence* of human beings on one another. In earlier hunting-and-gathering societies, individuals (or family groups) were relatively self-sufficient. In contemporary societies, where tasks are highly specialized, individuals and even families are very far from being self-sufficient and instead depend on the work of others on a day-to-day basis. It was Durkheim's view that a complex division of labor creates peace because competition between organisms of the same type is reduced:

> In the same city, different occupations can co-exist without being obliged mutually to destroy one another, for they pursue different objects. The soldier seeks military glory, the priest moral authority, the statesman power, the businessman riches, and the scholar scientific renown. (12, p. 265)

If we consider what is meant by Durkheim's use of the term *occupation,* we can see that it is somewhat different from the way in which occupational therapists and occupational scientists use the term. Durkheim is using the term to refer to what the *Chambers 20th Century Dictionary* terms "one's habitual employment, profession, craft or trade" (13). Virtually all the examples of occupations that he uses are based on what would now be called the *formal economy.* They refer to situations of paid employment. Presumably, the concept still can be considered to contain notions of goal-directed activities that were present in the occupational therapists' and occupational scientists' definitions. Goals that might be fulfilled by engaging in occupations in the formal economy might include earning wages and benefits, interacting socially with other people, and making a contribution to society.

Just as we noted that occupational therapists and occupational scientists introduce ideas that some occupations are valued more highly than others, Durkheim's analysis also introduces this aspect of occupation. Some occupations receive higher pay than others (professional basketball players earn more than kindergarten teachers), some occupations have more social status than others (university professors have more social status than dockworkers), and some occupations have better working conditions than others (secretaries have better working conditions than garbage collectors).

One of Durkheim's primary concerns, and one that many other social scientists after him shared, was that one's occupations should be based on one's talents and capacities and that there should be no obstacles to someone undertaking an occupation for which his[3] or her talents and capacities are fitting. This would constitute injustice in Durkheim's view and would become the basis for conflict in society.

Many other social scientists have picked up Durkheim's themes—the intricate division of labor that characterizes contemporary industrial societies, as well as the relationship of the occupational structure to social inequality and class conflict. Harry Braverman, for example, started a debate about the impact of technology in creating changes in the occupational structure of American society (14). He examined the American economy and argued that over time, occupations were becoming less and less skill based and that this skill was being transferred into machines, especially computers. For example, no longer does one need to hire a really accurate and skilled typist because the spell-checker in a word-processing program can quickly correct many of the mistakes. Braverman's work is intrinsically about the meaning of the changes associated with the decline of certain occupations and the rise of others, and he argues that with the loss of skill also comes a loss of status and bargaining power over wages for the majority of workers in the labor force.

Another avenue of investigation explored by many social scientists is concerned with the gender and ethnic composition of the occupational structure. Researchers have observed that occupations often have a strong gender or ethnic *typing*. Coal miners are most likely to be male; midwives are most likely to be female; professional ice hockey players are most likely to be Caucasian; reggae artists are most likely to be of Caribbean descent. The gender composition of occupations has been explored as social scientists try to understand the consequence of the existing patterns of social inequality and also investigate what changes are occurring over time. The racial composition of the occupational structure has been studied since the 1950s, with researchers trying to estimate the extent of racial discrimination in labor markets and its consequences for both individuals and communities (15). More recently, the gender composition of occupations has been of interest; in particular, to understand how successful women enter occupations that are traditionally male occupations (such as steelworker, engine mechanic, and doctor), and how successful men enter occupations that are traditionally female occupations (nurse, elementary schoolteacher, telephone operator) and how the traditional gender composition of occupations influences pay and stratification levels (16).

Social scientists in many countries have developed scales that measure **social class** or *social advantage*. These scales are based on occupations and are generally used to investigate levels of social inequality and social difference on a whole range of subjects: health and illness outcomes, voting patterns, wealth and income distribution, housing quality, propensity to obtain higher education, and so on. Examples include Canada's Blishen–McRoberts (17) and Pineo–Porter (18) scales, the United Kingdom's Registrar-General's Scale as well as the Cambridge scale, based on occupational, friendship, and marriage scores (19, 20).

To summarize the way in which social scientists use the concept of occupation, we can see that, once again, it emerges as a concept of fundamental importance. Occupations tend to have been viewed as arising from the work sphere, but in more recent years the boundaries have begun to be challenged as feminists have stressed the need to consider how women's occupations are defined, whether they are included, and in what detail they are enumerated (14–20). Social scientists have been very interested in how occupational structures change over time and what meanings this has for understanding the evolution of society and broad patterns of social inequality.

OCCUPATION IN GOVERNMENT STATISTICS

So widespread has been the focus on "occupation" as a category for research and government policy making that most governments around the world systematically and regularly collect statistical information about the occupations of the general population in the censuses, in labor force surveys, in general household surveys, and in health surveys. Many different constituencies of people use official statistics: researchers, policy makers, and even the business community. There is wide agreement across nations that "occupation" is of major interest when trying to understand trends in the labor market, health, consumption patterns, voting behavior, and general life advantages.

In the section on occupational therapists' and occupational scientists' use of the term "occupation," I noted that occupation could be defined by an occupational therapist in terms of a meaningful activity for an individual or social group, such as a family. When governments are collecting data, however, they go to great lengths to try to ensure that all the information that has been collected is classified in a way that is uniform from one analyst to the next if they give the same information. To ensure this kind of uniformity, national governments develop extensive classification manuals that define how occupations are to be coded so that information from one state or region can be reliably compared to information from another.

Government classifications are not arbitrary nor are they set in stone. Underlying any particular classification scheme is a whole set of assumptions that have been debated at length. Look for a moment at a small section of one widely used occupational classification scheme—the **International Standard Classification of Occupations (ISCO)**, which was introduced in 1988. Some countries have developed their own classification methods that are tailored to the types and detail of occupations found in the labor market and industrial structure of their own country. Creating such systems involves resource allocations that are often not a priority, especially for countries of the Southern Hemisphere. Many countries, therefore, rely on the International Labour Office's scheme. It was designed to be an international standard and to include occupations relevant in both Northern and Southern contexts, in industrial economies, and agricultural economies. This classification system is organized hierarchically. When analysts need to work with very general categories, they can use the major groups. If they need more detail, there are submajor groups (subdivisions of major groups) available. If they need even more detail, there are minor groups (subdivisions of submajor groups). If they need a fine level of detail, then there are unit groups (subdivisions of minor groups) available. Table 4-1 ■ illustrates how the first major group breaks down into smaller groups.

TABLE 4-1 *Major Group 1: Legislators, Senior Officials, and Managers*

Code			Title
1			**Legislators, senior officials and managers**
	11		**Legislators and senior officials**
	111		**Legislators**
		1110	Legislators
	112		**Senior government officials**
		1120	Senior government officials
	113		**Traditional chiefs and heads of villages**
		1130	Traditional chiefs and heads of villages
	114		**Senior officials of special-interest organisations**
		1141	Senior officials of political-party organisations
		1142	Senior officials of employers', workers' and other economic-interest organisations
		1143	Senior officials of humanitarian and other special-interest organisations
	12		**Corporate managers**
			(This group is intended to include persons who—as directors, chief executives or department managers—manage enterprises or organisations, or departments, requiring a total of three or more managers.)
	121		**Directors and chief executives**
		1210	Directors and chief executives
	122		**Production and operations department managers**
		1221	Production and operations department managers in agriculture, hunting, forestry and fishing
		1222	Production and operations department managers in manufacturing
		1223	Production and operations department managers in construction
		1224	Production and operations department managers in wholesale and retail trade
		1225	Production and operations department managers in restaurants and hotels
		1226	Production and operations department managers in transport, storage and communications
		1227	Production and operations department managers in business services
		1228	Production and operations department managers in personal care, cleaning and related services
		1229	Production and operations department managers not elsewhere classified
	123		**Other department managers**
		1231	Finance and administration department managers
		1232	Personnel and industrial relations department managers
		1233	Sales and marketing department managers

(continued)

TABLE 4-1 *Continued*

	1234	Advertising and public relations department managers
	1235	Supply and distribution department managers
	1236	Computing services department managers
	1237	Research and development department managers
	1239	Other department managers not elsewhere classified
13	**General managers**	
	(This group is intended to include persons who manage enterprises, or in some cases organisations, on their own behalf, or on behalf of the proprietor, with some non-managerial help and the assistance of no more than one other manager who should also be classified in this sub-major group as, in most cases, the tasks will be broader than those of a specialised manager in a larger enterprise or organisation. Non-managerial staff should be classified according to their specific tasks.)	
131	**General managers**	
	1311	General managers in agriculture, hunting, forestry/and fishing
	1312	General managers in manufacturing
	1313	General managers in construction
	1314	General managers in wholesale and retail trade
	1315	General managers of restaurants and hotels
	1316	General managers in transport, storage and communications
	1317	General managers of business services
	1318	General managers in personal care, cleaning and related services
	1319	General managers not elsewhere classified

Source: International Labour Organization, Bureau of Statistics (2008) ISCO-88 http://www.ilo.org/public/english/bureau/stat/isco/isco88/major.htm

How does an examination of the ISCO-88 classification deepen our understanding of occupation? As two experts in the development of occupational classification schemes clearly explain:

> ISCO-88 organizes occupations in a hierarchical framework. The lowest level unit of classification, a job, is defined as a set of tasks or duties designed to be executed by one person. Jobs are grouped into occupations according to the degree of similarity in their constituent tasks and duties. Thus, for example, the following jobs are grouped together in ISCO-88 to form the occupation unit group 3472: Radio, television and other announcers: News announcer, radio announcer; television announcer; disc jockey; media interviewer; newscaster. Although each job may be distinct in terms of the output required from the person who executes the constituent tasks, the jobs are sufficiently similar in terms of the abilities required as inputs into these tasks for them to be regarded as a single occupational unit for statistical purposes. (21)

In this example "occupations" are "sets of tasks or duties performed by a single individual," which are then grouped into occupations according to similarities of task and duty. Peter Elias and Margaret Birch (21) recognize that there may be differences in the tasks or duties from one person to another, but some generalization of content is made to distinguish an occupation. Although all of this looks very straightforward at first glance, the attempt to develop standardized occupational classification schemes has been rocked by major debates. Earlier, I noted that Townsend (9) made the point that occupations were gendered, and we observed that this gendering was not necessarily neutral in terms of the way in which occupations were valued (Box 4-1). Even though the meaning being assigned to the term *occupation* is somewhat different here with respect to its use in government statistics, major controversies have emerged that concern both the nature of gendering (or even sexism) inherent in the way that occupational classification schemes have been constructed and also the relationship of the categories to the more important issues of gendering of the occupational structure in various countries.

Feminist attention has been focused on the existence of some occupations in which there are large numbers of women—clerical worker is a classic example—but the occupations are insufficiently subdivided to capture the range of work that is entailed. Men's work, it is argued, has received far more attention from experts and is far more carefully described and subdivided into myriad fine categories. Sylvia Walby (22) has argued, "Workers with such significantly differing amounts of autonomy and authority as a typist in a pool and a managing director's secretary need to be distinguished."[4] Today, certainly far more attention is given to the formal, paid work of women, and those designing classification schemes are generally attentive to trying to capture the complexity of women's work in the same level of detail as that of men's work. Nevertheless, particularly when using older classification schemes, attention must certainly be given to the gendered assumptions inherent in the occupational classifications themselves.

A second area that has generated controversy concerns the inclusion or exclusion of certain categories of work from occupational classification schemes. In countries that use self-report categories for census data, for example, some respondents have identified their occupation as "prostitute." Prostitutes certainly perform paid work, and an interesting case can be made concerning the similarity and differences between what some would see as the "oldest occupation on earth" and other occupations with wider social acceptance. "Prostitute" does not, however, generally feature in occupational classification schemes and so responses like this would either be lost or recoded.

There have also been lengthy debates about whether "housewife" is an occupation that should be included in national occupational schemes. Housewives do not tend to get paid in wages, but rather make a contribution to the economic viability of households. Although most would see "housewives" as having much greater social legitimacy than "prostitutes," their relationship to labor markets is not as clear.

An examination of how government statisticians work with the concept of occupation shows that they are less open to "individual" definitions than the occupational therapists and scientists, and more concerned with providing definitions that are stable across large groups of people. In general, the focus is on paid employment, but there are also boundary issues as to what is work and what is not work, as the examples of prostitute and housewife illustrate. Finally, we see that the issue of levels of analysis comes up in this context also. Occupational therapists and scientists

BOX 4-1 Gender Issues in Culture and Classification

Japan is one nation that has undergone extensive cultural change during the last 50 years. Historically, the roles of men and women have been influenced by highly prescribed cultural expectations, to the point that nearly one-third of marriages in Japan are prearranged by families. Economics, culture, and communication have changed these practices and others, including more extensive participation by Japanese women in the workforce, who now comprise 40% of all workers (Figure 4-1■). The Japanese government has undertaken extensive policy initiatives and programs to promote gender equity in public employment. The division of labor in the home, however, is more difficult to change. A 1997 survey of married men indicated that over 50% are not inclined to share in housework, even if their working spouse earns a higher income. Yet some traditions in Japan, such as expecting wives to manage household finances, provide a degree of autonomy and responsibility that may reduce the attraction of those benefits for employment outside the home. Household work is an important economic role that may be inadequately reflected in economic and occupational classification schemes (23, 24).

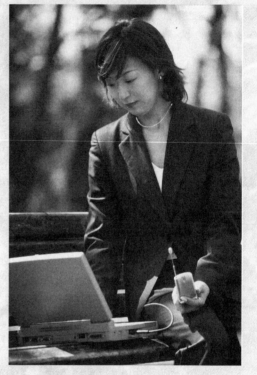

FIGURE 4-1 Cultural stereotypes concerning the roles of men and women in the workforce are slowly changing in Japan. (Photodisc/Getty Images)

struggle with boundary issues in terms of deciding where one occupation leaves off and another begins by introducing terminology such as *occupational scaffolding* or *suboccupation.* The government statisticians do something similar by introducing into classification schemes ideas about major unit groups (large occupational groupings) and minor groupings that are more detailed. Thus, we see that in both communities, the concept of nesting occupations within larger occupational groupings has been developed.

CHAPTER SUMMARY

This chapter has presented an analysis of the way in which the concept "occupation" is used in several different communities: occupational therapy and occupational science; sociology; and the community responsible for the production of official statistics. It is fair to say that in each community, "occupation" plays a central conceptual role. In the occupational therapy and occupational science communities, occupations were argued to be highly relevant to health and health recovery. In the sociological community and in government statistical bureaus, occupations were argued to refer to work or trades. The main focus of research and writing this chapter was on questions about the relationship of occupation to social advantage. More broadly, the question of whether or not the different traditions of usage in each community can usefully learn anything from one another about the nature of occupation is a question that has been posed by the editors of this book to the writers of the chapters and to you, the readers. This chapter represents an attempt to address this question from one perspective within sociology.

STUDY GUIDE

Study Guide Author: Linda Buxell

Summary of Main Points

This chapter contributes to our understanding of how we describe humans as occupational beings by representing various existing perspectives on the concept of occupation across disciplines. The perspectives of occupational therapy and occupational science, social science, and official statistical agencies are represented, contrasted, and compared.

Application to Occupational Therapy

Occupational therapy has been challenged to explain itself within the context and common knowledge of the idea of occupation as a job. This popular view of occupation as a job is often seen as a conflict with the view of occupation by the profession of occupational therapy. Rather than presented as a conflict, the alternate views are embraced as relevant to learn about and appreciate differences in understanding occupation. By contrasting and comparing these various perspectives, the uniqueness of occupational therapy is represented as complementary to the additional existing points of view.

Learning about and appreciating these various perspectives on occupation is supported as the means to promote thoughtful dialogue and understanding in the broader discussions about occupation and occupational therapy. These links are exposed as relevant and important in a complete view of the concept of occupation.

Individual Learning Activities

1. To apply the presented perspective on occupational therapy and occupational science:
    a. Choose a single occupation in which you engage on a daily basis. Write about this occupation and address the following dimensions of the occupation. How does it start? Why do you engage in it? What are the skills required to complete this occupation? What is the perceived value of this occupation in your family, community, greater culture? Would you categorize this occupation as play, work, or other? Is this occupation gendered? If so, how and why? How is this occupation linked to other occupations in which you engage? What would it mean if you could not do this occupation or your skills had changed so this occupation was done in a different manner? What would be required? What are your thoughts and feelings as you conduct this occupation? Is the doing of this occupation connected to others in your immediate or distant network? If so, how? For someone else to better appreciate the meaning of this occupation for you, what would they need to know?
    b. Using the preceding example of an occupation, illustrate the concept "suboccupation." What do you determine is a suboccupation, and what do you determine is the main occupation?
    c. Apply the term "scaffolding" to a past experience you had with an occupation. Describe the occupation and what occurred that represents the concept. Discuss.
    d. Describe how you think occupational therapy and occupational science define occupation.
2. To apply the presented perspective on the social science view of occupation:
    a. Write about the presented Durkeim argument, that the finer the division of labor the greater the interdependence among human beings. Provide an example of how this may or may not be experienced.
    b. Do you agree with the presented Durkeim view, that a complex division of labor creates peace due to less competition? Discuss.
    c. Contrast the meaning of occupation presented in the social science view to that discussed by occupational therapy and occupational science.
    d. Reflect on the idea of injustice in pursuit of occupation. Is it deprivation and injustice when someone is prevented from using their talents and skills? Who best determines how occupation is pursued or realized?
    e. Discuss how the social science view on occupation and composition of the occupational structure is linked to social inequality and class conflict.
    f. Describe a situation, an example of social advantage due to occupation.

Group Activity

To apply the presented perspective on the government statistics view on occupation:

a. Discuss why information on people's "occupation" is of major interest to policy makers and the business community.
b. Why is uniformity so important in gathering information on occupation? Discuss the drawbacks in this uniformity, with your now broader understanding of occupation.

c. Discuss how these classifications are hierarchical.
d. Review the International Standard Classification of Occupations (ISCO) and present an example of gendering. Respond to this with your own perspective.
e. Discuss the risk in not distinguishing occupations using this classification system.
f. Discuss in a group whether household work should be classified in ISCO.
g. Compare and contrast the concept of nesting occupations within larger occupational grouping across all three presented perspectives (occupational therapy and occupational science, social science and government classification).

Study Questions

1. Definitions of occupation by occupational scientists have all of the following ideas in common EXCEPT
   a. All occupations are viewed equally
   b. Occupations emerge from routine and everyday aspects of daily living
   c. Everyday living is a very complex process
   d. Occupations demonstrate worth and value in society
2. Emile Durkheim, who wrote the classic book *The Division of Labor in Society,* is regarded as a founding figure in this discipline
   a. Psychology
   b. Occupational science
   c. Anthropology
   d. Sociology
3. According to the International Classification of Occupations, the lowest level of classification is a
   a. Task
   b. Occupation
   c. Role
   d. Job
4. The three communities described in this chapter that have interest in occupations include all of the following EXCEPT
   a. Occupational therapy and occupational science
   b. Employers
   c. Social science
   d. Official statistical agencies
5. For the occupation, *driving a car,* the following is an example of a suboccupation.
   a. Changing the oil in the car
   b. Using public transportation
   c. Turning right in a stressful situation
   d. Finding an address on a map

REFERENCES

1. Wilcock, A. A. (1993). A theory of the human need for occupation. *Journal of Occupational Science: Australia, 1*(1), 17–24.
2. Sigert, H. E. (1944). *Civilization and disease.* Ithaca, NY: Cornell University Press.
3. Meyer, A. (1922). The philosophy of occupational therapy. *Archives of Occupational Therapy, 1*(1), 1–10.
4. Nelson, D. L. (1996). Therapeutic occupation: A definition. *American Journal of Occupational Therapy, 50*(10), 775–781.
5. Primeau, L. A. (1998). Orchestration of work and play within families. *American Journal of Occupational Therapy, 52,* 188–195.
6. do Rozario, L. (1994). Ritual, meaning and transcendence. The role of occupation in modern life. *Journal of Occupational Science: Australia, 1*(3), 46–53.
7. Howard, B., & Howard, I. R. (1999). Occupation as spiritual activity. *American Journal of Occupational Therapy, 51*(3), 181–185.
8. Christiansen, C., Clark, F., Kielhofner, G., Rogers, I., & Nelson, D. (1995). Position paper: Occupation. *American Journal of Occupational Therapy, 49*(10), 1015–1018.
9. Townsend, E. (1997). Occupation: Potential for personal and social transformation. *Journal of Occupational Science, 4*(1), 18–26.
10. Frank, G. (1992). Opening feminist histories of occupational therapy. *American Journal of Occupational Therapy, 46*(11), 989–999.
11. Litterst, T. (1992). Occupational therapy: The role of ideology in the development of a profession for women. *American Journal of Occupational Therapy, 46*(1), 20–25.
12. Durkheim, E. (1964). *The division of labor in society.* New York: The Free Press.
13. Kirkpatrick, E. (Ed.). (1983). *Chambers 20th century dictionary.* Edinburgh: W & R Chambers.
14. Braverman, H. (1975). *Labour and monopoly capital: The degradation of work in the 20th century.* New York: Monthly Review Press.
15. Jargowsky, P. A. (1996). Take the money and run: Economic segregation in U.S. metropolitan areas. *American Sociological Review, 61*(6), 984–998.
16. Blackburn, R. M., & Jarman, J. (2006). Gendered occupations: Exploring the relationship between gender segregation and inequality. *International Sociology, 21*(2), 289–315.
17. Blishen, B., & McRoberts, H. A. (1976). A revised socioeconomic index for occupations in Canada. *The Canadian Review of Sociology and Anthropology, 13*(1), 71–79.
18. Pineo, P., Porter, J., & McRoberts, H. (1977). The 1971 census and the socioeconomic classification of occupations. *Canadian Review of Sociology and Anthropology, 24*(4), 91–102.
19. Prandy, K. (1990). The revised Cambridge scale of occupations. *Sociology 24*(4), 629–655.
20. Stewart, A., Prandy, K., & Blackburn, R. M. (1980). *Social stratification and occupations.* New York: Holmes and Meier.
21. Elias, P., & Birch, M. (1994). *A guide for users. Establishment of community-wide statistics.* ISCO-88 (COM). Coventry, England.
22. Walby, S. (1986). Gender, class and stratification: Towards a new approach. In R. C. M. Mann (Ed.), *Gender and stratification* (pp. 23–39). Cambridge: Polity Press.
23. Martinez, D. P. (Ed.). (1998). *The worlds of Japanese popular culture: Gender shifting boundaries and global cultures.* Cambridge: Cambridge University Press.
24. Fujimura-Fanselow, K., & Kameda, A. (Eds.). (1995). *Japanese women: New feminist perspectives on the past, present, and future.* New York: The Feminist Press of the City University of New York.

Endnotes

[1]Lyrics from a song performed by Bob McGrath and the Anything Muppets on Sesame Street, written by Jeffrey Moss.

[2]Nelson defines occupational performance as "The person's voluntary doing in the context of occupational form" (3, p. 777). Occupational form is defined as "The composition of objective physical and sociocultural circumstances external to the person that influences his or her occupational performance" (p. 776). Occupational form, in this instance, would include the car, the map, the city streets, intense sunshine, the physical presence of the therapist in the front seat, and the therapist's words.

[3]Emile Durkheim was very much a product of the 19th century. His concern really was limited to men's talents and capacities and obstacles to men's mobility in the workplace. Durkheim's views about women's talents and capacities were informed by 19th-century anthropology that suggested that women had smaller brains than men and so on. He did, however, discuss the gender division of labor. Indeed, he saw this as one of the most fundamental divisions of labor on which a society is based.

[4]Note that this criticism is not being leveled at ISCO-88, but at the available British classifications of the time.

CHAPTER 5

What Do People Do?

Andrew S. Harvey and Wendy Pentland

There is a way in which the collective knowledge expresses itself, for the finite individual, through mere daily living a way in which life itself is sheer knowing.

Sir Laurens Van der Post, Venture to the Interior (1, p. 136)

OBJECTIVES

1. Discuss what and why people do what they do in terms of activities and occupations.
2. Identify types of occupations in terms of time use, including (a) necessary occupations, (b) contracted occupations, (c) committed occupations, and (d) free time occupations.
3. Explain the concept of roles and how they influence occupational behavior.
4. Describe factors influencing what people do and examine dimensions of occupational behavior.
5. Identify means of studying time use, and present the results of international time-use study.

KEY WORDS

Activities
Activity
Behavioral area
Committed occupations
Committed time
Contracted occupations
Contracted time
Free time
Free time occupations
Necessary occupations
Necessary time
Tasks

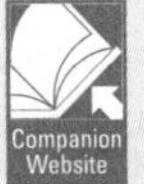

www.prenhall.com/christiansen

The Internet provides an exciting means for interacting with this textbook and for enhancing your understanding of humans' experiences with occupations and the organization of occupations in society. Use the address above to access the interactive Companion Website created specifically to accompany this book. Here you will find an array of self-study material designed to help you gain a richer understanding of the concepts presented in this chapter.

CHAPTER PROFILE

The understanding of human occupation is facilitated through the use of methods to conveniently describe and differentiate what people do from day to day. This chapter introduces terms and concepts that contribute to a taxonomy or classification of daily time use. It begins with an acknowledgment that the requirements of daily living provide a natural basis for naming and grouping occupations. The chapter recognizes characteristics of occupations that provide the basis for four generic categories. Social roles and individual projects are identified as other influences on time use and as means for characterizing occupational pursuit. The chapter concludes with a description of the factors that influence what people do with their time.

INTRODUCTION

We live life one minute, one hour, one day, one week, one month, and one year at a time. The years turn into decades and the decades into generations. At the same time, through memory, the minutes come back, the hours come back, the days come back, and the months, and the years, and the decades. During it all we spend our life doing. Occupation is what we do. It is what we are doing now, what we have done, and what we will do as time flows on. What we do is affected by what time it is on the clock and on the calendar, where we are, who we are with, and many other factors. This chapter introduces a way of looking primarily at what people do with their time with reference to their daily occupations. It suggests ways of thinking about occupations, ways of identifying and measuring them, and ways of generating insight into what we have learned from previous studies of daily living.

THE STRUCTURE OF DAILY OCCUPATIONS

Our interests in and ability to choose and engage in a variety of occupations defines us as individuals as we live our lives. When we look at what people do, then, we need to look at occupations beyond work. Through engagement in a variety of daily occupations, we express ourselves, find meaning in our lives, and adapt to life's challenges. Our doing in various occupations is our way of meeting our basic needs (e.g., survival, emotional, self-actualization) and coping with environmental demands (e.g., physical, social/cultural expectations).

Daily life consists of engaging in **tasks** to perform **activities** required by **occupations**. Each day we perform countless tasks that enable us to carry out occupations, that is to say, our activities of living. We sleep, wash, cook, eat, care for a child, work, study, play, talk, socialize, read, reflect, watch TV, listen to the radio, create, and engage in a wide range of other activities that help us fulfill our varied occupations.

For persons who study what people do, the terms *tasks, activities,* and *occupations* are not synonyms. In fact, they are used to represent a hierarchy of undertakings on which daily life is constructed. At the lowest level, tasks are undertaken as a means of accomplishing the activities that comprise an occupation. Hence, one gets out a pan, fills it with water, puts it on the stove, turns on the stove, waits until the water boils, adds eggs, and boils them. These tasks add up to the activity of boiling eggs. Boiling eggs, however, is one activity within the larger occupation of cooking. Using this hierarchy of language, there is little ambiguity in what the individual did. Within the occupation of cooking, there are many possible activities other than boiling eggs, such as preparing oatmeal, or toasting bread.

But what does the foregoing tell us about the occupational meaning of cooking? Actually, it tells us virtually nothing with respect to a broad classification discussed later that distinguishes occupations according to four categories labeled as necessary, contracted, committed, or free time. The person may be a chef preparing the eggs as part of a paid job. The person may be a father preparing the eggs for his children to meet his family commitment to them. The person may be a hobbyist who spends free time decorating eggs. Hence, inherently, tasks and activities are devoid of higher-level meaning until they have been put in the context of people's lives. Understanding what people do is important because tasks and activities have both desirable and undesirable effects on the individuals undertaking them and the environment around them.

The nature and structure of occupation is best understood by considering behavioral units (activities) and **behavioral areas** (activity groups) (2). An activity is an observable unit of behavior, for an individual, which has observable or determinable temporal beginning and end points (2). One sleeps, reads, talks, shops, buys, makes bread, and eats. Behavioral areas (activity groups) form a broad framework within which activities are organized (2). In essence, behavioral areas reflect occupations.

We may perform activities and occupations one at a time, or we may engage in two or three simultaneously. Hence, we may eat, or eat and watch TV, or cook, care for a child, listen to the radio, and wait on hold on the telephone. During our lifetimes we have a variety of occupational roles: child, student, spouse, parent, employed worker, unemployed worker, employer, manager, professional, grandparent, retiree, caretaker, or organization member. Often we will be involved in several occupations and occupational roles at a time: child/student, spouse/parent/student/friend. Our circumstances, beliefs, values, and attitudes are expressed through what we do. The occupations that we do each day and over the course of our lives sustain us; organize our lives; enable us to connect with, adapt to, and have some sense of control in our environment; allow us to express ourselves; and give us a sense of who we are.

Daily occupations not only define individual lives; they also define communities and cultures. In fact, we frequently use "doing"-based labels to describe whole groups and communities; hunter-gatherers, students, stay-at-home mothers or fathers, teachers, and mountain climbers. Through occupations we create communities (farming, professional associations, backpacking club, choir), and we transmit culture and beliefs from generation to generation through rituals and practices that themselves are made up of occupations. It has often been said "we are what we do." In this sense, knowledge of the occupations that humans choose to do each day reveals what their lives are really like and provides a window on their actual lifestyles and cultures, and indeed, over time, is evidence of social change.

CONCEPTUALIZING WHAT PEOPLE DO

This section outlines four ways of conceptualizing what people do: occupational roles, life projects, and meaning of activities and occupations.

Four Types of Occupations

In 1980, Aas (3) observed that in general terms, humans' lives are remarkably regular, similar, and systematic. On this basis he proposed that all human use of time, occupational behavior, falls into four categories based on the obligation or constraint inherent in the performance of the occupation. Aas proposed these four categories to be (1) necessary time, (2) contracted time, (3) committed time, and (4) free time. He hypothesized that humans allocate time on a priority basis to the first two categories of necessary time and contracted time, whereas the remaining two categories tend to get whatever time is left over.

Necessary Occupations

Occupations that comprise **necessary time** are those aimed at meeting basic physiological and self-maintenance needs. These occupations include eating, sleeping, resting, sex and personal care activities related to health, and hygiene such as bathing and grooming. Extensive research internationally reveals that time spent in **necessary occupations** does show some differences, but by and large it is remarkably stable across populations and cultures.

Contracted Occupations

Occupations occurring in **contracted time** are typically those involved in paid productivity or formal education. They are normally governed by an explicit contract extending over long periods including specified obligations relating to start time, finish time, and amount of pay or other reward. Participation in **contracted occupations** is normally performed in exchange for pay or some type of formal graduation or certification. Contracted time constrains committed and free time and to some extent necessary time. Aas (3) argued that one defining feature of contracted occupations [activities] is that they are normally required to be performed outside the home in the workplace, thus they clearly divide up the daily routine of human behavior. However, that was an observation made in the 1980s. With the recent surge in flexible work hours, teleworking, and home and mobile offices, contracted occupations are no longer restricted to an outside single "workplace" and no longer occur in the large discrete time blocks that they once did.

Committed Occupations

During **committed time, occupations** have a work or productivity character, but are typically not remunerated, and duration (hours) of work is often diffuse and unspecified. These include household work, meal preparation, shopping, child care, elder care, and home and vehicle maintenance. From an economist's standpoint, **committed occupations** involve nonmarket production. Committed time is unique from contracted and free time in that some people purchase the completion of these tasks as a service by paying others to do these occupations for them.

Free Time Occupations

Free time is the time that is left over after necessary, contracted, and committed occupations are completed. Because necessary time is generally not flexible, free time can be increased in the short term mainly by deferring some of one's committed responsibilities. Free time can be increased in the long term primarily by planning and organizing to reduce contracted time obligations (e.g., reducing work or studies to part time). Aas (3) was careful to distinguish leisure time from free time. He regarded leisure as a qualitative and personally defined experience of self-expression and engagement in satisfying occupations. Although free time is indeed leftover time, it does not necessarily consist entirely of leisure. **Free time occupations** can include occupations we feel forced to do to some degree, such as attend a neighborhood social or the office holiday party.

Occupational Roles

What people do can also be viewed in terms of their occupational roles (4). The term *role* refers to a pattern of behavior that involves certain rights and duties that an individual is expected, trained, and often encouraged to perform in a particular social situation. Role has been defined as "a culturally defined pattern of occupation that reflects particular routines and habits" (5). Our roles may be short term, such as a soccer game spectator, or of varied duration, such as child, parent, or spouse. Our roles may be discreet or overlap, congruent or in conflict with each other. Role conflict and role strain are relatively recent terms identified in the literature on stress and life balance. Any one occupation may be found in a number of roles, as in the egg cooking example described earlier. For example, parents maintain a household, and they nurture and read to children as part of their committed time. Nurturing and reading to children are also occupations that are typical for teachers, who occupy a role distinct from that of parent.

Occupational roles influence much of everyday behavior. Some occupational roles are chosen, others are thrust on us, and still others fall somewhere between choice and obligation. Clearly, engagement in occupational roles is dynamic, in that engagement and changes evolve across the life course (6–8). Some roles have powerful culturally prescribed "norms" in terms of whether and when one is expected to adopt them and how one is expected to operationalize the role. Tindale (9), in his research on work, family, and balancing time, discusses how the increase in two-earner families and greater involvement of women in paid work occupations has altered the timing and age at which women have children. These couples speak in terms of "on times" and "off times" to have children and assume the parent role. This seems similar to the on and off stage behavior described by Erving Goffman in his classic description of roles, *The Presentation of Self in Everyday Life* (10).

Cultural expectations can function as a form of *social clock* for occupational roles and underlie our judgments about what is *normal* and *deviant* in what people do. We use this information in turn to identify and target resources for both individuals and social problems. The messages we get about which roles to adopt and when are often very subtle and can be confusing. Examples include when widows, widowers or teenagers should begin dating or having sex and whether or not, or when, to have children. Whether and when to engage in other roles is much clearer for us and in fact may even be legislated, such as the age at which children start school or the age of mandatory retirement.

Shifts in the cultural expectations of people's engagement in occupational roles can reflect significant changes in a society and can profoundly affect others' role performance. An increase in women entering the workforce beginning in the 1960s, followed by recent evidence in Canada and the United States of a reversing trend in this practice (with many now opting to stay at home with children), is one example; increased integration and employment of people with disabilities is another example. Powerful recent demographic, cultural, economic, and value shifts during later life may be reflected in occupational trends, such as the abolishment of mandatory retirement, more older persons choosing to phase in retirement or continue working full or part time well past 65, and indeed discussions around what retirement really means in the current age. Environmental factors also shape and change role performance, which in turn modifies the complexion of society and culture. Consider the impact of computer technology on the existence and characteristics of certain roles (e.g., assembly-line worker, student, researcher, pilot, stock broker) as one example (11).

The nature of occupational roles typically varies and evolves over years and decades and may be determined by factors that endure throughout a lifetime or at least for major portions of it. People generally continue through their lifetimes within the gender role into which they were born. But virtually all other roles, such as child, student, spouse, parent, employed worker, unemployed worker, employer, manager, and professional, are taken on for varying periods throughout their lives. People remain the child, sometimes to their chagrin, as long as they have a parent alive. The duration of time as a spouse or parent revolves, to some extent, around marital and parental success or failure. Paid work roles revolve around choices and success in the labor market.

In addition to a number of factors already mentioned, how long individuals occupy certain roles depends on customary and legislated time requirements related to study and training, licensing, retirement legislation, and other time-related forces. Customs and legislation vary across occupations, sometimes in paradoxical ways. Hence, judges who can sit on the bench until they are 75 years old are given the power to decide whether employees—from government office workers to professors—must retire at the age of 65 (12, 13). Furthermore, the demands of many occupations dictate feasible durations of occupancy. For example, professional football players or firefighters would normally be expected to retire well before the age of 65 because these occupations become too physically demanding for maximum performance as people age.

There is endless variability in how people perform a given role and its inherent occupations. Some roles allow more choice and individual expression than others. Compare, for example, the daughter role or the watercolor artist role with the student or the bank teller role. Variability in role performance is a function of individuals' characteristics, circumstances, and environments. It is this potential for variation that allows humans personal expression and individuality and enables adaptation to life changes and challenges that otherwise might cause a sudden and unwanted role loss. Varying our "doing" allows us to adapt to life circumstances and continue in or adopt roles that are important for our survival and well-being and that of our community. Examples are modifying the way of "doing" the parent role to continue as a loving involved parent, despite acquiring a significant disability or being separated by many miles from one's children due to divorce or an overseas job.

The concept of looking at what people do in terms of occupational roles is embedded in all areas of our culture. People speak of taking on a new role, role loss, role balance, and role conflict. It can be argued occupational roles most profoundly influence what people do each day and, as such, who they are. Occupational behavior, or what people do within selected occupational roles, has received little attention. A review of time budget studies indicates that the major factors affecting daily occupational behavior include day of the week and personal characteristics such as sex, employment status, child responsibility, and the presence of children (14–19). Understanding the occupational behaviors intrinsic to specific roles will help us to identify the positive and negative impacts of role participation and can guide role modification efforts to improve participation and well-being.

Life Projects

Another way of conceptualizing and classifying what it is people do is to focus on the projects in which they engage. Little (20) suggested that at any point in time, an individual's occupational behavior is focused on several goals or projects. These life projects dictate what the person does with his or her time. Occupations can be grouped according to the life project with which they are connected. Ellegard (21) studies projects from the opposite direction yet makes the same point that activities and projects are connected. She argues that "when different activities of a particular person are related to each other by aiming at the same goal, they constitute a project" (p. 29).

The project may be relatively small and time limited, such as going to a movie. Or a project may be a major life occupation such as attending college or completing a health-care professional degree, having and raising children, or overseeing and ensuring a frail elderly parent's well-being over the last decade or more of life. In the instance of a smaller project such as attending the theater, the occupations would include arranging for a babysitter; buying tickets; bathing and dressing; executing transportation to the theater by walking, driving, or taking a bus or taxi; handling money; attending the show; and returning home. Conversely, on a larger scale, should an individual decide to enter university to study occupational therapy, this contracted occupation will have a profound effect on their activities, the decision will commit possibly 80% of their activities, context, and occupations during the next 2 to 3 years.

Obviously, we choose some life projects, whereas we do not choose others, such as recovery and learning to live following a traumatic spinal cord injury or caring for our disabled child or demented elderly parent. Research suggests that increased life satisfaction is associated with spending most of one's time on projects that the individual chooses, values highly, and whose requirements fall within the individual's abilities (22). Other aspects of the life project occupations that have been studied are the *cross impact* or extent to which individuals perceive their various projects to be complementary to or in conflict with each other (22).

Ellegard (21) shows that, within the household, projects can be approached in different ways. Hence, in caring for the household and household members, there are at least two different strategies, the *division of labor* strategy and the *work-sharing* strategy (21). Clearly, the activities carried out by household members will be greatly affected by the strategy adopted. A poignant reflection is that, in a single-parent household, neither strategy is possible because opportunities for dividing the labor or work-sharing are very different for the single parent.

Important factors to consider when examining the impact of life projects on health and well-being are choice and personal control and the impact that individuals' life projects have on their immediate community and society. In particular, understanding behavior in terms of projects can facilitate community and social response to given problems. For example, child-care facilities need to be concerned not only with the care of children while they are there, but also with relevant timing and transport needs and demands placed on parents. The concept of life projects seems to be a useful framework for understanding what people do and for assisting people to construct meaningful satisfying lives.

Meaning of Activities and Occupations

An alternative approach to understanding activities and occupations is to view them in terms of what they mean to the persons doing them. Elchardus and Glorieux (23) see meaning as arising from the motivation of the doer to perform the occupation and the criteria used to evaluate performance in it. They identified seven general meanings of time: (1) time devoted to *satisfaction of physiological needs* (for example, medical, hygienic, dietary); (2) *personal gratification,* that is, time yielding pleasure; (3) *duty,* time spent as an obligation so as to avoid punishment; (4) *instrumental behavior,* exemplified by time spent traveling to get to work; (5) *affect/solidarity,* time with others to strengthen relationships; (6) *obligation,* based on one's perception of how he or she should behave; and (7) *killing time,* none of the foregoing. Elchardus and Glorieux then decided that the seven categories could be reduced to four. They folded duty, affect/solidarity, obligation, and instrumentality into one factor they called *social meaning* (23, p. 247). Hence, they arrived at four meanings, namely: physiological needs, personal gratification, killing time, and social meaning. In analysis relating these to a variety of occupational coding schemes, they concluded that, although such schemes seemed to capture variation in the meaning of activities, the schemes did not allow one to infer motivations, and thus if one wanted to determine meanings of activities, it was necessary to do so explicitly.

FACTORS INFLUENCING WHAT PEOPLE DO

Many disciplines and theories of human behavior have begun to recognize and examine the complex interactions between individual characteristics (intrinsic) and the environment (extrinsic) that result in human occupational behavior.

Human "doing" influences both individual and community health and well-being. To facilitate healthy and satisfying occupational behavior, we must understand those factors that influence "doing." Why humans do what they do is an incredibly complex concept to explain. Simply stating what an individual did, and ignoring context, gives us only a shallow understanding of occupational behavior. The context within which an occupation is performed gives it a culturally based meaning and provides the basis for assigning it to a specific area deemed to represent a particular form of behavior. Next we examine three sets of contextual factors that influence and describe what people do: intrinsic factors, extrinsic factors, and contextual factors.

Intrinsic and Extrinsic Factors Influencing Occupational Behavior

One set of forces shaping behavior can be classified as intrinsic and extrinsic factors. These can independently or interactively influence occupational behavior. Intrinsic (to the individual) factors are those that are innate in the individual, such as physical/organic factors and psychological traits. Extrinsic factors are external to the individual and include resources (social support, income), the environment (physical, social, political), and cultural influences. Table 5-1 ■ lists some of these factors. Many, although not all, of the intrinsic factors tend to be fixed and more difficult to change. Conversely, factors in the environment can change and evolve or can sometimes be escaped from, eliminated, or modified (24).

The International Classification of Functioning, Disability and Health, published by the World Health Organization (11), identified an extensive list of environmental factors that influence human behavior. They include social networks, family structure, political systems and government, legal systems, economic organizations, health and social services, educational services, public infrastructure services, community organizations, social rules, values and attitudes, land development, and technology. Extrinsic or environmental factors that influence what we do include *zeitgebers,* which are cues that influence our occupational behavior to the extent that our natural free-running rhythms will resynchronize in response to these *zeitgebers.* Physical *zeitgebers*

TABLE 5-1 *Factors Influencing What People Do*

Factors Intrinsic to the Individual
• Personality/temperament • Preference • Skills, abilities, knowledge • Basic needs (e.g., Maslow) • Health/chronic illness/disability • Biological rhythms • Age, gender, socioeconomic status • Values/attitudes/meaning we give to what we do/spirituality
Factors Extrinsic to the Individual
• *Zeitgebers* (physical and social), etc. • Temporospatial environment • Socioeconomic environment and social support • Cultural environment • Physical environment • Circumstance • Resources (time, money, space)

Source: Drawn from Christiansen and Baum (24).

include daylight, nightfall, and noises. Social *zeitgebers* include mealtimes, bedtime rituals, and start times for work and school.

Circumstances also influence what we do. Things happen to us that we have no or little control over, such as disability, death of a spouse, relocation of a family due to one member's job, or nonacceptance at a training program or university. Societal circumstances may profoundly affect our occupational behavior such as economic recession or depression, famine, an epidemic, or war.

Dimensions of Occupational Behavior

At any given time an individual must be doing something that can be considered his or her *primary activity* even if it is just resting or reflecting. The term **activity** will be used here to link with current literature, but the discussion is actually about occupations as defined in this book.

Numerous contextual factors facilitate or constrain activities and occupational behavior (4). This section identifies a variety of contextual factors (secondary activities, time, location, with whom and for whom the activity is done, tension, enjoyment, and technology) and contextual constraints (capability, authority, and coupling) that facilitate or impede involvement in "activity" (and occupational behavior).

Secondary activities are activities undertaken simultaneously with a primary activity. Virtually anything can be done along with something else, but typically a relatively few activities account for the major share of the total number identified. Secondary activities take on meaning when we recognize that individuals have multiple senses and generally use them concurrently. An individual can be watching soccer on TV, listening to the play-by-play commentary on the radio, and drinking a beer, all with the same friends. All of these activities—TV viewing, radio listening, drinking, and socializing—are concurrent. It makes no sense to try to time slice, allocating one-quarter of the time to each. Unquestionably, it is the mix of activities and contexts that provides life with meaning and richness. This is so often the case that time survey respondents find it difficult to report only one activity at a time.

Time has several dimensions beyond duration. In particular, timing and sequence play an important part in individual behavior. Activities are not randomly distributed. Rather, in a given society, most activities follow a predominant pattern in terms of when they occur and in what order. This is true of various scales of time measurement. Dominant patterns exist on a daily basis too: getting out of bed, work and schooling, meals, and even free-time occupations. Similarly, there tend to be weekly, monthly, annual, and life course patterns and rhythms (25–27). Whereas any one individual may deviate from such patterns, they cannot easily avoid being affected by them. People who work in the evening have greatly reduced access to cultural events that take place only in the evening. Shopping has to be carried out before meals can be prepared, and they must be prepared before they are eaten. Then meal cleanup follows. In fact, a great deal of activity and occupation involves routines (28). It is argued that the temporal order is a major stabilizing factor in daily living. Hence, any study of activities and occupations cannot ignore temporal dimensions such as timing and sequence.

Location is a fundamental activity and occupation dimension. A person may be doing several things simultaneously, with several different people, or working under several motives, but they can only be in one place at a time. Typically, location is defined generically in terms of home, work, restaurant/bar, other public places, or mode of travel. Some studies have captured in which room in the house each activity and occupation occurred.

Being able to identify work locations is important as an indication of socialization and community participation (29). Research shows specific activities and occupations occur in a wide range of locations. For example, although productive work time may be traditionally viewed as all time spent at the paid workplace, teachers' paid productive time often invades their home and family life (30, 31).

Time–space diaries have captured not only activities but also the specific geographic location of activities on a one-tenth-kilometer map grid (32). Specific geographic location information is also a significant contextual dimension of activities and occupations, and there is an extensive body of literature in this area. It includes the study of direction and distance of travel, speed of travel (33, 34), and diurnal patterns of geographic space, for example, the temporospatial rhythm of a city.

With whom, or social contact, is an important contextual dimension of occupational behavior (18, 29). Activity and occupational behavior may be a solitary undertaking, or it may involve family members, friends, work/school colleagues, or various other people. The company we keep can have a significant effect on the nature of our experience.

For example, in Canada in 1992, the workplace provided the major source of time with others. Persons employed in a workplace spent more time with persons other than family (about one-half of total time) than individuals working at home or elsewhere (29). Furthermore, individuals at the workplace only spent about one-half as much of their time with family members when compared with persons working only at home (29). Clearly, work arrangements have an impact on social contact time.

For whom an activity is performed provides information for understanding an individual's motivation for performing an activity. Information on who is involved is particularly useful in studies of voluntary activity and instrumental material services in a helping network (35). In an Australian study, "for whom" information was captured in terms of self, family, friend/neighbor, community, and other persons (36). Another study of teachers provided a broader choice, including, as well as the above, various types of students, administrators, and the community (31). For whom an activity is done is particularly useful in determining whether it can or should be considered as work.

Tension, time pressure, or stress, often associated by the popular press with concerns about balancing work and family life, have become contemporary issues of interest to occupational scientists and other researchers interested in occupations. Tension or stress is typically captured by means of a graded scale ranging from no tension to great tension or stress. There is evidence that a subjective sense of time pressure is grounded in objective reality with individuals carrying heavier work burdens (paid and unpaid) reporting higher perceived time pressure (37).

Enjoyment or *satisfaction* influences motivation for activities, encourages occupational engagement, and is a reflection of the meaningfulness of occupational behavior. Enjoyment is strongly associated with free time or leisure occupations (38). Not only are different activities considered as leisure by different people, but the same activity may be leisure at one time and not at another for the same person (39, 40).

Technology, manifest in facilities and equipment, influences occupational behavior at a number of levels. It includes, among other items, household equipment and facilities available and means of travel, media, and communication technology. Access to such facilities and equipment reduces the time required to do various activities or gives one the ability to do more in the same amount of time. Access to automobiles and cell phones significantly increases an individual's ability to interact with others and their surroundings. How the technology affects behavior is unclear. It may lead people to spend less time doing laundry or it may lead them to change their clothes more often. A cell phone may lead to less travel or to more. Thus, although there is a relationship between technology and occupational behavior, the nature of the relationship is unclear and variable.

Contextual Constraints Influencing Occupational Behavior

Hagerstrand (41) provides further insight into individual occupational behavior by suggesting that activities are subject to three types of constraints: capability, authority, and coupling constraints.

Capability constraints limit the activities of an individual because of biological construction and/or the tools at one's command (41). Necessary occupations, such as eating and sleeping, are examples of capability constraints. They are subject, most directly, to the forces of circadian rhythms. Variations in such constraints will result from socioeconomic factors such as age, sex, employment status, family status, and income.

Authority constraints refer to the degree of control that exists over something that is considered a control area or domain. Such domains are organized in a hierarchy with smaller ones (for example, Dad's favorite chair) protected only by immediate power or custom, and larger ones (for example, private property and national territory) protected by law and, if necessary, armed force. Store opening hours, work hour legislation, and similar devices represent an exercise of authority over domains that impinge on individual occupational behavior, both obligatory and discretionary. Many such constraints are likely to be reflected in an examination of the occupational context.

Coupling constraints "define where, when and for how long the individual has to join other individuals, tools and materials" (41, p. 20). For example, drivers of armored trucks for transporting currency and bank receipts are coupled with their vehicles and may be required to work with an armed guard on the job. This would be an example of a coupling constraint. Thus the concept of coupling constraints adds additional contextual elements: necessary objects, "other individuals" or, more commonly, "social contacts." Ellegard (21), drawing on the time–geographic approach of Hagerstrand, explores behavior in terms of activity purpose, temporal flow of the day, social contact, and geographic context. Her work highlights the fact that projects are manifest in a flow of activities and goal-oriented occupational behavior and may not be a continuous act but intermittently undertaken as time flows on.

WHY STUDY WHAT PEOPLE DO?

Try to generate a list of questions about what people do. Such a list can be endless because there are so many things to know and so many areas of daily life to consider. This endless list of questions about what people do, about their occupations, has prompted the authors of this book to introduce occupations in a new and creative way. Box 5-1 lists some examples of common yet important questions that ask about occupation. What would your list of questions look like? Such a list of "occupational questions" could go on and on. The list in Box 5-1 represents a sample of the kinds of questions that can be asked about the everyday occupations of people that account for how they spend their time. Likely, you can add to it.

The questions in Box 5-1 should provide insight into why it is important to study what people do. How people spend their time, that is to say, the tasks, activities and occupations they engage in, is central to each and every question presented. Such questions are important to people in many disciplines, including sociologists, childcare specialists, economists, environmentalists, home economists, human resources personnel, marketing specialists, media specialists, nutritionists, psychologists, sleep researchers, traffic planners, and others who want to understand the lives of those with whom they work. Of course, they are also of particular interest to occupational scientists and occupational therapists for whom occupation is the primary domain of concern.

BOX 5-1 A Sampling of Some Questions to Answer About Daily Occupations

- What is a balanced life?
- What is occupational balance?
- Are people working longer hours, or is leisure increasing?
- Which people are leading balanced lives?
- Is stress related to long hours at work?
- Is stress the result of trying to do too many things at once?
- Is the gender division of labor changing?
- Who works from home (telecommutes)?
- Is religious involvement increasing or decreasing?
- What is the value of housework, volunteer work, do-it-yourself work?
- What is the real pattern of work hours?
- Are parents spending more or less time with their children?
- How much time are people spending on the Internet?
- What is the relationship between childhood activity patterns/time use and increasing childhood obesity? Are people becoming "couch potatoes"?
- Are retirees becoming more active? What activities and occupations are behind the pattern of household energy use?
- How long do people engage in occupations while exposed to toxic fumes in traffic or parking garages?
- Do students work longer hours than regular job holders?
- Are individuals and families more likely to engage in occupations alone, thus becoming more isolated from others?
- Who is watching television?
- When are they watching?
- Are we eating mostly fast food?
- Do the open hours of child-care and shopping facilities put undue pressure on workers?
- Are people time poor?
- Who is still engaged in occupations other than sleep at midnight?
- Are people getting enough sleep?
- Who are the volunteer workers?
- Who is taking care of elderly people?

Planning and policy making, in any endeavor, require knowledge of what *is*. And daily activities or occupations are a major facet of what is. Eastern European countries, lacking a market economy, long looked to time-use studies to provide insight into what people did and needed. Western countries, on the other hand, have depended on the market economy to provide the signals for what is wanted and needed. However, it has become increasingly obvious that market production is only a part of the full economy. Work done by parents, homemakers, volunteer workers, caregivers, and others is nonmarket production. In fact, governments are using time-use data to quantify the extent of nonmarket production. They are quantifying and valuing time spent in activities and occupations in the nonmarket sectors of the economy and society. In short, time-use and occupational analyses help people who are planning and enacting policy.

In this chapter, it has been shown that tasks, activities, and occupations can be viewed in a variety of ways. It has also been described that occupations are contextually dependent and subject to a number of influences and constraints. Moreover, there are many reasons for wanting to know what people do. However, the question, *What do people do?* has not yet been answered. That question will be addressed after looking at how to learn about what people do. You are encouraged to use Chapter 3 to understand the varieties of ways in which one can study occupation. Here, the focus is on studying time in relation to occupation.

HOW IS HUMAN TIME USE STUDIED?

Occupations occur in time and over time, and they occur in sequence. To understand them at any point on the continuum, we must observe occupations in some manner. But how can we do that? Have you ever stopped to reflect on what you are doing? Seldom do we reflect on our actions; we just act. Have you ever asked yourself, "What am I doing?" or "Why did I do that?" If you have, it is likely because you reached a point where your actions were routine, and you suddenly realized you acted without thinking. If we do not know what we are doing, how can we know what someone else is doing? The answer to both questions is the same. We can record and reflect on what we do and on the environment in which our actions occur.

Strategies for recording what we do include keeping a diary, a day planner, or simply jotting things down on a calendar, personal digital assistant (PDA), or smart phone. Later, reflecting on what we have written, we can see what we did and hence gain insight into what we were doing: our occupations. But what would we write? What information would be relevant in understanding what we were doing? Recording our tasks in excruciating detail would be counterproductive. Our challenge is to create a line drawing, not a snapshot, by abstracting from myriad tasks on any given day to yield a meaningful set of activities carried out within the framework of our occupations, occupational roles, occupational projects, and meaningful behavior.

What people record is only a small part of the complex detail of daily events. I write in my day planner, "11:30 am meet Joe at Lucy's—call first." Obviously, there is much information assumed in that statement. What have I assumed? I know why I am meeting Joe, I know or can find out where Lucy's is and how to get there, and whom to call and the number. I know Lucy's is a restaurant. All this and more is taken for granted as I make my note. When I actually meet Joe at Lucy's, I will have phoned and then traveled by some means to Lucy's. I will be there with Joe. Quite likely I will be eating lunch, and because Joe runs a summer college painting business, I am discussing going to work for him. I finish at 12:30 p.m. What would an observer see? How can one capture the information needed to understand what I am doing?

A person could shadow me, carry a notebook, and record all the things I do and details about them, which is known as *observation* (42, 43). Or one could give me a questionnaire asking me a series of questions known as *stylized questioning* about what I did (44). For example, one might ask, "How many hours a week do you work at a paid job?" Both of these approaches would provide some picture of what I was doing. Of course, it would be very costly to follow me around—and an observer may not see all I do in the same manner that I see it. Alternatively, a person might ask a series of many stylized questions, which, although somewhat informative, fail to capture the stream of what I am doing (my occupational behavior). Additionally, stylized questions tend to yield incomplete and inaccurate recording of a full day's or week's activities.

Fortunately, a proven technique is available that enables one to capture the needed information. *Time-use studies* are specifically designed to capture the flow of activities inherent in occupation and the context in which they are carried out. Time-use studies are about life, minute by minute, day by day. They are not snapshots, they are line drawings. They provide a skeletal representation of what one does. Using a diary format, an individual records, in sequence, each activity or occupation they engage in, usually 20 to 30 per day, and the context in which that activity or occupation was carried out. Literature to guide an individual in undertaking time-use studies exists (19, 45).

To understand more fully what people do, it is necessary to capture in time diaries a variety of dimensions focused on occupations and their contexts. Individuals often engage in multiple occupations at once, giving rise to the need to capture in a diary simultaneous occupations, described in current literature as primary and secondary activities. Additionally, as indicated earlier, a number of contextual dimensions influence activities and occupational behavior. These include location, social contact (with whom), for whom, tension, and technology. A combination of these and other relevant dimensions, depending on the issue of concern, needs to be captured in specific diary studies. Figure 5-1 ■ shows a prototype diary to be completed by an individual. It incorporates several of the dimensions discussed earlier.

The earliest published accounts of time-use studies appear to have been conducted in the early 1900s in the United Kingdom (46) and the United States (47). Then in the 1920s, time-use research emerged in Europe in conjunction with early studies of living conditions of the working class in response to pressures generated by industrialization. Household time-allocation studies date from 1915 in the United States (48). Over time, various investigations examined shares of activities such as paid work, housework, personal care, leisure, and so on in the daily, weekly, or yearly time budget of the population. They also examined how time use varied among population groups such as workers, students, and housewives. Most commonly, activity has been captured by stylized questions, asking respondents to estimate how much time they allocated to various activities. However, in view of a number of shortcomings of this approach, time diary studies have flourished since the 1960s and since the Multinational Time-Use Study (49). The Multinational Time-Use Study

What you did from midnight until 9 in the morning?

What did you do?	Time used	What else were you doing?	Where?	With whom?	For whom?

FIGURE 5-1 Prototype Time-Use Diary

(MTUS) was first developed in the early 1980s in England with the development of a data set that consolidated the approaches used by several nations into a single data set with common time-use categories or variables.

WHAT DO PEOPLE DO?

Most of us are used to thinking about what people do in terms of how we spend time during the day. The clock (mechanical and biological) and calendar run much of our lives, and we are used to scheduling our time. We can talk readily about our experience with time-related concepts such as having enough, too little, and saving or spending time. Consequently, much of what we know about what people do comes from time-use studies that have asked large groups of people to recall the activities that occupied their time in a given period, usually a 24-hour day.

As noted earlier, diary studies exist for many countries around the world as well as many population subgroups such as seniors, women, teachers, and persons with disabilities. Actual activities are recorded, as well as considerable contextual information. Objective information about participation in an activity such as when, where, or with whom it was performed, as well as subjective information such as how the person felt while engaging in the activity, is sometimes captured. The activities reported are then grouped or classified into major areas that generally reflect occupational behavior and can be examined within or across groups or populations and over time.

When examining the time-use data presented later in this chapter, the reader should realize two things. First, the data, unless otherwise noted, refer to time spent in primary activities; that is, the main activity the person was doing. Second, the average times presented in the tables are dependent on the prescribed coding definitions used. By coding the information, scientists gain the ability to compare groups and to see differences and changes in behavior over time. Coded data are important for assessing impacts of numerous factors ranging from individual (aging, disability, sex) to environmental (cultural expectations, social programs, poverty, war). Obviously individuals might not code their activities and occupations in the same way. What is one person's work may be another's leisure, or what feels like leisure to an individual at one time may feel like work at another time (39, 40). Depending on the intended use of the information, it is important to recognize that the purpose and meaning an individual ascribes to his or her occupations will be critical, especially when considering issues such as the relationships between occupational behavior and health and well-being. As noted elsewhere, contextual information is used to help code data as closely as possible to its meaning for respondents.

Time diary data provide a simple way of understanding daily life. On average during 2005, male Canadians allocated 4.7 hours per day to paid work, compared with 3.1 hours for females (Table 5-2 ■). The higher average for males can be explained by two key observations: those men who worked on any given day spent slightly longer hours than did females at paid work (9.1 compared to 7.9 hours, respectively), and a higher proportion of men than females engaged in paid work on an average day, 51% and 40%, respectively (Table 5-2). Across the whole population, the only activity taking more time per day than paid work is sleep, at 8.2 and 8.4 hours for males and females, respectively.

What more is there to life than working and sleeping? Well, there is television, the third largest use of daily time for both males and females, averaging 2.2 and 1.9 hours per day, respectively. For both men and women, socializing (1.7 and 1.8 hours), other personal activities (1.2 and 1.4 hours), and eating meals (1.0 hours each) are ranked next in explaining how time is used.

The remainder of time in a day is allocated over a broad range of activities as individuals fulfill their roles and pursue their occupations. What is particularly interesting to note in Table 5-2 is the small amount of time, overall, that is allocated to paid work, particularly by women. The data clearly reflect the need to view occupation broadly from a population perspective because this reveals social trends beyond individual experiences.

Time Use Across Countries and Over Time

Table 5-3 ■ compares differences in national time use between countries and over time. These sorts of compilations can be powerful evidence of stability or changes in social/cultural behavior. The daily time allocation to necessary, contracted, committed, and free time differs very little among countries. Calculated over all persons and all days of the week and nine different countries or years, contracted hours per day ranged between 2.9 and 4.8 hours per day (Table 5-3). Austria, which registered 4.8 hours in contracted time in 1992, has a large agricultural sector.

There is further evidence of major differences in time use that emerges between the sexes in contracted and committed time. Men register 3.3 more hours in Australia (1992) and 2.3 more hours in the Netherlands (1995) on contracted time in comparison with women, who register 3.8 and 1.9 (respectively) hours more on committed time (Table 5-3). However, gender differences in necessary and free time are far smaller between men and women. Women register between 0.1 and 0.5 hours (6 to 30 minutes) more per day on necessary time, and men register between 0.1 and 1.0 hours (6 to 60 minutes) more free time per day.

Time Use Across Subpopulations

Figure 5-2 ■ presents the time allocations to the four occupational areas for various role groups of the 1998 Canadian population defined in terms of gender (M, F), age

TABLE 5-2 *Allocation of Primary Activity Time and Participation Rates by Sex, Canada, 2005*

Activity Group	Population		Participants		Participation Rate	
	Male	Female	Male	Female	Male	Female
	(Hours per day)		(Hours per day)		(Percent)	
Total work[1]	7.8	7.8	8.3	7.9	97	99
Paid work	5.0	2.5	8.2	7.1	50	36
Unpaid work[2]	2.7	4.4	3.2	4.6	87	96
Personal care	10.2	10.6	10.2	10.6	100	100
Free time	6.0	5.6	6.1	5.7	97	97
1. Paid work and related activities	4.5	2.8	9.1	7.7	51	36
Paid work	4.1	2.5	8.8	7.1	50	35
Activities related to paid work	0.1	0.5	0.7	0.5	9	6
Commuting	0.4	0.3	0.9	0.8	45	32
2. Household and related work	2.4	4.1	2.8	4.3	85	95
Cooking/washing up	0.4	1.1	0.7	1.3	63	85
Housekeeping	0.3	1.0	1.5	1.8	22	59
Maintenance & repair	0.2	0.1	2.7	2.0	9	4
Other household work	0.4	0.4	1.6	1.1	27	33
Shopping for goods & services	0.7	0.9	1.8	1.9	38	47
Child care	0.3	0.6	1.8	2.4	16	24
3. Civic and voluntary activities	0.3	0.4	2.0	1.9	17	19
4. Education and related activities	0.5	0.6	6.0	6.3	9	9
5. Sleep, meals, and other personal	10.2	10.6	10.2	10.6	100	100
Night sleep	8.0	8.2	8.0	8.2	100	100
Meals (excl. restaurant meals)	1.1	1.1	1.2	1.2	92	91
Other personal activities	1.1	1.4	1.2	1.4	94	96
6. Socializing and restaurant meals	1.9	2.0	3.0	2.8	62	70
Restaurant meals	0.3	0.3	1.6	1.5	20	18
Socializing (in homes)	1.2	1.4	2.5	2.3	49	61
Other socializing	0.3	0.3	2.7	2.3	12	12
7. TV, reading, other passive leisure	2.9	2.6	3.3	3.1	87	84
Watching television	2.4	2.0	3.0	2.7	80	75
Reading books, magazines, newspapers	0.4	0.5	1.3	1.4	30	34
Other passive leisure	0.1	0.1	1.1	1.1	9	9
8. Sports, movies, other entertainment events	0.2	0.2	2.6	2.8	6	6
9. Active leisure	1.1	0.8	2.6	2.2	41	39
Active sports	0.6	0.4	2.3	1.7	26	22
Other active leisure	0.5	0.5	2.4	2.1	21	22

Source: Statistics Canada, General Social Survey, 2005. <http://www40.statcan.gc.ca/l01/cst01/famil36b-eng.htm> and <http://www40.statcan.gc.ca/l01/cst01/famil36c-eng.htm> extracted December 9, 2008

[1]Groups 1 to 4.

[2]Groups 2 and 3.

TABLE 5-3 *Daily Time Allocation, Selected Countries, and Years (in hours per day)*

	Necessary			Contracted		
	Total	**Male**	**Female**	**Total**	**Male**	**Female**
Canada, 1998	10.4	10.2	10.6	4.0	5.0	3.1
Canada, 2005	10.6	10.4	10.8	4.5	5.2	3.7
USA, 1998	10.3	10.1	10.5	4.5	5.4	3.9
USA, 2003	10.5	10.2	10.7	4.2	5.0	3.4
USA, 2004	10.6	10.5	10.7	4.2	4.9	3.5
USA, 2005	10.7	10.5	10.8	4.1	4.9	3.4
Australia, 1992	10.7	10.3	10.4	4.8	6.6	3.3
Australia, 1997	11.1	11.0	11.2	3.7	4.8	2.7
UK, 1995	10.4	10.1	10.7	3.0	4.0	2.2
UK, 2000	10.8	10.7	11.0	2.9	3.5	2.3
Netherlands, 1995	10.5	10.2	10.7	3.7	4.9	2.6
Netherlands, 2000	10.9	10.6	11.0	3.1	4.2	2.3
Norway, 1990	10.1	10.0	10.3	3.9	4.7	3.1
Norway, 2000	10.2	10.0	10.3	3.9	4.6	3.2
France, 1999	12.1	11.9	12.2	3.4	4.2	4.6
Slovenia, 2000	10.8	10.7	10.8	2.9	3.4	2.4
South Africa, 2000	11.6	11.5	11.6	3.7	4.8	3.0

	Committed			Free Time		
	Total	**Male**	**Female**	**Total**	**Male**	**Female**
Canada, 1998	3.5	2.6	4.2	6.6	6.7	6.5
Canada, 2005	3.4	2.7	4.2	5.5	5.7	5.3
USA, 1998	3.8	2.9	4.5	5.3	5.6	5.2
USA, 2003	4.0	3.1	4.6	5.5	5.7	5.3
USA, 2004	3.8	2.8	4.6	5.5	5.8	5.2
USA, 2005	3.7	2.8	4.6	5.5	5 8	5.2
Australia, 1992	4.0	2.0	5.8	5.8	6.0	5.9
Australia, 1997	4.0	2.8	5.1	5.3	5.5	5.1
UK, 1995	3.5	2.5	4.4	7.0	7.4	6.7
UK, 2000	3.4	2.6	4.2	6.8	7.1	6.5
Netherlands, 1995	3.4	2.4	4.3	6.4	6.5	6.4
Netherlands, 2000	3.6	2.5	4.4	6.2	6.4	6.0
Norway, 1990	3.5	2.6	4.3	6.5	6.6	6.3
Norway, 2000	3.4	2.7	4.1	6.5	6.6	6.3
France, 1999	3.4	2.4	4.4	4.5	4.9	4.2
Slovenia, 2000	3.9	2.9	4.8	6.2	6.8	5.8
South Africa, 2000	3.5	2.1	4.7	3.4	3.8	3.0

Source: Calculated from the Multinational Time-use Study (MSTU) data files for the selected countries and years.

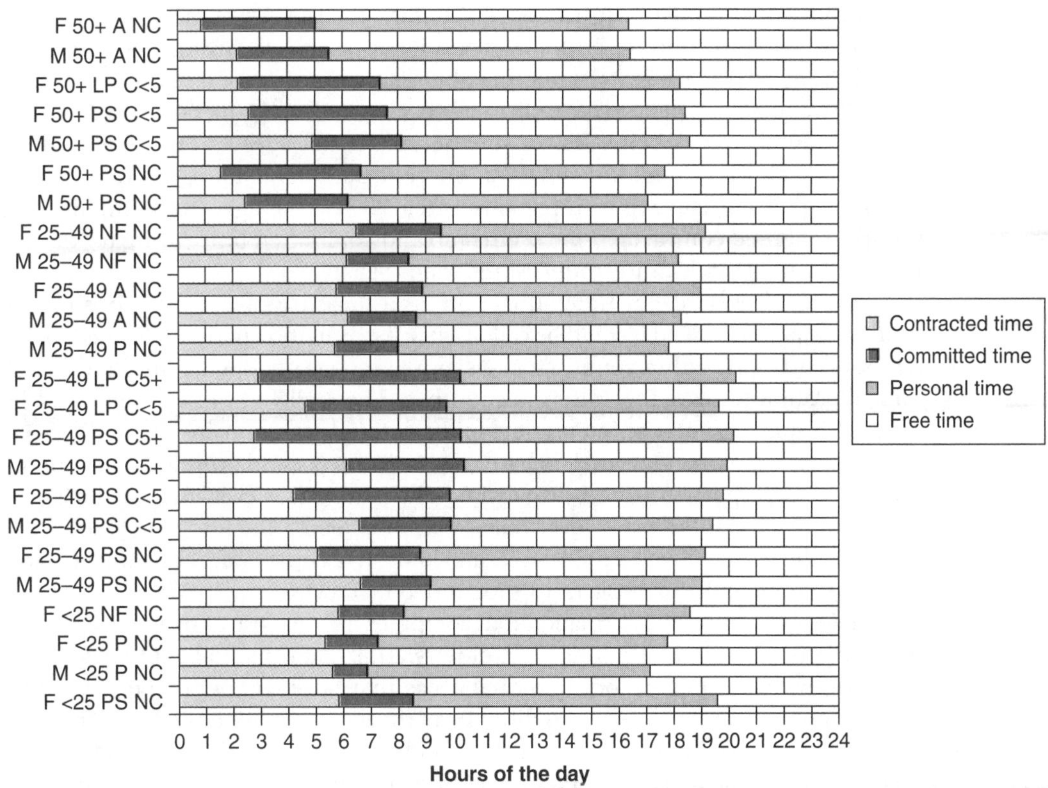

FIGURE 5-2 Time Allocation by Occupation, Canada, 2005
Source: Harvey, Marshall, and Frederick, 1991.

(< 25 to 50+), living arrangements (A, alone; PS, partner or spouse; P, parent; LP, lone parent; NF, nonfamily) and child status (C< 5, child under 5; C5+, child 5–14; NC, no child). The groups presented in Figure 5-2 are not exhaustive of all role groups but represent meaningfully sized groups in the sample. Figure 5-2 shows the great variation in occupation across the various defined role groups.

Of the 13 groups presented in the 25- to 49-year-old age group, all but 4 allocated an average of about 6 or more hours per day (42 hours per week) to contracted (paid) activities (Figure 5-2). The 4 groups registering fewer hours consisted of female (F) lone parents (LP) with children 5+ years old (C5+); the same group with children under 5 years old; females living with partner/spouse (PS) with a child under 5; and same group with no children (NC). Although contracted time was low for these groups, in general they exhibited the highest combined contracted and committed time, often referred to as *productive time*, registering about 10 hours per day (70 hours per week). Additionally, males, aged 25 to 49 living with a spouse/partner and children either under or over 5 years of age, registered about 10 hours per day. These same groups, male and female, can be seen to have the least free time, approximately 4 hours per day. In contrast, both males and females, age 50+, living alone (A) with no children (NC), have 7 hours per day (49 hours per week) of free time.

A life course perspective for individuals is reflected in Figure 5-2, with economically productive work being less in younger and older ages and more in middle adulthood. This is evident in Figure 5-2, where the subpopulations are ranked bottom to top by age, starting with persons under 25 years of age. In the middle age group, combined contracted time on the job and committed time caring for household and family significantly reduces free time available.

This brief overview of time allocation, as a measure of occupation, shows a fundamental fact, indeed it could be called a law: The variation in time allocated to different occupations within countries varies more among subpopulations than overall time allocation varies across different countries. The reality of this view emerged in the Multinational Time-Use Study in the mid-1960s (50) and remains true today. Societies appear, at an aggregate level, to have very similar needs and provide similar opportunities with respect to occupational time allocation. However, the burdens and opportunities are differentially distributed within societies. The foregoing also vividly illustrates the extent to which the allocation of time in occupational behavior is affected by at least some of the intrinsic factors identified in Table 5-1.

Table 5-4 ■ presents information that compares the time use of three specific subpopulations (the general population, elderly adults, and mentally/physically disabled individuals) in four occupational areas that have frequently been used in occupational research. These areas differ from the four areas identified earlier in the following ways: Productive time consists of both contracted and committed time as used earlier, and sleep is included in necessary time in the Aas (3) classification.

Individuals with mental and/or physical disabilities, relative to their general population counterparts, spend slightly more time on personal care (Table 5-4). Elderly

TABLE 5-4 *Allocation to Occupations for Different Populations, Canada, 1998 (in hours per day)*

	General Population		Elderly (65+)		Mentally/Physically Disabled	
	Male	Female	Male	Female	Male	Female
Personal Care	0.7	0.9	0.7	1.0	0.8	1.0
Productivity	7.6	7.5	4.2	4.6	5.5	5.7
Leisure	6.2	5.9	8.3	8.0	7.6	7.0
Sleep	8.1	8.4	8.7	8.7	8.4	8.7

Source: Statistics Canada, General Social Survey, Cycle 19: Time Use (2005) - Public Use Microdata File, Catalogue 12M0019XCB.

adults are less productive and have more leisure and sleep time than the general population. In general, the differences between men with a disability and elderly persons are less when compared to the general population. Research is needed to help us understand the implications of the differences, why they exist, and if they should be altered and how.

Studies also exist of other subpopulations such as homemakers (51), industrial workers (52), employed mothers (53, 54), and people with disabilities (19, 55, 56) that provide insights into the conduct of time-use studies. As well, there are studies of general populations, such as those conducted in Canada and Australia (57, 58).

The Context of Doing

Time spent in primary activities or occupations, as shown earlier in Table 5-2, reveals powerful similarities and differences in what people do, despite the aggregate similarities across the world. However, the amount of time we spend in various activities and occupations tells us very little about the quality of someone's life. It is more the attributes of engagement in the activity or occupation that have a bearing on quality of life, well-being, and health. These include the objective and subjective contexts, whether we are in a suitable location, whether we are with people we like or don't like, time pressures, personal control (whether we are doing the activity because we want to or have to), the meaning of the activity for us, and whether we have the skills to perform the activity or such advanced skill that we are bored in that activity (59). It is this contextual information that begins to give us a sense of what occupational engagement contributes to individuals and their society.

Secondary Activity and Occupation

Individuals often engage in concurrent activities and occupations in addition to their primary activities and occupations. Data from a 1997 Australian time-use study provide some insight into this phenomenon (58). It shows that a short but not inconsequential list of activities accounts for most secondary activities. The top five most frequent secondary activities accounted for 80% of all such episodes (Table 5-5 ■). Communication, media, and child-related activities dominate secondary activities. These are important dimensions of daily life and social involvement that are missed if studies do not collect secondary activity and occupation data. Some activities and occupations can be virtually totally missed if secondary ones are ignored, with minding children and caregiving heading the list of those often ignored. Minding children (child care) was recorded in diary episodes as a secondary activity far more frequently than as a primary activity in the Australian 1997 time-use study (60).

Secondary time can be significant. A study of teachers in Nova Scotia, Canada, found that one-fifth of a teacher's paid work time is considered to be a secondary activity, 10.2 hours per week from a total of 52.4 (31). This interpretation was made by listing as secondary activities such things as grading while supervising students or preparing materials for class while watching TV.

TABLE 5-5 *Secondary Activities, Australia, 1997*

	Episodes (*N*)	% of Total	Cumulative %
Communication (casual, leisure)	34,238	22.93	22.93
Listening to radio	32,524	21.78	44.70
Minding children	22,848	15.30	60.00
Watching TV	20,710	13.87	73.87
Playing/reading with child	9,101	6.09	79.96
Using audio/visual media	3,557	2.38	82.34
Drinking/nonalcohol	2,414	1.62	83.96
Reading newspaper	2,346	1.57	85.53
Listening to records	1,858	1.24	86.78
Reading (not further defined)	1,458	0.98	87.75
Meal preparation	1,209	0.81	88.56
Eating	1,185	0.79	89.35
Thinking	959	0.64	90.00
Other secondary	14,940	10.00	100.00
Total Secondary	149,347	100.00	100.00
Total Primary Only	256,786		
Total Episodes	406,133		

Source: Calculated from Australian Bureau of Statistics, *Australian Time Use Study,* 1997.

Location

The main location for activities and occupations is the home. In 2005, Canadian females averaged 17.2 hours per day at home, whereas Canadian males averaged 15.9 hours at home (Table 5-6 ■). The second major site of activities and occupations was the workplace, where females averaged 2.6 hours and males 3.8 hours. Males and females spend almost equal hours per day in transit (1.3 and 1.2, respectively) and 0.8 hours per day each in someone else's home. Hence, although there were very notable differences in the activities and occupations of males and females, the location of behavior is very similar.

With Whom

Excluding sleep and personal care time, Canadian males spent 6.5 hours a day and Canadian females 6.3 hours a day alone in 2005 (Table 5-7 ■). Female members were more likely than male members to spend time only with household members, 5.7 hours compared with 5.3 hours. Women spent nearly twice as long (1.7 hours compared to 1.0 hours) as men with household children under the age of 15. Males and females shared roughly the same amount of time each day with friends living outside the household (1.6 and 1.4 hours, respectively). Time for which social contact was not considered applicable, namely, sleep and personal care time, plus time spent alone, accounted for 16 hours per day. There was little difference between females, 15.9 hours, and males, 16.1 hours. In essence, this left only about 8.0 hours per day of stated social contact.

TABLE 5-6 *Average Hours per Day Spent at Various Locations, Canada, 2005*

Location of Activity	Total (Hours per day)	Male	Female
At respondent's home	16.5	15.9	17.2
At workplace	3.2	3.8	2.6
At someone else's home	0.8	0.8	0.8
At another place:	2.2	2.2	2.2
Restaurant or bar	0.3	0.3	0.2
Place of worship	0.1	0.0	0.1
Grocery store	0.1	0.1	0.2
Other store or mall	0.3	0.2	0.3
School	0.4	0.4	0.4
Outdoors away from home	0.3	0.4	0.3
In transit:	1.2	1.3	1.2
As an automobile driver	0.8	0.9	0.6
As a passenger in an automobile	0.2	0.1	0.3
Walking	0.1	0.1	0.1
Taking bus or other public transit	0.2	0.1	0.2

Source: Statistics Canada, General Social Survey, Cycle 19: Time Use (2005)-Public Use Microdata File, Catalogue 12M0019XCB.

TABLE 5-7 *Average Hours per Day Spent with Various Other Persons, Canada, 2005*

Social Contact During Activity	Total (Hours per day)	Male	Female
Alone	6.4	6.5	6.3
With household members:	5.5	5.3	5.7
Spouse or partner	3.4	3.5	3.2
Child(ren) under age 15	1.4	1.0	1.7
Parent(s) or parent(s)-in-laws	0.3	0.3	0.3
Other members including children age 15 and over	0.5	0.4	0.5
With persons outside the household:	5.0	5.2	4.8
Respondent's child(ren) under age 15	0.1	0.1	0.1
Respondent's child(ren) age 15 and over	0.1	0.1	0.2
Parent(s) or parent(s)-in-laws	0.2	0.2	0.3
Other relative(s)	0.6	0.5	0.7
Friend(s)	1.5	1.6	1.4
Other person(s)	2.5	2.8	2.2
With household members only	4.5	4.3	4.7
With persons outside the household only	4.7	4.9	4.4
Social contact not applicable to activity (includes sleep)	9.1	9.0	9.3

Source: Statistics Canada, General Social Survey, Cycle 19: Time Use (2005)-Public Use Microdata File, Catalogue 12M0019XCB.

The Social Environment

Although it is informative to understand where and with whom activities and occupations are carried out, it can be more meaningful to understand the interaction between these contextual dimensions. A meaningful way to explore the relationship between social contact and location can be cast in terms of social environment (29). The social environment is one's social circle, consisting of those people with whom an individual comes in contact, and social space, the locations occupied by persons. Looked at in this way, Canadians spend about 10% more time alone at home than do individuals in Norway and Sweden, 31.2%, compared with 21.9% and 21.2%, respectively (Table 5-8 ■).

In contrast, little difference is seen among Canada, Norway, and Sweden in the amount of time spent alone in transit, about a half percent of total time per day. With respect to family time, both Norwegians and Swedes spend a larger proportion of their time at home with their family than do Canadians. In terms of time in the community, both Canadians and Norwegians spend approximately 20% of their time there, whereas in Sweden the figure is less than 15%. The lesson to be learned here it is that different people play out their day-to-day lives in somewhat different social

TABLE 5-8 *Social Environment in Selected Countries*

	Social Space					
Social Circle	**Home (%)**	**Workplace (%)**	**Community (%)**	**Transit (%)**	**Total (%)**	**Total (minutes)**
Canada 1992						
Alone	31.2	3.1	3.4	3.5	41.2	390.0
Family	19.9	0.4	5.2	2.5	27.9	263.9
Others and multiple	3.8	14.5	11.1	1.4	30.9	291.8
Total	54.8	18.1	19.7	7.4	100.0	945.6
Norway 1990						
Alone	21.9	7.4	3.3	3.2	35.8	345.4
Family	26.1	0.6	6.2	2.6	35.6	343.0
Others and multiple	4.1	13.4	9.4	1.8	28.6	276.0
Total	52.2	21.4	18.9	7.5	100.0	964.5
Sweden 1991						
Alone	21.2	5.2	2.7	3.7	32.7	335.1
Family	26.5	0.4	2.2	1.9	31.0	317.3
Others and multiple	5.8	18.7	9.4	2.3	36.3	371.9
Total	53.5	24.3	14.3	7.9	100.0	1024.4

Source: Harvey and Taylor, 2000 (29).

TABLE 5-9 *Communications Technology, Australia, 1997*

Mode	Number of Events	Percent
In person	14,866	48.39
Mobile phone	39	0.13
Fixed phone	7,165	23.32
Written	6,486	21.11
Fax	62	0.20
PC	1,816	5.91
Undescribed	286	0.93
Total	30,720	100.00

Source: Calculated from 1997 Australian Time-Use Data, Australian Bureau of Statistics (36).

environments. As well as understanding why people do certain activities and occupations, it is also necessary to understand the context in which they engage in them.

Technology

Technology plays a role in everyday life in many ways. We can observe in Table 5-6 that in 2005 Canadians spent 1.0 hours per day in a car either as driver or passenger and only 0.2 hours per day on public transit.

The 1997 Australian time-use study provides insight into the use of communications technology (58). Nearly one-half of recorded communication was done in person, as illustrated in Table 5-9 ■. Approximately one-fifth of reported communication was written, and slightly more than one-fifth was by phone. The data reflect relatively little use of computers and an infinitesimal amount of mobile phone and fax use. These numbers could reflect one of two things. On the one hand, the use of mobile phone, fax, and other communication means may have been underreported in the diaries. Underreporting is a real possibility because using a mobile phone may often be a very short activity. On the other hand, the low numbers could reflect reality in the face of hype. Often, much is made about the length of time spent on cell phones, the Internet, and dealing with e-mail. Data on technology use are often derived from market surveys that rely on extremely biased samples in a manner that leaves the impression that a phenomenon is much greater than it is. Determining which explanation is more valid would constitute a worthwhile study. Of course, households have far more technological equipment in the form of appliances, tools, entertainment equipment, and more. Far too little research has been carried out to help us understand the strengths and follies of such technological advancements.

CHAPTER SUMMARY

This chapter discussed a variety of ways of conceptualizing what people do and the factors that influence and characterize human occupational behavior. Measurement of human time use is well developed and applied across numerous disciplines. We have briefly reviewed some of the methods of recording and measuring time use in activities and occupations. Each affords us unique information about human doing and will proscribe different approaches to the understanding, assessment, and facilitation of health and well-being.

Finally, data were presented and compared on the use of time among various groups and across countries. We have noted that, in reality, paid work accounts for a rather small portion of time in activities and occupations on a lifetime basis. This suggests that it is important to view occupation in a broad manner so as to identify and understand all occupations in which people engage and how they interrelate in life from one day to a lifetime. We have also noted that activities and occupations vary much more among subpopulations in a given country than they do in total across countries. This suggests that populations as a whole, reflected by the countries, have very similar occupational needs. It further suggests that these needs are met, in each case nationally, by a division or sharing of work and responsibility determined by some of the forces identified in this chapter and elsewhere in this text. Although the chapter has tended to focus on individual human occupation, many of the constructs discussed can be applied to the occupational behavior of communities and groups.

STUDY GUIDE

Study Guide Author: Kristine Haertl

Summary of Main Points

The concept of doing is central to occupational science. As indicated by the authors, "Occupation is what we do." An examination of human occupational behavior in the context of time contributes to our understanding of individual and collective cultures and means by which we create meaning in life. Personal roles and contextual influences shape our occupational engagement and time use. An understanding of time use in relation to what, how, and why people do what they do is vital to a number of scientific disciplines, including occupational science.

Application to Occupational Therapy

Occupational therapists have a core concern for occupation, and thus how occupation is used over time. Knowledge of how and why people do what they do in the context of time is, thus, foundational to occupational therapy services. Classic occupational therapy questions in interviewing individuals, families or communities refer to time use: What did you do during the day? the last week, month, year? How did you spend your day? What do you need and want to do with your time? What would you like to or need to do today? How much time is spent in self-care, paid work, school, play, productivity, leisure, sleep or other occupational categories? Occupational therapists analyze time use in considering how occupational participation in particular time segments influences personal health and well-being. In addition to interviewing clients about time, occupational therapists use many evaluation methods to analyze time: inviting clients to keep a time log, diary or chart of occupations for a day, week or more; engaging clients in drawing or otherwise constructing time charts to portray time use; videotaping occupational participation in time chunks and inviting discussion about how and why decisions and choices were made about participation in particular times and places. These and other strategies are similar to the time use study methods outlined in the chapter, with the added use of the information to assist in planning, implementing and evaluating occupational therapy services. Strategies are developed to enhance patterns of time use and develop occupational patterns that contribute to individual and societal life satisfaction. With goals such as using blocks of time for discovering meaningful occupations or re-engaging in occupations in light of occupational deprivation, lack of occupational development or other challenges, intervention programs may be aimed at the micro/personal level and look at barriers and supports to successful occupational participation, or at the community and societal level in considering how policies, structures, and resources are developed to enhance communal lifestyle and occupational engagement.

Occupational therapists embrace the importance of time use through occupational engagement as the core focus for this profession. Understanding personal, family, group, community, organizational, or population time use and patterns of occupational engagement are foundational to creating an evidence-based practice to enhance health, well-being, and equitable participation in society for all. Cultural differences in time use must be understood as well as individual and contextual influences on occupational performance and engagement. Use of occupational classifications and other occupational taxonomies help occupational therapists to address time use (e.g., necessary time, contracted time, committed time, and free time) and how people construct diverse meanings in everyday life.

Individual Learning Activities

1. Create and follow a time-use chart or time diary for 1 week. Upon completion of the chart, categorize items into the four uses of time as identified by Aas (necessary time, contracted time, committed time, and free time. Within this chart, also indicate that which you consider leisure time (note, not all free time is leisure time). Following completion of your diary, write a three- to four-page paper reflecting on these questions:
   a. Briefly summarize your time-use patterns. Did anything surprise you regarding the way you spent your time?
   b. What are your current roles and how do they influence your patterns of time use?
   c. Is there anything you would change about your patterns of time use? If so, what?
   d. Do you believe your time-use patterns contribute to your overall health and well-being? If not, what could you do to enhance well-being through changes in your patterns of time use?
2. Imagine yourself in 20 years, create a daily time-use chart including how you believe you will spend your time, what types of necessary, contracted, committed, and free time you have. Write a brief reflection on how your time use will likely remain the same and how it will differ in time.

Group Learning Activity

As a group, take a field trip around your community. Write observational notes on structures, places, and environments observed and how they contribute to or detract from time use and occupational engagement. How does your community influence the choices in what you do during the early morning, day, evening, night? Following your trip, prepare a 20-minute presentation on your findings. Discuss observations of things, structures and environmental aspects that seem to contribute to occupational engagement in healthful ways and areas that seemed to detract from healthful occupational engagement. If you were presenting to your community board, what recommendations would you make for improvements that would encourage healthy time use in everyday occupations?

Study Questions

1. In considering Aas's conceptualization of time use, formal education would fall under which of the following?
   a. Necessary time
   b. Contracted time
   c. Committed time
   d. Free time
2. Aas distinguished between leisure time and free time.
   a. True
   b. False
3. A pattern of behavior that involves certain rights and duties that an individual is expected, trained, and may be encouraged to perform in a particular social situation.
   a. Occupational behavior
   b. Roles
   c. Zeitgebers
   d. Human performance
4. Social support and income would be considered what type of factors influencing occupational behavior?
   a. Intrinsic
   b. Extrinsic
   c. Fixed
   d. None of the above
5. Capability constraints:
   a. Limit the activities of an individual because of the biological construction and/or tools he/she can command
   b. Refer to the degree of control that exists over something that is a control area or domain
   c. Defines where, when, and for how long the individual has to join other individuals, tools, and materials
   d. All of the above

REFERENCES

1. Van der Post, L. (1951). *Journey to the interior.* New York: Morrow.
2. Harvey, A. S., & Neimi, I. (1994). An international standard activity classification (ISAC): Toward a framework of relevant issues. In *Fifteenth reunion of the International Association for Time Use Research.* Amsterdam: NIMMO.

3. Aas, D. (1980). Designs for large scale time use studies of the 24 hour day. In *It's about time.* Sofia: Institute of Sociology at the Bulgarian Academy of Science.
4. Harvey, A. (1982). Role and context: Shapers of behavior. *Studies of Broadcasting, 18,* 70–92.
5. Canadian Association of Occupational Therapists. (1997). *Enabling occupation: An occupational therapy perspective.* Ottawa: Author.
6. Ickes, W., Knowles, E. S., & Kidd, R. F. (Eds.). (1982). *Personality, roles and social behavior.* New York: Springer-Verlag.
7. Mancuso, J. C., & Sarbin, T. R. (1985). The self-narrative in the enactment of roles. In T. R. Sarbin & K. E. Scheibe (Eds.), *Studies in social identity* (pp. 233–253). New York: Praeger Publishers.
8. Marks, R. R. (1977). Multiple roles and role strain: Some notes on human energy, time and commitment. *American Sociological Review, 39,* 567–568.
9. Tindale, J. (1999). Variance in the meaning of time by family cycle, period, social context, and ethnicity. In W. Pentland, A. S. Harvey, M. P. Lawton, & M. A. McColl (Eds.), *Time use research in the social sciences* (pp. 155–182). New York: Kluwer Academic/Plenum Publishers.
10. Goffman, E. (1959). *The presentation of self in everyday life.* New York: Doubleday.
11. World Health Organization. (2001). *International classification of functioning, disability and health.* In *ICIDH-2.* Geneva: Author.
12. Canada. Supreme Court of Canada. (2001). About the court. In http://www.scc.csc.gc.ca/aboutcart/judges/aboutjusticies_e:html.
13. McKinney, V. (1990). *McKinney v. University of Guelph* (p. D/171). Supreme Court of Canada.
14. Cheek, N. H., & Burch, W. R. (1976). *The social organization of leisure in human society.* New York: Harper and Row.
15. Forbes, W., Singleton, J., & Agavani, N. (1993). Stability of activities across the lifespan. *Activities, Adaptation and Aging, 18*(1), 19–28.
16. Harvey, A. S., Elliot, D. H., & Procos, D. (1977). *Sub-populations relevant to the study of the use of time: A working paper.* Halifax, Nova Scotia: Dalhousie University–Regional and Urban Studies Center.
17. Lounesbury, J. W., & Hoopes, L. L. (1988). Five year stability of leisure activity and motivation factors. *Journal of Leisure Research, 20*(2), 118–134.
18. Schneider, A. (1972). Patterns of social interaction. In A. Szalai (Ed.), *The use of time: Daily activities of urban and suburban populations in twelve countries.* Amsterdam: Mouton & Company.
19. Pentland, W., Harvey, A. S., Lawton, M. P., & McColl, M. A. (Eds.). (1999). *Time use research in the social sciences.* New York: Kluwer Academic/Plenum Publishers.
20. Little, B. R. (1983). Personal projects: A rationale and method for investigation. *Environment and Behavior, 15,* 273–309.
21. Ellegard, K. (1993). Activities in their every-day context: Using individual diary data to set forth the complex pattern of people's activities in their every-day life. In *Time use methodology: Toward consensus.* Rome: Italian National Statistical Institute.
22. Palys, B. R., Palys, T. S., & Little, B. R. (1983). Perceived life satisfaction and the organization of personal project systems. *Journal of Personality and Social Psychology, 44,* 1221–1230.
23. Elchardus, M., & Glorieux, I. (1993). Towards a semantic taxonomy classifying activities on the basis of their meaning. In *Time-use methodology: Toward consensus.* Rome: Italian National Statistical Institute.
24. Christiansen, C., & Baum, C. M. (1997). Person–environment–occupational performance. In C. Christiansen & C. M. Baum (Eds.), *Person–environment occupational performance: A conceptual model for practice* (2nd ed., pp. 47–70). Thorofare, NJ: Slack Inc.

25. Maric, D. (1997). *Adopting working hours to modern needs: The time factor in the new approach to working conditions.* Geneva: International Labour Office.
26. Zuzanek, J., & Smale, B. (1994). Life cycle variations in across-the-week allocation of time to selected daily activities. *Society and Leisure, 15*(2), 559–586.
27. Frederick, J. A. (1995). *As time goes by: Time use of Canadians. General survey.* Ottawa: Statistics Canada (Housing, Family and Social Division).
28. Cullen, I., & Godson, V. (1975). Urban networks: The structure of activity patterns. *Progress in Planning, 4*(1), 1–96.
29. Harvey, A. S., & Taylor, M. E. (2000). Activity settings and travel behavior. *Transportation, 27,* 53–73.
30. Drago, R. (1999). New estimates of working time for elementary school teachers. *Monthly Labor Review, 4,* 31–40.
31. Harvey, A. S., & Spinney, J. (2000). *Life on and off the job: A time use study of Nova Scotia teachers.* Halifax: St. Mary's University Time Use Research Program.
32. Elliot, D., Harvey, A. S., & Procos, D. (1976). An overview of the Halifax time-budget study. *Society and Leisure, 3,* 145–159.
33. Goodchild, M., & Janelle, D. (1982). Diurnal patterns of social group distributions in a Canadian city. *Economic Geography, 59*(4), 403–425.
34. Janelle, D. G., & Goodchild, M. F. (1983). Transportation indicators of space–time autonomy. *Urban Geography,* No. 4, 4.
35. Blanke, K., & Schafer, D. (1993). What for whom? Experience from the diaries of the pretest of 1991/1992. In *ISTAT time use methodology: Toward consensus.* Rome: Italian National Statistics Institute.
36. Australia Bureau of Statistics. (1988). *Time use survey of Australia: User's guide.* Canberra: Australian Commonwealth Government Printer.
37. Zuzanek, J., Beckers, T., & Peters, P. (1998). The "harried leisure class" revisited: Dutch and Canadian trends in the use of time from the 1770s to the 1990s. *Leisure Studies, 17*(1), 1–19.
38. Robinson, J. P. (1977). *How Americans use time: A social psychological analysis of everyday behavior.* New York: Praeger Publishers.
39. Shaw, S. (1985). The meaning of leisure in everyday life. *Leisure Sciences, 7*(1), 1–23.
40. Sorokin, P., & Berger, C. Q. (1939). *Time budgets of human behavior.* Cambridge, MA: Harvard University Press.
41. Hagerstrand, T. (1970). What about people in regional science? *Papers and Proceedings of The Regional Science Association, 24,* 7–24.
42. Skjoensberg, E. (1989). *Change in an African village: Kefa speaks.* West Hartford, CT: Kumarian Press.
43. Altman, R. M. (1974). Observational study of behavior: Sampling methods. *Behavior, 48,* 227–267.
44. Ho, T. J. (1979). Time costs of child rearing in the rural Philippines. *Population and Development Review, 5*(4), 643–662.
45. Harvey, A. S., Szalai, A., Elliot, D. H., Stone, P. J., & Clark, S. (1984). *Time budget research: An ISSC workbook in comparative analysis.* New York: Campus Verlag.
46. Pember-Reeves, M. (1913). *Round about a pound a week.* London: Bell.
47. Bevans, G. E. (1913). *How working men spend their spare time.* Unpublished doctoral dissertation, Columbia University.
48. Bailey, I. (1915). A study of management of farm homes. *Journal of Home Economics, 7,* 348.
49. Szalai, A. (Ed.). (1972). *The use of time.* The Hague, Netherlands: Mouton.

50. Converse, P. E. (1972). *The social organization of leisure in human society.* New York: Harper and Row.
51. Walker, E., & Woods, M. E. (1976). *Time use: A measure of household production of family goods and services.* Washington, DC: Center for the Family, American Economics Association.
52. Zuzanek, J. (1980). *Work and leisure in the Soviet Union: A time budget analysis.* New York: Praeger Publishers.
53. Michelson, W. (1985). *From sun to sun: Daily obligations and community structure in the lives of employed women and their families.* Ottawa: Rowman and Allanheld.
54. Robinson, J., & Bianchi, S. (1997). The children's hours. *American Demographics, 19*(12), 22–24.
55. Ujimoto, K. (1987). Organizational activities, cultural factors and well-being of aged Japanese Canadians. In D. E. Gelfand (Ed.), *Ethnic dimensions of aging* (pp. 145–160). New York: Springer.
56. Klumb, P., & Baltes, M. (1999). Time use of old and very old Berliners: Productive and consumptive activities as functions of resources. *Journal of Gerontology, 54B*(5), 271–278.
57. Harvey, A. S., Marshall, K., & Frederick, J. (1991). *Where does time go?* (Catalogue 11-612E, no. 4). Ottawa: Statistics Canada.
58. Marshall, K., & Frederick, J. A. (1997). *How Australians use their time.* (Report 4153.0). Canberra: Commonwealth of Australia, Bureau of Statistics.
59. Csikszentmihali, M., & Larson, R. (1987). Validity and reliability of the experience-sampling method. *Journal of Nervous and Mental Disease, 175*(9), 526–536.
60. Harvey, A. S., Australian Bureau of Statistics. (2000). *Use of context in time use research.* Paper given at Expert Group Meeting on Methods for Conducting Time-Use Surveys, New York, United Nations Secretariat–Statistics Division.

CHAPTER 6

Occupational Development

Jane A. Davis and Helene J. Polatajko

OBJECTIVES

1. Describe the role of occupation in human development.
2. Explain the authors' proposed Interactional Model of Occupational Development (IMOD).
3. Describe the systematic change in occupational behavior at the micro, meso, and macro levels.
4. Discuss the four major viewpoints on development: preformationist, maturationist, environmentalist, and interactionist and how they influence occupational development.
5. Describe the influence of person, occupation, environment, and interaction determinants on the course of occupational development.
6. Discuss the changing course of occupational development across the life span.

KEY WORDS

Active participation
Continuity theory
Environmentalist viewpoint
Interactionist viewpoint
Mastery
Maturationist viewpoint
Multiple determinicity
Multiple patternicity
Multiple variation
Preformationist viewpoint
Tabula rasa

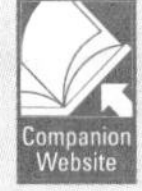

www.prenhall.com/christiansen

The Internet provides an exciting means for interacting with this textbook and for enhancing your understanding of humans' experiences with occupations and the organization of occupations in society. Use the address above to access the interactive Companion Website created specifically to accompany this book. Here you will find an array of self-study material designed to help you gain a richer understanding of the concepts presented in this chapter.

Parts of this chapter have been adapted from Davis, J. A., & Polatajko, H. J. (2006). The occupational development of children. In S. Rodger & J. Ziviani (Eds.), *Occupational therapy with children: Understanding children's occupations and enabling participation* (pp. 136–157). Oxford, UK: Blackwell Publishing. Reproduced with permission.

CHAPTER PROFILE

Watson (1928) assumed that genetic factors place no restrictions on the ways that environmental events can shape the course of a child's development and claimed that by properly organizing the environment he could produce a Mozart, a Babe Ruth, or an Al Capone. (1, pp. 5–6)

In this chapter the reader will be asked to consider whether Watson's perspective has merit. In other words, the reader will be asked to consider the nature and course of **occupational development**. Human growth and development have been studied for more than a century. Although a variety of domains have been investigated, there has not been a specific, systematic investigation of human *occupational* development. In this chapter, the authors present a framework of occupational development that has been constructed from the existing developmental literature. First the authors present perspectives on occupation and on development. Then the Interactional Model of Occupational Development (IMOD) will be proposed as a way of explaining three interactive levels of occupational development—micro, meso, and macro. Finally, a discussion of the ages and stages of occupational development across the life span is offered.

INTRODUCTION

Human growth and development has been a focus of study for more than a century. By its very nature, such study is an interdisciplinary enterprise concerned with various aspects of human development. Textbooks on development typically describe changes in a number of areas, including changes in body size and shape; motor, cognitive, and language skills; and social, sexual, moral, and personality domains. However, occupational development is rarely specifically included among these, with one of the few exceptions being the literature on career development, where the concept of occupation is narrowly defined in terms of economically productive work.

Nevertheless, many of the descriptions of development found in the literature are stated in terms of what people ***do*** at various ages and stages of life, in other words, in terms of occupation. This can be seen vividly in Shakespeare's profile of the ages and stages of life in *As You Like It,* a romantic comedy written in the late 16th century:

> All the world's a stage
> And all the men and women merely players;
> They have their exits and their entrances;
> And one man in his time plays many parts;
> His acts being seven ages. At first the infant,
> Mewling and puking in the nurse's arms.
> Then the whining school-boy, with his satchel
> And shining morning face, creeping like snail
> Unwillingly to school. And then the lover,
> Sighing like a furnace, with a woeful ballad
> Made to his mistress' eyebrow. Then a soldier,
> Full of strange oaths and bearded like the bard,

Jealous in honour, sudden and quick in quarrel,
Seeking the bubble reputation
Even in the cannon's mouth. And then the justice,
In fair round belly with good capon lined,
With eyes severe and beard of formal cut,
Full of wise saws and modern instances;
And so he plays his part. The sixth age shifts
Into the lean and slipper'd pantaloon
With spectacles on nose and pouch on side,
His youthful hose, well saved, a world too wide
For his shrunk shank; and his big manly voice,
Turning again toward childish treble, pipes
And whistles in his sound. Last scene of all,
That ends this strange eventful history,
Is second childishness and mere oblivion,
Sans teeth, sans eyes, sans taste, sans everything.

Shakespeare, As You Like It, Act II, scene vii

Similarly, the developmental literature provides information that can be used to construct a framework for occupational development. Theories of human development that are consistent with an occupational perspective can be used to create an integrative model of occupational development. The purpose of this chapter is to present such a model. The reader is introduced to a framework of human occupational development, relevant theories, a potential model of occupational development, and a preliminary discussion concerning the ages and stages of occupational development across the life span.

AN OCCUPATIONAL PERSPECTIVE ON DEVELOPMENT

An Occupational Perspective

Humans are occupational beings; they derive meaning in their lives through what they do. "Doing" is central to human life. As Fidler and Fidler (2) noted, "Doing is viewed as enabling the development and integration of the sensory, motor, cognitive, and psychological systems; serving as a socializing agent, and verifying one's efficacy as a competent, contributing member of one's society" (p. 305). Ultimately, "occupation is the crucible in which our identities are formed" (3).

Humans in all cultures engage in a wide variety of occupations, which are shaped by individuals' innate cognitive, affective, and physical abilities and the environments in which they live, work, and play. The specific occupations in which people engage are influenced by their abilities, preferences, values, lifestyles, and by the obligations, expectations, and possibilities afforded by the physical, cultural, social, and institutional environments in which they act. Interactive relationships are assumed to exist among person, occupation, and environment, each influencing the other two and causing the other two to change. To quote Wilcock, "occupation has the potential to change the world or the species and this provides the mechanism for human survival and development which in turn impacts and maintains health and well-being and offers the individual the ability to adapt to their environmental demands" (4, p. 35).

The performance of those occupations is considered to be "the result of a dynamic, interwoven relationship between persons, environment, and occupation over a person's life span" (5, p. 181). Occupational performance is influenced by a person's emotions, physical abilities and skills, and ability to process information. The developmental literature indicates that individual performance in these domains changes and develops across the life span. Because competent performance can only be achieved when there is a match among the abilities of the individual, the demands of the occupation, and the supports of the environment (6, 7), a person's ability to engage in and master occupations can be presumed to change and develop throughout life.

A Perspective on Development

Human development has been of interest since the time of Aristotle (8), who observed: "What makes men good is held by some to be nature, by others habit or training, by others instruction" (9, p. 975). Since that time, people have attempted to more fully understand developmental influences. In the 20th century, a concerted effort was made to gain scientific knowledge. Theories and research on human development expanded within a variety of disciplines, including psychology, anthropology, sociology, biology, and history, leading to the formation of a distinct body of knowledge.

Until recently, developmental research has focused almost exclusively on the first 20 years of life. Thus, concepts of human development have been essentially concepts of "child" development. In the last few decades, however, greater emphasis has been placed on understanding development in adulthood and old age. It is now generally accepted that human development is a lifelong process, including both the concepts of child development and adult development and aging (10–15).

Humans go through a lifelong process of change and development. These two terms, *change* and *development,* are often used interchangeably; yet, there are significant differences in their meaning. Although "development involves change, not all change is developmental" (16, p. 5). The differences between the two terms involve the notions of (a) reversibility, (b) distinctiveness, (c) length of time, and (d) growth and maturation. For example, the emergence of facial hair in a young man is the result of developmental maturation, whereas shaving off a beard involves a change that is not developmental, because it is easily reversed, can reoccur, happens within a few minutes, and does not add to what has already happened. As a lifelong process, unlike most changes, development is not easily reversed, is distinct in nature from prior occurrences, occurs over long periods of time, and is influenced by growth and maturation.

Historically, there have been four major viewpoints on how human development occurs: **preformationist, maturationist, environmentalist,** and **interactionist.** The major difference among them relates to the relative emphasis each viewpoint places on the concepts of maturational, environmental, and interactional influences on an individual's development. The *preformationist view,* popular from the Middle Ages to the latter part of the 18th century, viewed little children as miniature adults (17) who acquired all their lifetime characteristics at conception, including body shape and personality. *Maturationists* believed that a person's genes dictated human development. Therefore, heredity alone was thought to direct the course and nature of a human's development. *Environmentalism* had its origins with John Locke, an English physician and social philosopher from the mid-17th century, who believed that all individuals were born empty of influence (sometimes referred to as ***tabula rasa,*** Latin for "blank slate") and that they developed due to their different life experiences. According to this view, environment alone affects development.

The *interactionist view* holds that individuals are involved in a reciprocal interactive relationship with their environment that ultimately delineates human development across the life span. Individuals bring their genetic makeup, or *genotype,* to this dynamic relationship. Their genotype dictates a certain outward expression of human characteristics, or *phenotype;* however, it is constrained by the environment, which is thought to play a significant role in an individual's development. As individuals grow and mature, the nature of this interactive relationship stays the same. However, the phenomena involved may change and build on previous occurrences, making development a cumulative experience (18).

The strength of the interactionist perspective is that it draws on concepts from both maturationism and environmentalism, influenced by developmental research during the last few decades. Arnold Gesell (19, 20) used the term *maturation* to mean developmental changes that are caused or directed by genes. He believed that children's development unfolds due to the action of the genes with the environment playing a supportive but limited role in children's development. Maturation is said to occur in fixed sequences, such as those seen in embryonic change in which there is an exact order of biological development. This sequential development continues after birth, with maturational changes seen from infancy through puberty to old age.

Although Gesell believed that genes are the main regulatory mechanism for development, he also believed that individuals are products of their environment. As individuals age, the rates of developmental change increasingly vary as the influence of the environment shapes development. Children require positive influences of the social and cultural environments to realize their full potential within society. Gesell and Ilg (20) believed that developmental potential is maximized when socializing forces have a goodness of fit with the unfolding maturation of the individual.

Most current researchers lean toward an interactionist perspective, agreeing that both genetics and the environment play important roles in development. The unanswered question seems to be, *What role does each factor play in the individual's development?* It is currently believed that the influences of the person and the environment act together, making it extremely difficult to determine the unique influences of each on human development. Researchers have attempted to determine how much each factor contributes and have found this question extremely difficult to answer. Consequently, some investigators have shifted their study from *How much?* to *How* genes, the environment, and their interaction influence development (21–25).

INTERACTIONISM AS A FRAMEWORK FOR OCCUPATIONAL DEVELOPMENT

The interactionist perspective that now pervades the field of development fits well with an occupational perspective, which is to focus attention on occupations and the influences of personal traits and experiences, as well as environmental conditions on the occupations of individuals, families, groups, communities, organizations, or populations. Thus it follows that interactionism could provide a framework for understanding and defining human occupational development. Further, there is good evidence to support applying an interactionist perspective to occupational development. Consider, for example, the story from the 1790s of Victor, the Wild Boy of Aveyron (26), which depicts the pervasive negative effect on all aspects of development from being raised apart from civilization. The more recent story of Genie, a young girl who was confined to a crib for most of her 13 years (27), shows a similar pervasive negative developmental effect from severe prolonged deprivation. The stories from orphanages have demonstrated that less-severe deprivation of shorter duration also has detrimental effects. However, these experiences also demonstrate that the effects are influenced by the duration of the deprivation and may be reversed through exposure to richer occupational environments (28).

An Interactionist Definition of Occupational Development

The Canadian Association of Occupational Therapists' definition of occupational development alludes to an interactionist perspective: "the gradual change in occupational behaviors over time, resulting from the growth and maturation of the individual in interaction with the environment" (5, p. 40). This definition provides a starting point for an interactionist definition and suggests three levels of occupational development: micro, meso, and macro.

The gradual change in occupational behaviors can be understood in terms of the development of occupational competence of the individual—that is, progression along the continuum from novice to mastery, in the performance of given occupations. From this **micro** perspective, occupational development is considered at the **level of the occupation**, with a beginning, a progression, and an endpoint that can be viewed as occurring somewhere along the continuum from novice to mastery. The expectation is that an individual moves through this progression at a specific rate and sequence. The development of occupational competence is an iterative process, with the progression from novice toward mastery repeated again and again, with the addition of each new occupation.

The gradual change can also be understood in terms of an individual's occupational repertoire—that is, the array of occupations an individual has at a specific point in their life course. From this **meso** perspective, occupational development is considered at the **level of the individual** with changes having multiple patterns and no specific endpoint. Rather, occupational repertoires change continuously throughout the life span, sometimes expanding, and sometimes shrinking. There is no a priori determination of the number or specifics of the occupations that will constitute an individual's repertoire, either at a particular point in time or across the life course. However, it is anticipated that a repertoire will develop, and that the development will continue throughout the life span.

Finally, the gradual change in occupational behaviors can be understood in terms of humankind's occupational possibilities—that is, the set of occupations that exist in any given place and at any given time across the evolution of the occupational human that provide opportunities for engagement and participation. From this **macro** perspective, occupational development is considered at **the level of the species** with change occurring constantly across evolution. As with development at the level of the individual, there is no a priori determination of the number or specifics of the occupations that the species will have at any given point in time or place. It is simply anticipated there will be a continuous development of a large variety of occupations, and that the development is in keeping with the species' needs, environments, and possibilities.

Taking all three levels together, occupational development is defined as the systematic process of change in occupational behaviors across time resulting from the interaction of person, environment, and occupation at the level of the occupation, individual, and species.

An Interactional Model of Occupational Development

The Interactional Model of Occupational Development (IMOD) (29) has been proposed as a means of describing the interactional nature of the change in human occupation at the micro, meso, and macro levels. The IMOD portrays the systematic change in occupational behaviors as occurring, across time, as the outcome of the interactions of person(s), occupations, and environments. The IMOD is based on the premise that interactionism is a key mechanism for occupational development at all three levels. The three variables of interactional occupational development are (1) occupational behavior, (2) time, and (3) interaction (see Figure 6-1■). Occupational behavior is depicted as three circles, composed of two intersecting circles representing person(s) and occupation, respectively, inside a larger third circle, representing the environmental context. Change is depicted by the expanding arc, in which the principles of interactionism appear as a backdrop. The circles representing occupational behavior are shown at two points in time; the one on the right is larger than the one on the left to indicate change over time. The measure or metric for time in the figure is dependent on the level of occupational development discussed: For micro level it is the time required to develop competence in one occupation, for the meso level it is the life span, and for the macro level it is the human evolutionary span.

Occupational Competence Development: Micro—at the Level of the Occupation

The most frequently discussed level of occupational development in the literature is at the level of the occupation (i.e., development of competence in a single

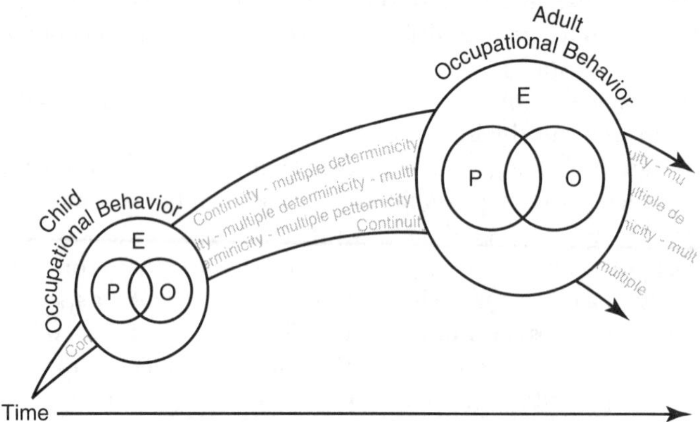

FIGURE 6-1 Interactional Model of Occupational Development (IMOD)

occupation) or in the component skills that subtend occupational competence (e.g., mature grasp or social skills). The key focus of micro occupational development is on how domain-specific development establishes the capacity for occupational performance. Much of the literature that addresses development and aging describes the occupations that can be expected, whether due to maturational expectations or societal expectations, at various ages and stages and the skills required for their performance. Frequently the behaviors noted for each age and stage are occupational in nature. The infant explores objects in many different ways: mouthing, banging, dropping, and throwing. The toddler develops independence in self-care tasks such as self-feeding and hand washing. The young child begins school, and the youth attends university or begins employment. The older adult is often viewed as engaging in less work occupations and increased leisure occupations due to retirement.

There have been some attempts to theorize about the development of occupational competence in children. Case-Smith (30) created a Model of the Development of Child Occupations, which she conceptualized as the interaction among individual abilities, occupations, and environments. She used this model as an outline to discuss the qualitative changes in the play occupations of children during infancy and early and middle childhood. She discussed the child's development in the cognitive, psychosocial, and sensorimotor domains and how these interact with the play environment.

Humphry (31) drew on dynamic systems theory to create a Model of Developmental Processes, which explicates the interaction of person and environment in developing occupational competence. She identified four fundamental aspects of occupational development: (1) intentional actions, (2) mechanisms for generating occupational behaviors, (3) sociocultural niche—children are more inclined to imitate culturally relevant occupations, and (4) engagement in occupation as a condition for developmental changes. Although modeling and imitation are considered to be large contributors to occupational development, Humphry invites attention to the role of intention or purpose as a key to occupational development. She implies that without knowledge of the intention, or a representation of what the occupation should look like, development of competence would be difficult, at best. For example, when an adult man decides to learn how to ice skate, he does so knowing what ice skating looks like and has an idea of the intention of the occupation. Without that knowledge, he would have a difficult time knowing how to begin.

Similar to Humphry (31), Edwards and Christiansen (32) discussed occupation as both a product of development and a facilitator of the process of development, offering a belief that occupation shapes and is shaped by development. They viewed growth, maturation, and learning as three key factors in development and occupation and the domains of development as acting in a reciprocal, interactive manner to facilitate further changes in the individual across the life span. Edwards and Christiansen provided a broad-based discussion of occupational development in which they highlighted domains of development and key theorists—Freud, Piaget, Kohlberg, Havighurst, Erikson, Levinson, Watson, Bandura, and Baltes—whose work, they believe, can inform understanding of changes in occupational behavior. Unfortunately, most of these theorists overemphasize the association between intrinsic changes in the individual and the development of new behaviors; therefore, they are limited in their ability to explain fully the complexities of occupational development, as they neglect the influence of the environmental context or sociocultural niche (31).

Occupational Life Course Development: Meso—at the Level of the Individual

In 1784, K. L. Reinhold wrote,

> The disposition to everything that man can become in the world is the direct work of nature. What man has actually become is the result of all the situations from his cradle onward, through which he had to pass. (33, p. 70)

The authors of this chapter believe, as Reinhold did, that occupational performance (5, 34) and occupational competence (6, 7) result from the dynamic interaction of the individual, the occupation, and the environment. Further, the interaction is viewed as bidirectional, meaning that not only does the person respond to change in the environment, but also that people adapt the environment to suit their needs. This perspective is similar to the interactionist perspective on development. Thus, it follows that the changes observed in type, meaning, and form of occupations across the life span are expressed as a function of the growth, maturation, and experiences of the person in "progressive, mutual accommodation, throughout the life span, between a growing human organism and the changing immediate environments in which it lives" (35, p. 514). These expressions are known within the field of biology as *phenotypes,* which are the observable qualities of a person, or the way he or she appears, feels, or thinks. Kurt Lewin, as presented in Conger & Galambos, (36) believed that past experiences played an important part in one's development across the life span. By adapting a widely known formula derived from Lewin's field theory, which is expressed as $B = f(PE)$, meaning behavior (B) is a function of the person (P) and his or her environment (E), we can characterize occupational development from an interactionist perspective as $OD = f(PoE)$, where O signifies an active process that directs time and attention toward an occupation. It should be noted that occupation is not simply the result of an interaction between a person and his or her environment. Rather, occupations result from an intentional and particular behavior by a particular person in interaction with particular aspects of the environment.

Principles of Occupational Life Course Development

At the level of the individual, the studies into the nature and course of developmental change provide us with a number of principles that can be used to understand meso occupational development. Although the principles of development are described differently for childhood/adolescence[1] and adulthood/aging,[2] they have a number of similarities that allow for them to be brought together as three overarching principles of occupational development across the life course. These principles are *continuity, multiple determinicity*, and *multiple patternicity*, and they provide a model of occupational life course development, as shown in Table 6-1 ■.

Continuity Development is a continuous, lifelong process, occurring across different life stages (18), starting at conception and continuing until death, with no specific age or stage seen as dominant. From personal experience, it is clear that occupations do not occur at only one age or stage. Occupations emerge at various points across the life course with different occupations developing at different rates and involving

TABLE 6-1 *Principles of Human Development*

Child/Adolescent Development	Adult Development and Aging	Occupational Life Course Development
Active child	Continuity	Continuity
Behavioral reorganization	History and context	Multiple determinicity
Continuity/discontinuity	Mastery	*Person determinants*
Expanding environments	Multidirectionality	Heredity
Interaction of heredity and environment	Multiple causality	Learning/plasticity
	Plasticity	Active participation
Learning/plasticity	Trajectories and transitions	*Occupation determinants*
Motivation		*Environment determinants*
Intention		Physical and social
		Historical and cultural
		Interaction Determinants
		Multiple patternicity
		Multiple variation
		Changing mastery

different skills (Figure 6-2 ■). Often an individual's occupational repertoire will contain similar occupations across many stages of life; however, the occupations also change throughout life. Many of these changes occur in concert with changes in growth, maturation, and aging. Individual life pathways are comprised of periods of both growth and decline, or occupational transitions, across the life course. Thus, occupational development is a lifelong process involving the "expansion, culmination and contraction in activities and accomplishments" across the life span (37, p. 11).

Continuity theory (38), taken from the literature on adult development, holds that, as they age, adults adapt to changes in their life situations. Atchley (38) found that many older adults maintain consistent activity engagement, or occupational engagement, far into older adulthood: "The key is to conceptualize continuity as the persistence of general patterns rather than as sameness in the details contained within those patterns" (38, p. 2). Changes in physical, psychosocial, and cognitive readiness and interest lead to occupational changes. Thus, changes in occupations across the life span can mirror developmental changes.

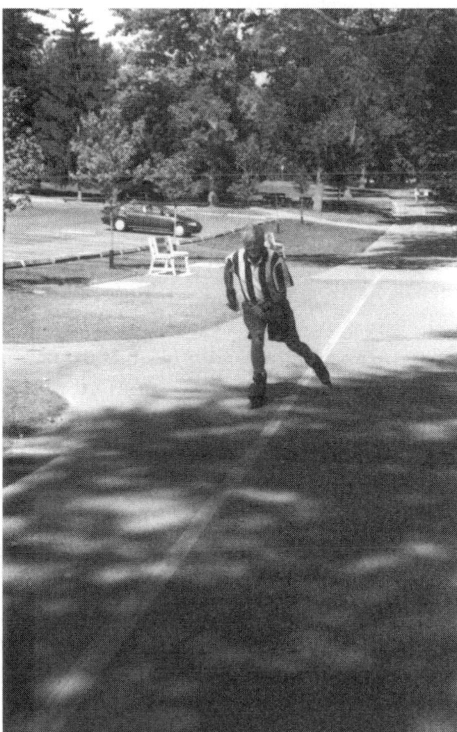

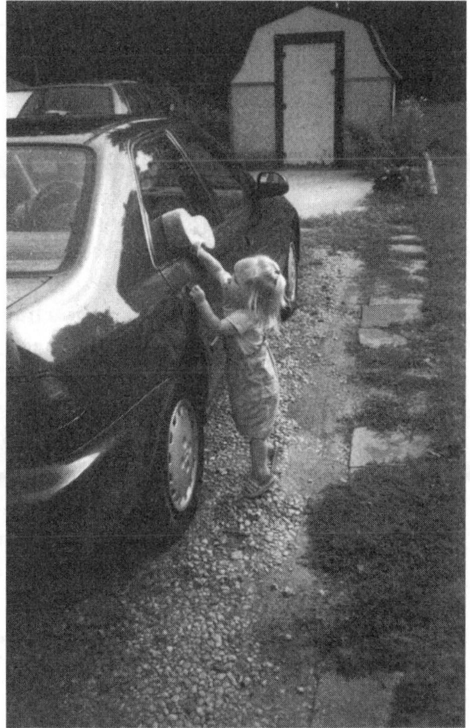

FIGURE 6-2 New occupations can occur at any age.

Multiple Determinicity The interactionist perspective holds that no single factor (e.g., heredity or environment) determines development. Proponents of this perspective argue that all factors are relevant to occupational development and that occupational development is governed by multiple determinants. This is referred to here as the principle of **multiple determinicity**.

The multiple factors that are the determinants of occupational development have some relation to those of human development (see Table 6-1); however, they also relate to occupational performance and competence. The multiple determinants of occupational development are organized under the headings of person, occupation, environment, and interaction.

Person Determinants The three person determinants of occupational development are (1) heredity/genes, (2) learning/plasticity, and (3) active participation/motivation.

Heredity/genes: It was once held that individuals were born to their occupations; hence, a son was expected to "follow in his father's footsteps." In some cultures, last names indicated the work of the family (e.g., Smith for a metalworker, and Cooper for a barrel maker), as though type of work was a result of genetic predisposition. It is still argued that Mozarts are born, not made. This would suggest widespread belief in the concept that occupational development is governed by the genetic makeup of the individual.

The belief in a heredity predisposition to occupations is now creeping into the career counseling field as witnessed by the popularity of such books as *Do What You Are* (39). In addition, supportive evidence for this perspective has emerged from studies of identical twins. Wright (40) discussed the well-publicized findings of twins James Springer and James Lewis, who were reared apart and reunited at age 39. The twins were found to have many similarities in personality and in occupations: "Both Lewis and Springer enjoyed carpentry and mechanical drawing. Both had worked part time in law enforcement" (40, p. 44). However, this is clearly not true for all twins. There are numerous examples of identical twins, even those reared together, who do not engage in the same occupations, or in the same way (41). As Plomin and colleagues (22) have pointed out, it is now recognized that genes do not "program the unfolding of development" (p. 15), but rather that development is governed by the interaction of genes and environment. Thus, genes influence development but do not control it. Scarr and McCartney (42) suggest that heredity influences the individual's development in two ways, through its expression as phenotypes, and through its influence on the choices of environment an individual makes.

Scientists have recently mapped the human genome and have begun to determine the role of over 30,000 genes in the unfolding of human life (43). For example, research on Williams syndrome, a rare genetic condition, demonstrates the variable influence that genes can have on occupational development. Although individuals with Williams syndrome cannot tie their shoes, write their name, or perform simple addition, they are avid readers and have extraordinary musical abilities. These individuals demonstrate a great love of music, a wider range of emotional responses to music than typically observed, a higher incidence of perfect pitch, and strong musical rhythm (44, 45, 46).

Child prodigies also demonstrate exceptionally mature abilities in the performance of specific occupations at a young age (typically before the age of 10). Both innate mental and physical capacities and temperament and personality factors, such as persistence, passion, and commitment, influence their occupational development (47). Often seen as precocious, child prodigies are found most commonly to have superior abilities in music (such as playing the violin and piano and singing), chess, and visual arts (47).

As Plomin (21) pointed out, although genes influence development, they cannot do it alone. Without the influence of learning, active participation, an enabling environment, and occupational exposure, an individual will not develop these skills.

Learning/plasticity: The genetic makeup with which an infant is born endows that infant with abilities, interests, and temperament that influence development and interactions with environments. It "defines what can be learned, when it can be learned, how likely behaviors are to occur, and what is reinforcing" (25, p. 1335). Learning governs the interaction between the person and the environment and regulates the course of development (36). It "is the process by which behavior or the potential for behavior is modified as a result of experience" (36, p. 31). Learning occurs in all aspects of life, involving occupations with social, spiritual, religious, play, work, leisure, and survival purposes. Cultural systems and societal structures are created for the transfer of information to infants and children (48) to allow for development of behaviors that "fit" with societal expectations. Because each child is born with different capacities, the development of competence in each occupation will be unique. The ease of learning signifies the fit among the child's innate and developing capacities, the child's environments, and the occupations being learned. These occupations will form the basis for his/her occupational repertoire.

The ability to learn is a function of *neural plasticity,* a neuroscientific term referring to the "ability of the central nervous system to adapt structurally or functionally in response to environmental demands" (49). The degree of change that the central nervous system can undergo is age dependent; that is, the degree of change decreases with increasing age. Learning is thought to occur more readily in early life when plasticity is greatest and, especially, the first year of life when the human brain undergoes a fast rate of growth. The human brain triples in size from the time of birth to maturity (50). The growth in brain size is paralleled in general by an increase in occupational competence.

Humans are totally dependent at birth, incapable of survival without the care of adults. This level of dependence is greater than that of other species and it lasts for a longer period. Yet, at maturity, humans are the most technologically and cognitively advanced species, having acquired a vast myriad of skills. This dramatic change in occupational competence is the result of the interaction of growth, maturation, and learning. Over the life span, as human abilities develop, humans learn to feed themselves, protect themselves from the elements, navigate their environments, explore their world, express their individuality, and be creative. Plasticity allows for this change in the phenotype of the individual, the overt expression of behavior resulting from the interaction of genotype and environment (51). Thus, learning/plasticity is an important determinant of the development of occupational competence.

Active participation/motivation: It is now generally believed that children are active participants in their own development, shaping, controlling, and directing their life course from birth. It is known that children are born, not as a *tabula rasa,* as Locke hypothesized, but with many abilities and a distinct temperament (52). The active child, with innate and unique predisposition and physical, emotional, and cognitive capacities, affects the environment in which the child interacts, thus acting as an agent in her/his own development, by selecting the pathways he/she wishes to follow (14).

Because occupation involves active doing, it follows that occupational development at all ages must demand the **active participation** of the individual. Across the life span, individuals act on their environments (23). Active participation can be affected, to varying degrees across the life span, by physical, emotional, or cognitive capacities, depending on the fit of one's capacities with the occupational and environmental demands and societal attitudes. Active participation remains essential throughout life. For example, it has been shown that in the later stages of life, engagement in occupation can help maintain health and one's capacities, by slowing down physical and cognitive decline (53), and warding off emotional difficulties.

In the absence of opportunity for active participation or human agency (e.g., in deprived environments), occupational development can become stunted or abnormal. This is tragically evident in the story of Genie (27), who was "locked away in almost total isolation for her entire childhood. At night she was placed in a kind of straitjacket and caged in a crib with wire mesh sides and a cover" (15, p. 160). Not only was Genie's confinement a form of environmental deprivation, but occupational deprivation (see Chapter 12) as well, because "she could only move her hands and feet and had virtually nothing to do every day of her life" (15, p. 178). When she was found at 13 years of age, Genie had not developed any of the typical occupations of her age group. In fact, she did not even have the typical skills of a toddler; she could not stand erect or walk and was not toilet trained. The influence of active participation is extremely apparent in the story of Genie. One aspect of active participation is the motivation of an individual to do.

An individual's motivation toward initiating a behavior, which refers to an individual's "needs, goals and desires that provoke them to action" (36, p. 35), also affects development by influencing further acquisition of additional behaviors. Without a motive or motivation to develop, stagnation could occur in certain areas of development within an individual, possibly affecting health and well-being. Active participation in an occupation is influenced by the individual's motivation toward engaging in the occupation. The stronger the motivation an individual has for an occupation, the more likely it is that the person will engage in the occupation and acquire the necessary competencies for the occupation to develop. For example, the only thing that young Wayne Gretzky ever wanted to do was to skate and play hockey. He started skating at age 2 and by age 5 "he lived on the backyard rink, carrying the puck in and out of pylons made from Javex bleach containers, or any other plastic jug we could find, working on his skating and puck control. Sometimes you had to argue to get him to come in at night" (54, p. 56).

Motivation stems from an understanding of the intent of the occupation and having a desire to experience that intent. From early on, very young children show motivation to engage in occupations, beyond simple imitation. Although it is difficult to know what is motivating the very young child, each child appears to exert and strive for an individual occupational intention (31). Their desired intention motivates them to learn to perform an occupation by gaining an understanding of why they would want to perform it. Children often construct new ways of being successful in fulfilling their intentions, demonstrating their active participation in their occupational development.

Although it is commonly believed that children are primarily motivated to do fun things, studies have shown many other motivators for children's active occupational participation. In her analysis of historical literary works, Davis (55) found twelve motivating factors leading children to participate in occupations, including: wanting to know everything about everything, trying to outdo one another, sense of accomplishment, pleasing and assisting one another, and wanting to be a grown-up. Also Morrow (56) found that children ages 11 to 16 participated in paid work to buy consumer goods, to do something outside school, and to feel confident, independent, and more "adult." Many of these were supported by the findings of a pilot study by Wiseman, Davis, and Polatajko (57), which examined the factors that influenced why children do (or stop doing) occupations. They uncovered numerous motivating factors for the children: feels good, positive reinforcement, being good at it, curiosity, desire to teach or help others, feeling of responsibility, and competition.

Occupation Determinants Humans are distinct from other species largely because of the things they do. Historically, occupations were focused on immediate survival needs (4); however, as occupations and historical conditions evolved, the purposes of occupations expanded to encompass other human needs (e.g., creativity, socialization, relaxation, and accumulation of material goods). Occupations are constantly being transformed and new ones created, due to technological advances and cultural and societal demands, expanding humankind's occupational possibilities.

Two factors appear to influence an individual's uptake of occupational possibilities: occupational exposure and occupational expectations. As individuals develop and age, they are exposed to occupations by the people and conditions around them. Within society, occupational possibilities are always changing, thus occupational exposure can occur at any time across the life span. Individuals see what others do and this may provide them with the motivation to initiate and develop those occupations. Motivation occurs when there is a fit between an individual's abilities, his or her environment, and the occupation. In some instances, individuals appear to have an innate drive to do certain things regardless of exposure (57), a notion that is supported when reflecting on how the tens of thousands of occupational possibilities that exist today were created. However, for the most part, individuals are not likely to develop occupations unless they are exposed to them. Although individuals may be exposed to many different occupations, society's occupational expectations and the contexts required for their engagement limit their ability to participate in all of them. Occupational expectations are constructed by a society or culture and pertain to who should be engaging in what occupations at what age and which occupations are culturally and socially sanctioned. These three interrelated occupational determinants, (i.e., possibilities, exposure, and expectations), play a central role in the development of an individual's occupational repertoire.

Environment Determinants The role of the environment in development has been discussed in the child/adolescent literature under the principles of "expanding environment" and "interaction of heredity and environment," and in the adult development and aging literature under "multiple causality" and "history and context." Embedded in these principles are discussions of the physical, social, cultural, and temporal environments.

Physical and social: Humans exist in a physical and social context. Learning from experience gained through interaction with the physical and social environments occurs across the life span, but note that different aspects of learning can occur at different periods of the life span, at different rates, and to varying degrees.

From birth on, the size of the individual's world is ever increasing. When infants are born, their environment includes what they can see, hear, taste, smell, and touch. Yet, their ability to use these senses to engage in occupations is limited in infants due to their immaturity at birth. Their interactions with their environments are restricted to the immediate situations, although many broader environments affect their care. As infants become mobile, they begin to explore their space more broadly. As children grow and mature, they are able to interact to a greater extent with more physical and social environments that influence their development. In early childhood, as independence increases, children begin to move into their neighborhoods and communities close to home. Once they enter school, they spend increasingly more time away from their home environments at progressively greater distances. For the independent adult, no geographical limitations are placed on the environment in which they operate. They can even fly to the moon.

Since the discovery of Victor, the "wild boy" of Aveyron, in the 1790s (26), researchers have recognized that the physical and social environmental contexts can significantly alter development. This young boy had spent much of his childhood living in the wild, isolated from society. Victor, at the age of 12, had none of the occupational skills typical of his age group, which is similar to the state of Genie. However, unlike Genie, Victor had not been occupationally deprived and had developed a number of skills that allowed him to survive alone in the wild. He could find food, climb trees, and run at a great speed, although he did so on all fours. These occupations, not typical of childhood at the time, were developed in response to environmental demands and enabled him to survive. Elder (58, 59) found similar environmental effects in a study in which he examined children of the Great Depression. His findings suggested that economically deprived environments had greater implications for middle-class children and their parents than for working-class children (59). However, there were also many common elements in the changes of individuals' occupations across socioeconomic status. Boys developed a greater role in paid employment, and girls had an increased role in household duties and child care, while the mothers left the home to engage in paid work. Using the longitudinal data of the Terman study of talented California men, which began in 1922, Crosnoe and Elder (18) attempted to uncover whether and how one's "family environment in childhood and adolescence were related to patterns of adjustment and functioning in the later years" (p. 648). They found that the family's socioeconomic status during childhood predicted whether as adults the men in the study would be career focused decades later. Thus, it is clear that the specific occupations people develop are, at least in part, environmentally determined.

The importance of the environment for occupational development has been repeatedly corroborated by reports from orphanage studies, where young children have undergone environmental deprivation. The more recent experiences with children from orphanages have shown that the detrimental effects of environmental deprivation are reversible to some extent. However, this is dependent on the length of deprivation and the age at which it occurred (28), as well as the child's exposure to toys and attention from caregivers (60). This evidence would suggest that the environment interacts with the maturational stage of the child in determining occupational development.

Historical and cultural: The physical and social environments in which humans live are constructed by their historical and cultural contexts. Although pioneers such as Margaret Mead and Lev Vygotsky (Box 6-1) have increased awareness of the importance of society and culture on development (61–63), the extent to which history influences sociocultural development, and hence human development, has been given less consideration. Originally, Bronfenbrenner (35) identified four aspects of the human environment that influence development: *microsystem, mesosystem, exosystem,* and *macrosystem.* More recently, he added a fifth structure to his General Ecological Model, the *chronosystem,* which "encompasses change or consistency over time not only in the characteristics of the person but also of the environment in which that person lives" (64, p. 1646). This system recognizes the importance of examining the influences of environmental changes due to historical developments and their contribution to cultural shifts. Historical and cultural influences on human development are typically widespread and difficult to reverse.

Only recently has the importance of history, or the temporal context, been discussed as having a substantial effect on development (14, 18). Research is now showing how the historical period in which an individual lived, for example, the Industrial Revolution, World War I, the Great Depression, or during the invention of the personal computer, has influenced occupational development (59, 65). Although difficult to tease apart from other influences, Elder (59) suggests that children who grew up during the Great Depression were influenced substantially by this historical event with respect to their occupational outcomes. Historical events, due to their widespread nature, are believed to become a part of broad societal structures and cultural experiences, producing permanent changes in many aspects of life (18, 59). Similarly, Davis and colleagues (65) suggested that broad sweeping historical beliefs, such as those associated with the Enlightenment, and historical changes, such as technological developments, have extensive influences on the occupational development of children. Other deeply ingrained social structures, such as racism, ageism, and classism, are now commonly believed to have the potential to provide significant barriers to the occupational development of many individuals.

BOX 6-1 Lev Semenovich Vygotsky

An Interactionist's View of Cognitive Development

Lev Semenovich Vygotsky (1896–1934; Figure 6-3 ■) was a Russian educator who became a psychologist. He was raised in a provincial town in Belorussia and from 1913 to 1917 studied philosophy, history, and law in Moscow. He returned to his birthplace (Gomel) from 1917 to 1924 to teach literature and psychology at several schools and colleges. During this time he also wrote extensively about language, poetry, learning, and drama. Most of Vygotsky's work about language development in children was not translated and published in the Western world until the 1960s, decades after his death. Vygotsky gave a paper in 1924 that so impressed those attending that he was invited to join the Moscow Psychological Institute, where he continued his research and writing until his death.

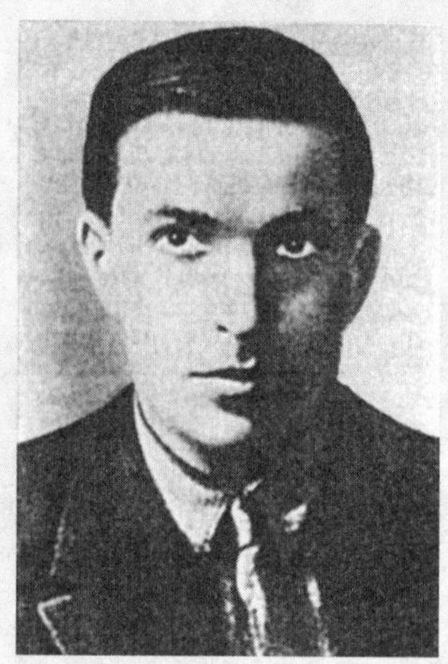

FIGURE 6-3 Lev Semenovich Vygotsky
(Felicia Martinez/PhotoEdit. Courtesy of Robert Solso.)

Vygotsky's most well-known work, *Mind in Society* (63), provided two important concepts that continue to influence our understanding of child development. Vygotsky theorized that cognitive development occurs in humans based on the use of language, which provides an internal dialogue from which the mind can interpret the surrounding world. With this view, it seemed clear to him that culture, experience, and a child's interactions with things (objects, events, and particularly people) in the immediate surroundings were instrumental to the child's understanding of the world. Indeed, social processes were at the heart of Vygotsky's understanding of mental development.

Two of his related concepts, in particular, have continued to influence those interested in human development and learning from a practical standpoint. The first is known as the *zone of proximal development*. Vygotsky (63) maintained that the learner follows the teacher's (parent, grandparent, sibling) example and gradually develops the ability to do certain tasks without help or assistance. He called the difference (or space) between what a child or learner can do with help and what he or she can do without guidance the *zone of proximal development*.

This notion led to a second concept that inspired a teaching and training approach now called *scaffolding*. Scaffolding is based on the belief that humans can acquire skills through a step-by-step process that improves their competence by providing means by which an individual can complete a task with gradually decreasing amounts of support as the individual moves toward a goal of independent performance. Vygotsky's developmental concepts seem highly appropriate for understanding occupational development because they emphasize person, environment interactions, and opportunities for mastery that take place in everyday situations.

Historical trends and circumstances shape culture and influence the individual's development of values, beliefs, preferences, lifestyles, and skills. "Cultures define what is desirable to be learned, what is to be believed, and how to behave" (25, p. 1335); in other words, cultures shape human occupation (Figure 6-4 ■). Two studies examining the influence of culture on children's occupational participation found that Mayan and Ugandan children's occupations were different from North American children's occupations (66–68). Sedgwick and colleagues (68) provide an example of the influences of cultural environments on occupational development in childhood. They found that children in Uganda performed different occupations than those children in North America, at different ages and in different ways. At very young ages, Ugandan children helped with chores around the home, including selling vegetables, sweeping, collecting water, and caring for younger siblings. Children played with toys made from old containers and tires that had been discarded. Bazyk and colleagues (66) found that Mayan culture had very different values and expectations associated with play than those of North American culture, demonstrating how culture influences the development of play occupations.

Dominant cultural beliefs about behavior and occupational participation are often depicted in policy, media, and academic texts. Since the late 1960s,

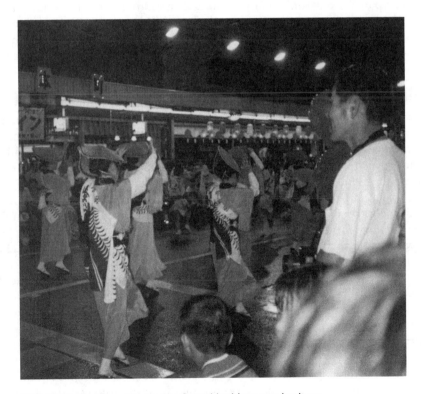

FIGURE 6-4 Occupations are shaped by history and culture.
(© by Jane A. Davis, 2002.)

the cultural representation of aging and later life in North America has shifted away from emphases on social isolation, structured dependency, and lack of roles and passivity to emphases on opportunity, self-fulfillment, self-reliance, and continued self-development. Along with policy changes, this shift has led to changes in the perceived occupational potential and ideal occupations for older adults and their associated developmental goals. Increasingly, in North American society, self-development is viewed as continuing into later life, and occupations are promoted as vehicles for the discovery and development of new skills and aspects of the self (38, 69, 70).

Interaction Determinants The interactionist perspective brings into focus the notion that the interaction between person and environment is, in itself, a determinant of development. The person and environment "interpenetrate one another in such a complex manner that any attempt to unravel them tends to destroy the natural unity of the whole and to create an artificial distinction between organism and environment" (71, p. 316). The interaction determinant is considered to be so important in the developmental process that it serves as the name for the perspective, as a whole.

The question regarding development is no longer whether the person's genetic makeup or the environment determines its unfolding; rather, it is how the interaction occurs and to what extent it plays a role in development. Evidence is being accumulated to suggest that this interaction is not simply additive (21), but operates in complex ways. Scarr and McCartney (42) hypothesized that people make their own environments based on their genetic makeup. Along with this idea, Scarr and Ricciuti (72) proposed the notion of "a good enough environment" (p. 19), which they feel is the "typical" environment available to most children in most cultures. It is proposed that the typical environments in which most children are raised contain many variables that provide the basics for "normal" human development expected within particular sociocultural and economic conditions. According to Scarr and Ricciuti, the "good enough environment" provides individuals with environments from which they can choose experiences that "match" their genetic makeup. However, similar to the belief of Gesell (19, 20) outlined previously, Scarr and Ricciuti (72) noted that this theory requires that the environment be varied and allow for opportunities that match the individual's genotype; infants and people who are limited in making their own choices about occupations cannot be expected to develop the typical capacity for making occupational choices.

Scarr and McCartney (42) suggest that if the genotype and environment do not match, the effects of either can be greatly diminished. For example, if a child has innate talent for drawing, it is unlikely to be realized unless the child is exposed to a rich and supportive artistic environment. Hence, as an adult, the engagement in a drawing-related occupation, either for work or leisure, may never be realized. This suggests the need for a goodness of fit between the individual's genotype and the environment to develop one's occupational potential. This seems especially important for children, whose occupational exposure may be under the control of the adults in their lives. The story of Maryanne (73), whose parents have a developmental delay, provides an interesting example. Maryanne was not exposed to music or singing until her aunt came to care for her when she was in her mid-teens. She found that she not only had a love of music but that her abilities were well suited to singing. In 2000, at the time of filming the story of Maryanne, she was singing in a choir with aspirations to study music therapy. Her desired occupational pursuit was to bring together her love of music with her devotion to individuals with developmental delays.

The goodness of fit concept is similar to the concept of a "just right challenge," which proposes that the environment and occupation must present the appropriate challenge to be engaging (74), to allow "flow," or a feeling of enjoyment (75). Extending this concept into the realm of development, it would seem likely that there needs to be a "just right environment" that matches the individual's genotype, to allow for, and to support each individual's optimal occupational development and occupational competence.

The active child shapes her/his environment, which enables the interaction of the child's genetic makeup with her environment, hence affecting development throughout life. The ongoing effects of experiences are determined, in part, by the individual's characteristics and other social, cultural, physical, and institutional environmental elements (Box 6-2). Controversy does remain as to whether early or late life experiences have a greater impact on development, because it is believed that the genetic unfolding of different characteristics occurs at different times throughout the life span.

Multiple Patternicity It is presumed that the patterns of occupational development mirror those of general human development. Two forms of **multiple patternicity** are suggested: one, **multiple variation,** characterizing the nature and direction of the patterns of occupational development, and the other, **mastery,** characterizing the patterns of proficiency across the life span.

Multiple Variation The principle of multiple variation is that development is neither smooth nor unidirectional, involving both decline and growth. Different aspects of development show different patterns at different times (Figure 6-5■). This is the principle of continuity/discontinuity in the child/adolescent literature. The principles of multidirectionality, trajectories, and transitions in the adult development and aging literature describe the pattern of gains and losses across the life span. These principles are combined here under the title of multiple variation to denote not only the patterns of growth, development, and decline seen in occupations across the life span, but also the variation in rate, characteristics, quality, quantity, complexity, and specialization involved in the patterns of change.

A typical life course or pathway is seen as following a trajectory, which is modified by various transitions through life (14). Trajectories are continuations of development, whereas transitions are periods of change or disruption in the trajectory. Potential occupational transitions or milestones, such as baby's first step, starting kindergarten, the first camping trip away from home, graduating from school, getting the first job, or retiring from a lifelong career, are extremely dependent on individual characteristics. Hence, each individual shows multiple variation in occupational life course development.

BOX 6-2 A Word About Gender and Occupational Development

Gender has become a predominant topic in the discussion of health, work, and occupational choice. The impact of one's gender on the occupational development of that individual can be seen throughout cultures. Levinson (76) discusses the concept of gender splitting, "the creation of a rigid division between male and female, masculine and feminine, in human life" (p. 38). He believes that gender splitting occurs in virtually every culture, although the patterning may be different. Levinson states that for years, women's lives have centered around the "domestic sphere." "It has been the key source of their identity, meaningful activity, and satisfaction, as well as dissatisfaction" (p. 39). He feels that there has been a gender revolution occurring that is reducing this gender split. Women are being "impelled, by powerful social forces as well as inner motivations, into the public, occupational world. And men are, much more slowly, becoming involved in family life and accepting the entry of women into all sectors of the occupational system" (p. 45).

Although changes have occurred over time with respect to the available occupational pathways through which both men and women can develop, an occupational division does still exist among their self-care, productivity, and leisure occupations. Sports and many business and management occupations are still male dominated, whereas caretaking professions and homemaking activities remain the main occupations of women. The interaction of the individual's gender with the demands of society is seen to affect the occupational development of each individual. As the demands of society are being altered and the dominant discourses are shifting, changes in occupational development are being seen.

The patterns of occupational development parallel the development of the components that support occupational performance and competence (e.g., elements of cognitive, affective, and physical function). For example, the development of competence in reading is influenced by an individual's cognitive and language skill development. Gymnastic prowess is enabled by physical growth and motor development; and accomplishment in team sports requires social development as well as physical and motor skills.

Muir (76) described four patterns that characterize the development of various attributes, abilities, and skills. These are *continuous,* gradually increasing with age (e.g., height, weight); *step,* increasing in a stop-and-start manner (e.g., mobility, cognition); *inverted-U shape,* first increasing, then reaching a plateau, and then decreasing (e.g., visual acuity, coordination); and *U shaped,* first decreasing, then being absent, and then increasing, (e.g., the step reflex, auditory localization function). Therefore, occupational development can be continuous, step, inverted-U, or U shaped. It is believed to occur in both continuous and discontinuous patterns.

Using in-depth interviews to examine the occupations that children do, Wiseman and colleagues (57) found that the pattern of occupational engagement varied

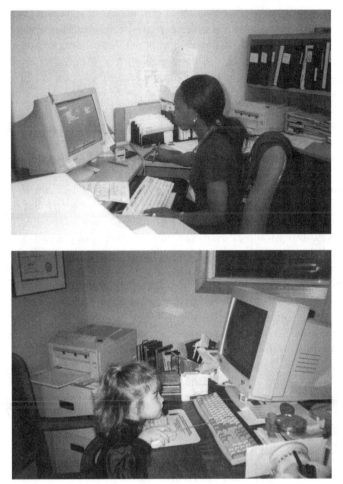

FIGURE 6-5 Multiple variation: occupational similarities at different ages and for different reasons.
(© by Jane A. Davis, 2002.)

widely among children. In some cases children as young as 6 years of age had abandoned occupations that older children were still continuing. As well, some children had continued with such occupations as drawing and painting pictures since toddlerhood. Thus, none of the patterns described by Muir completely characterize the occupational life course. Hence, the occupational life course is described as having multiple variations.

Mastery The principle of mastery is taken from the adult development and aging literature. It refers to the observation that levels of proficiency change as a result of maturation, experience, and skill.

People are thought to have a natural drive for mastery, which "requires an individual to integrate his behavior and develop skill in performing certain tasks" (78, p. 92). The concept of mastery is addressed in the child/adolescent literature under the principles of behavioral reorganization and learning/plasticity, that is, the increase in specialization, complexity and integration of behavior, and skill acquisition, respectively. The term *mastery* is preferred here because it is more congruent with the concept of interactionism, which is central to occupational development. The authors propose that mastery is not static in that it changes across the life span along a continuum from novice to mastery, hence the phrase *changing mastery*. Changing, rather than increasing, describes mastery in a manner to allow for the principle of multiple variation discussed earlier, that is, that change in occupational development is not unidirectional.

The development of mastery begins in infancy, when behaviors are very global in their intent. Crying, for example, is used by infants as a general form of communicating discomfort, hunger, tiredness, or boredom. Behaviors that have an unspecified or global intent during infancy, such as crying and reaching or grasping, become more specialized and distinct in nature as the child gains control of primitive reflexes and develops voluntary movement patterns. The skills that are typically first developed in infancy appear to be "virtually released" through interaction with the environment and are quickly and easily mastered (79). In comparison, mastery of learned skills is dependent on the development of these "prewired" skills and proceeds at a much slower rate. Increasingly, skills are performed to meet specific goals, showing greater usefulness in their intent. For example, as children develop language and other forms of communication skills, their crying becomes more specialized in its form, intention, and usefulness.

Along with the notion of specialization, behaviors also become more complex during development. The discrete features of children's behaviors increase in quantity and become more refined and skilled, demonstrating a higher-quality behavior (Box 6-3). The increased quality is due, in part, to the increased integration of the cognitive, emotional, and physical components of behavior. As children develop, these components show greater interplay. This can be seen in children's increasing sophistication in toy use; for example, banging blocks on a table top in comparison to constructing a fort out of blocks.

Each phase of development across the life span sees the emergence and disappearance of mastery of a variety of occupational skills. The term *mastery* appears in the adult development and aging literature primarily in reference to the level of competency achieved in a career. However, mastery can refer to a high level of skill or proficiency in any everyday occupation. Those occupations that require a low level of skill, such as dressing or eating, are mastered more often by more people than those occupations that are highly challenging and require a high level of skill, such as a major league baseball home run hitter. When an individual masters a skill, control and power are achieved over a task or situation. "The instinct to master one's environment has a biological foundation, which is a function of man's attempt to control or change some portion of his environment through the combined use of his intellectual and neurological processes" (78, p. 92).

At birth, babies are totally dependent on caregivers for basic necessities. Through interactions with their developing child, caregivers provide opportunities for learning and adaptation. In infancy, primitive reflexes are reorganized into simple voluntary movement patterns. Preschool children are focused on mastering the foundational skills required for occupational competency in their elementary school years. Throughout adolescence and adulthood, the number of occupations over which

BOX 6-3 Robert J. Havighurst

Changing Mastery

After obtaining a PhD in the area of physical chemistry, Havighurst shifted his career focus to the fields of aging and experimental education. In his work, Havighurst defined the principal developmental tasks of six age periods from infancy to later maturity. He felt that schooling was created to enable children to successfully achieve certain developmental tasks constructed by society, so that the children could progress to the next stage of development. Havighurst believed that nature provided individuals with the possibilities for the acquisition of occupations, which he called developmental tasks, including walking, talking, reading, and kicking a ball (80). However, he recognized that possibilities are only realized when learning is related to the developmental tasks of interest. Havighurst felt that this learning was influenced by the needs of the individual in interaction with the demands of society.

As individuals grow, they typically acquire additional physical and psychological abilities. The infant's legs grow larger and stronger, enabling crawling and walking. The child's nervous system grows more complex, enabling reasoning and the understanding of complex subjects such as arithmetic. The individual also finds herself/himself facing new demands and expectations from the surrounding society. The infant is expected to learn to talk, the child to learn to subtract and divide. (80, p. 5)

Hence, Havighurst felt there were three sources of developmental tasks: (1) physical maturation, (2) sociocultural pressure, and (3) personal values and aspirations (which Havighurst believed emerged from the interaction of organic and environmental forces). In interaction, these three sources affect, to varying degrees, the development of different developmental tasks [occupations] across the life span, such as walking and reading; the three sources also influence task [occupational] choice, that is, what type of paid work or what leisure tasks [occupations] one chooses to perform.

mastery is achieved increases as does the quality and complexity of the occupations. In late adulthood, there is no longer a general trend to the mastery of new occupations. Great individual difference is seen, with many individuals taking up new occupations, or hobbies, after retirement, whereas others reduce the number of occupations in which they engage (16), and still others maintain their old interests and skills, using them for engagement in different forms of similar past occupations (38, 81, 82) (Figure 6-6 ■).

The Ages and Stages of Occupational Life Course Development

The ages and stages of human development have been catalogued in various sources and in various ways. Among the best-known and most detailed accounts of ages and

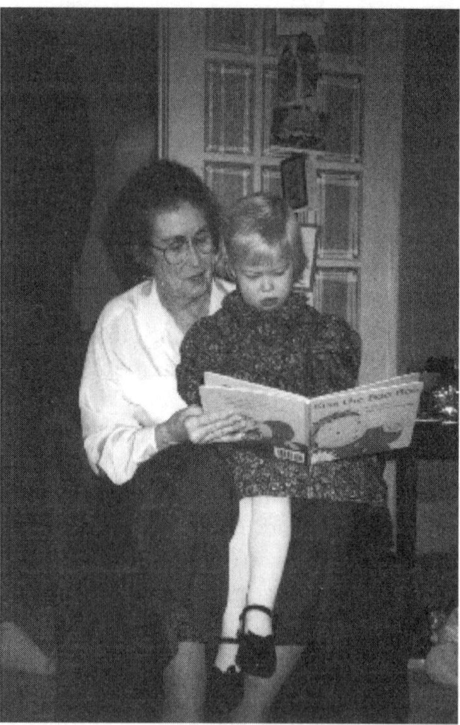

FIGURE 6-6 Grandmother and granddaughter reading: an example of an intergenerational occupation.
(© by Jane A. Davis, 2002.)

stages of development are those provided by Gesell (83). Through careful observation and detailed study, Gesell and his colleagues developed detailed behavioral norms of infant and early childhood development that are still applicable today for the sociocultural groups that he studied. Many of these descriptions focus on what children do, that is, children's occupations at various ages and stages (e.g., at 5 years old children skip using feet alternately, copy triangles, dress and undress independently, and play dress up). Thus, the temptation would be simply to adopt these as descriptions of the ages and stages of occupational development. However, this temptation must be avoided.

Descriptions of human development emanated from a focus on neuromotor development. Although it can be seen as an indicator of neuromaturational preparedness for various occupations at various ages and stages (e.g., skipping at 5 years) it must be kept in mind that occupational engagement is not solely the result of neuromaturation. Rather, occupational engagement results from the interaction of person, occupation, and environment. Thus, not all 5-year-old children, although maturationally prepared, will skip in all cultures or environments. As a person ages, maturation is less significant, and social and cultural environmental factors are more significant in influencing occupational development. Indeed, as Elder (59) has shown, socioeconomic circumstances can influence the occupational development of entire generations throughout their life course.

To date, no attempt has been made to create a Gesell-type description of occupational development. It may be that this is neither possible nor desirable; it may be that because of the interactional nature of occupational development, no clear ages and stages cross environments or contexts. This would, none-the-less, be an interesting undertaking for occupational developmentalists. Sources such as Gesell provide a suggestion of what the indicators of occupational development might be, at least in childhood (see Table 6-2 ■). This table indicates potential indicators of the ages and stages of occupational development of children in the North American context. The reader is cautioned that this profile is in need of empirical validation and is offered only as a point of departure for those interested in examining occupational development across the life span in various conditions.

Occupational Evolutionary Development: Macro—at the Level of the Species

Humans have engaged in a vast array of occupations at various points in history; some persist today, whereas many have changed. The development of these occupations across the course of human history is referred to as macro occupational development. The occupations of humans across evolution have been of considerable interest to scholars, particularly anthropologists, for some time, and countless descriptions of macro occupational development are available, albeit not under that rubric. Indeed, the study of the evolution of the human species has been tied to occupation, so much so that evolutionary eras are known by their key occupations (e.g., hunters/gatherers and agriculturalists).

Wilcock (4), a key proponent of understanding human occupation across time, drew heavily on the existing literature to create a comprehensive description of human history from an occupational perspective. Wilcock described occupational changes that occurred at each evolutionary era (see Table 6-3 ■). She proposed that human biological evolution and occupational evolution have a reciprocal relationship influenced by the environmental context. The evolution of human occupation has matched the evolution of human biological capacities, and they in turn have provided humans with the capability to create further occupational possibilities and construct the necessary tools and materials to enact those occupations.

Davis and colleagues (65) added to this literature with their study of literary works written between 1650 and 1990. They found evidence of both change and continuation. Over this 340-year period, some occupations, such as coal collecting, essentially disappeared in North America. New occupations, such as the playing of computer games, emerged, and some occupations remained throughout, such as playing with balls or dolls. Most significantly, the continuation or transformation of old occupations and the addition of new occupations over time was influenced by dominant sociocultural beliefs, values, and discourses (65). Similarly, Bing (84, see also Chapter 1, Box 1-1), describing the evolution of occupations as they relate to historical beliefs, argued that numerous variables contribute to macro-level occupational development. He stated that historical beliefs alone have not determined occupational behavior; technological advances have also altered the amount of time spent in work and leisure occupations.

TABLE 6-2 *Ages and Stages of Occupational Development*

Age	Stage	Characteristic Occupations	
(YRS.)		Self-Care	Productivity/Leisure
0–1	Infancy	■ Opens mouth when spoon with food is present ■ Removes food from spoon with mouth ■ Sucks and chews on crackers ■ Eats solid food ■ Crawls across floor on hands and knees, without stomach touching floor ■ Opens doors that require only pushing and pulling	■ Shows interest in novel objects or new people ■ Reaches for familiar person ■ Picks up small objects with hands, in any way ■ Transfers object from one hand to the other ■ Picks up small objects with thumb and fingers ■ Plays with toys or other objects alone or with others ■ Plays with very simple interaction games with others ■ Uses common household objects for play ■ Shows interest in activities of others ■ Imitates simple adult movements, such as clapping hands or waving good-bye, in response to a model
1–2		■ Drinks from cup of glass unassisted ■ Feeds self with spoon ■ Indicates wet or soiled pants or diaper by pointing, vocalizing, or pulling at diaper ■ Sucks from a straw ■ Feeds self with fork ■ Removes front-opening coat, sweater, or shirt without assistance ■ Walks as primary means of getting around ■ Climbs both in and out of bed or steady adult chair	■ Participates in at least one game or activity with others ■ Rolls ball while sitting ■ Climbs on low play equipment ■ Marks with pencil, crayon, or chalk on appropriate writing surface
2–3	Toddler	■ Feeds self with spoon without spilling ■ Urinates in toilet or potty chair ■ Bathes self with assistance ■ Defecates in toilet or potty chair	■ Imitates a relatively complex task several hours after it was performed by another ■ Engages in elaborate make-believe activities, alone or with others

		■ Asks to use toilet ■ Puts on "pull-up" garments with elastic waistbands ■ Puts possessions away when asked ■ Walks up stairs, putting both feet on each step ■ Walks downstairs, forward, putting both feet on each step ■ Runs smoothly, with changes in speed and direction ■ Opens door by turning and pulling doorknobs	■ Jumps over small objects ■ Screws and unscrews lid of jar ■ Pedals tricycle or other three-wheeled vehicle for at least 6 feet ■ Builds three-dimensional structures, with at least five blocks ■ Opens and closes scissors with one hand
3–4	Early childhood	■ Brushes teeth without assistance ■ Helps with extra chores when asked ■ Washes and dries face without assistance ■ Puts shoes on correct feet without assistance ■ Answers the telephone appropriately ■ Dresses self completely, except for tying shoes ■ Walks down stairs with alternating feet, without assistance	■ Climbs on high play equipment ■ Cuts across a piece of paper with scissors
4–5		■ Summons to the telephone the person receiving a call, or indicates that the person is not available ■ Sets the table with assistance ■ Cares for all toileting needs, without being reminded and without assistance ■ Puts clean clothes away without assistance when asked ■ Cares for nose without assistance ■ Dries self with towel without assistance ■ Fastens all fasteners	■ Completes non-inset puzzle of at least six pieces ■ Draws more than one recognizable form with pencils or crayons ■ Cuts paper along a line with scissors ■ Uses eraser without tearing paper ■ Unlocks key locks ■ Shares toys or possessions without being told to do so ■ Follows rules in simple games without being reminded ■ Follows school or facility rules
5–6		■ Assists in food preparation requiring mixing and cooking ■ Ties shoelaces into a bow without assistance ■ Bathes or showers without assistance	■ Cuts out complex items with scissors ■ Catches small ball when thrown from a distance of 10 feet, even if moving is necessary to catch it ■ Rides bicycle without training wheels, without falling ■ Follows community rules

(continued)

TABLE 6-2 *(continued)*

Age	Stage	Characteristic Occupations	
(YRS.)		Self-Care	Productivity/Leisure
6–8	Late child-hood	■ Uses fork, spoon, and knife competently ■ Initiates telephone calls to others ■ Dresses self completely, including tying shoelaces and fastening all fasteners ■ Makes own bed when asked ■ Fastens seat belt in automobile independently ■ Uses basic tools ■ Sets table without assistance when asked	■ Plays more than one board or card game requiring skill and decision making ■ Makes or buys small gifts for caregiver or family member on major holidays, on own initiative
8–10		■ Sweeps, mops, or vacuums floor carefully, without assistance, when asked ■ Orders own complete meal in restaurant ■ Dresses in anticipation of changes in weather without being reminded. ■ Tells time by 5-minute segments ■ Cares for hair without being reminded and without assistance ■ Uses stove and microwave oven for cooking ■ Uses household cleaning products appropriately and correctly	■ Returns borrowed toys, possessions, or money to peers, or returns borrowed books to library ■ Uses appropriate table manners without being told ■ Watches television or listens to radio for information about a particular area of interest
11–12		■ Correctly counts change from a purchase costing more than a dollar ■ Uses the telephone for all kinds of calls, without assistance ■ Cares for own fingernails without being reminded and without assistance ■ Prepares foods that require mixing and cooking, without assistance	■ Goes to evening school or facility events with friends, when accompanied by an adult ■ Initiates conversations on topics of particular interest to others

12–15	Adolescence and adulthood	■ Uses a pay phone ■ Straightens own room without being asked	■ Has a hobby ■ Repays money borrowed from caregiver
16–18+		■ Makes own bed and changes bedding routinely ■ Cleans room other than own regularly, without being asked ■ Sews buttons, snaps, or hooks on clothes when asked ■ Budgets for weekly expenses ■ Manages own money without assistance ■ Plans and prepares main meal of the day without assistance ■ Takes complete care of own clothes without being reminded ■ Budgets for monthly expenses ■ Sews own hems or makes other alterations without being asked and without assistance ■ Has checking account and uses it responsibly	■ Participates in nonschool sports ■ Watches television or listens to radio for practical, day-to-day information ■ Holds full-time job responsibly ■ Earns spending money on a regular basis ■ Performs routine household repairs and maintenance tasks without being asked

Source: Adapted from Sparrow, S.S., Balla, D. A. & Cicchetti, D.V. (1984) (65).

The primary source for this profile has been the Vineland Adaptive Behavior Scales, which provide descriptors of personal and social behaviors of individuals, from birth to adulthood, in four domains: communication, daily living skills, socialization, and motor skills. The items in the table were selected from the scale on the basis of their relevancy to occupation and must be treated as preliminary, requiring empirical validation.

TABLE 6-3 *The Evolution of Human Occupations*

Evolutionary Age	Human Occupations
Hunters/Gatherers	Humans hunt, gather, and scavenge for food Simple stone tools are developed to help with survival Sharing or social interaction does not occur As groups get larger food-sharing develops, and occupations are divided up among group members
Agriculture	Shift from hunting/gathering occupations to farming occupations Farmers begin to plant own food, remain in one place with larger groups of people Both women's and men's occupations change to accommodate farming Possible reasons for this shift: Climatic changes that produced physical environments conducive to agriculture Increases in population requiring different means of sustainability Development of occupational capacity or competence, which led to increased skills, development of new occupations
Industrialization Town and City Workers	Producing goods for others' consumption begins Occupations are still about survival needs; however, many individuals receive remuneration for their work and services instead of creating the food and shelter themselves Paid work is valued More social occupations emerge as groups became larger Occupational specialization occurs whereby the individual does small parts of a larger occupation, repetitively
Postindustrialization	Work becomes primarily something people do to earn money to buy food and material things Occupations change from those of production to service Technological development begins to drive occupational development instead of human nature and needs

Source: Based on information found in Wilcock (1998). Reprinted with permission from Davis & Polatajko, 2006.

Interaction of the Three Levels of Occupational Development

Similarly to Bronfenbrenner's Ecological Models of Human Development (63), the three levels of occupational development are subsumed one inside the other. Occupational competence development occurs at the level of one occupation; however, it takes the development of many different occupations across an individual's life course to form an occupational repertoire and, ultimately, to understand his or her occupational life course development, including how each occupation has shaped the others. Both the micro and meso levels of occupational development are embedded within the macro level of occupational evolutionary development. An individual's occupational life course development can only be understood within the context of broad historical understandings of occupational development or evolutionary development. Thus, all three levels hold an important place within the **Interactional Model of Occupational Development.**

CHAPTER SUMMARY

The purpose of this chapter was to present the reader with a framework for understanding human occupational development, relevant theories and research, a new Interactional Model of Occupational Development (IMOD), and a discussion of the ages and stages of occupational development across the life span. The authors have presented a framework for occupational development, taking the perspective that occupation is "everything people do to occupy themselves" (5, p. 181). This perspective was discussed from the concept of the human as an "occupational being" interacting in the environment and requiring engagement in occupation as a mechanism for development across time.

The perspective on development outlined a brief history of the views taken in the study of human development, and development was discussed in relation to the term *change* to enable a clearer understanding of the concept. The interactionist perspective on development was proposed as the perspective of choice because it is consistent with the identified perspective on occupation. This concept was used as the basis for the construction of the Interactional Model of Occupational Development (IMOD), which encompasses the levels of occupational development: the micro, the meso, and the macro.

At the micro level, ideas were presented for understanding how competence is developed within a single occupation. It was proposed that competence development occurs along a continuum from novice to mastery. At the meso level, relevant principles were incorporated from the child/adolescent development literature[1] and the adult development and aging literature[2] to provide an understanding of occupational life course development. Three principles of occupational development from an interactionist perspective were proposed: *staged continuity, multiple determinicity,* and *multiple patternicity.* These principles were described in relation to the IMOD and the formula OD = *f*(PoE). As well, a discussion about the ages and stages of occupational development was initiated, and the beginning of a potential profile of the ages and stages of early occupational development was provided. At the macro level, recent ideas, which pertained to the occupational evolutionary development of the human species, were presented. It was proposed that occupational possibilities are constantly changing due to humans' interaction with their environments and changes in the biological and cultural nature of the human species.

34. Baum, C. M., & Christiansen, C. H. (2005). Person-environment-occupation-performance: An occupation-based framework for practice. In C. H. Christiansen, C. M. Baum, & J. Bass-Haugen (Eds.), *Occupational therapy: Performance, participation, and well-being* (pp. 243–268). Thorofare, NJ: Slack.
35. Bronfenbrenner, U. (1977). Toward an experimental ecology of human development. *American Psychologist, 32,* 513–531.
36. Conger, J. J., & Galambos, N. L. (1997). *Adolescence and youth: Psychological development in a changing world* (5th ed.). Don Mills, ON: Addison-Wesley Educational Publishers.
37. Kimmel, D. C. (1990). *Adulthood and aging.* Toronto, ON: John Wiley.
38. Atchley, R. C. (1999). *Continuity and adaptation in aging: Creating positive experiences.* Baltimore: The Johns Hopkins University Press.
39. Tieger, P. D., & Barron-Tieger, B. (1995). *Do what you are: Discover the perfect career for you through the secrets of personality type* (2nd ed.). Toronto, ON: Little-Brown.
40. Wright, L. (1997). *Twins and what they tell us about who we are.* Toronto, ON: John Wiley.
41. Segal, N. L. (1999). *Entwined lives: Twins and what they tell us about human behavior.* Toronto, ON: Penguin Books.
42. Scarr, S., & McCartney, K. (1983). How people make their own environments: A theory of genotype environment effects. *Child Development, 54,* 424–435.
43. International Humane Genome Sequencing Consortium. (2001). Initial sequencing and analysis of the human genome. *Nature, 409*(6822), 860–921.
44. Don, A., Schellenberg, G., & Rourke, B. (1999). Music and language skills of children with Williams syndrome. *Child Neuropsychology, 5,* 154–170.
45. Lenhoff, H., Perales, O., & Hickok, G. (2001). Absolute pitch in Williams syndrome. *Music Perception, 18*(3), 491–503.
46. Williams Syndrome Foundation. (June 22, 2004). *Nightline transcript: Two fathers, two scientists: A father's love: When everything you do is not enough.* (Televised on Friday, October 9, 1998). Retrieved January 24, 2005, from http://williamssyndrome.org/multimedia/niteline.htm
47. Feldman, D. H., & Goldsmith, L. T. (1986). *Nature's gambit: Child prodigies and the development of human potential.* New York: Basic Books.
48. Newman, P. R., & Newman, B. M. (1997). *Childhood and adolescence.* Pacific Grove, CA: Brooks-Cole.
49. Jacobs, K. (1999). *Quick reference dictionary for occupational therapy* (2nd ed.). Thorofare, NJ: Slack.
50. Leakey, R., & Lewin, R. (1992). *Origins reconsidered: In search of what makes us human.* Toronto, ON: Doubleday.
51. Bogin, B. (1999). *Patterns of human growth* (2nd ed.). New York: Cambridge University Press.
52. Saudino, K. J., & Eaton, W. O. (1991). Infant temperament and genetics: An objective twin study of motor activity level. *Child Development, 62,* 1167–1174.
53. Schaie, K. W. (1994). The course of adult intellectual development. *American Psychologist, 48*(1), 304–313.
54. Gretzky, W., & Taylor, J. (1984). *Gretzky: From the back yard rink to the Stanley cup.* Toronto, ON: McClelland & Stewart.
55. Davis, J. A. (2000). *Historical development of children's occupations during late childhood from the 1650s to the 1990s.* Unpublished master's thesis, The University of Western Ontario, London, Ontario, Canada.
56. Morrow, V. (1994). Responsible children? Aspects of children's work and employment outside school in contemporary UK. In B. Mayall (Ed.), *Children's childhoods observed and experienced* (pp. 128–143). London: Falmer Press.

57. Wiseman, J. O., Davis, J. A., & Polatajko, H. J. (2005). Occupational development: Why children do the things they do. *Journal of Occupational Science, 12*(1), 26–35.
58. Elder, G. H., Jr. (1992). The life course. In E. F. Borgatta & M. L. Borgatta (Eds.), *The encyclopedia of sociology.* New York: Macmillan.
59. Elder, G. H., Jr. (1999). *Children of the great depression: Social change in life experience.* Chicago: University of Chicago Press. (Original work published 1974)
60. Morison, S. J., Ames, E. W., & Chisholm, K. (1995). The development of children adopted from Romanian orphanages. *Merrill-Palmer Quarterly, 41*(4), 411–430.
61. Harkness, S. (1992). Human development in psychological anthropology. In T. Schwartz, G. M. White, & C. A. Lutz (Eds.), *New directions in psychological anthropology* (pp. 102–122). Cambridge: Cambridge University Press.
62. Damon, W. (1989). Introduction: Advances in development research. In W. Damon (Ed.), *Child development today and tomorrow* (pp. 1–13). San Francisco, CA: Jossey-Bass.
63. Vygotsky, L. S. (1978). *Mind in society: The development of higher psychological process* (M. Cole, V. John-Steiner, S. Scribner, & E. Souberman, Eds.). Cambridge, MA: Harvard University Press
64. Bronfenbrenner, U. (1994). Ecological models of human development. In T. Husen & T. N. Postlethwaite (Eds.), *The international encyclopedia of education* (2nd ed., pp. 1643–1647). New York: Elsevier Science.
65. Davis, J. A., Polatajko, H. J., & Ruud, C. A. (2002). Children's occupations in context: The influence of history. *Journal of Occupational Science, 9*(2), 54–64.
66. Bazyk, S., Stalnaker, D., Llerena, M., Ekelman, B., & Bazyk, J. (2003). Play in Mayan children. *American Journal of Occupational Therapy, 57*(3), 273–283.
67. Gaskins, S. (1999). Children's daily lives in a Mayan village: A case study of culturally constructed roles and occupations. In A. Göncü (Ed.), *Children's engagement in the world: Sociocultural perspectives* (pp. 25–61). New York: Cambridge University Press.
68. Sedgwick, A, Polatajko, H. J, & Davis, J. A. (2003). *Children's occupations: A naturalistic study of Ugandan children.* Poster presented at Canadian Association of Occupational Therapists Conference, Winnipeg, Manitoba. May 26, 2003.
69. Gilleard, C., & Higgs, P. (2000). *Cultures of ageing: Self, citizen and the body.* London: Prentice Hall.
70. Laliberte-Rudman, D. (2005). Understanding political influences on occupational possibilities: An analysis of newspaper constructions of retirement. *Journal of Occupational Science, 12*(3), 149–160.
71. Hall, C. S., & Lindzey, G. (1970). *Theories of personality* (2nd ed.). New York: Wiley.
72. Scarr, S., & Ricciuti, A. (1991). What effects do parents have on their children? In L. Okagaki & R. J. Sternberg (Eds.), *Directors of development: Influences on the development of children's thinking* (pp. 3–23). Hillsdale, NJ: Erlbaum.
73. Puchniak, T. (Director). (2000). Is love enough? In A. Handel (Producer), *Witness.* Ottawa, ON: Canadian Broadcasting Corporation (CBC).
74. Yerxa, E. J., Clark, F., Frank, G., Jackson, J., Parham, D., Pierce, D., et al. (1989). An introduction to occupational science: A foundation for occupational therapy in the 21st century. *Occupational Therapy in Health Care, 6*(4), 1–17.
75. Csikszentmihalyi, M. (1975). *Beyond boredom and anxiety.* San Francisco: Jossey-Bass.
76. Levinson, D. J. (1996). *The seasons of a woman's life.* New York: Knopf.
77. Muir, D. (1999). Theories and methods in developmental psychology, In A. Slater & D. Muir (Eds.), *The Blackwell reader in developmental psychology* (pp. 3–16). Malden, MA: Blackwell Publishers.
78. Osipow, S. H. (1968). *Theories of career development.* New York: Meredith Publishing Co.
79. Bruner, J. S. (1973). Organization of early skilled action. *Child Development, 44,* 1–11.

80. Havighurst, R. J. (1972). *Developmental tasks and education* (3rd ed.). New York: David McKay.
81. Laliberte, D. (1993). *An exploration of the meaning seniors attach to activity.* Unpublished master's thesis. The University of Western Ontario, London, Ontario, Canada.
82. Laliberte-Rudman, D., Cook, J., & Polatajko, H. J. (1997). Understanding the potential of occupation: A qualitative exploration of seniors' perspectives on activity. *American Journal of Occupational Therapy, 51*(8), 640–650.
83. Gesell, A. (1928). *Infancy and human growth.* New York: Macmillan.
84. Bing, R. (2005). The evolution of occupation. In C. H. Christiansen, C. M. Baum, & J. Bass-Haugen (Eds.), *Occupational therapy: Performance, participation, and well-being* (pp. 24–40). Thorofare, NJ: Slack.
85. Sparrow, S. S., Balla, D. A., & Cicchetti, D. V. (1984). *Vineland adaptive behavior scales—interview edition—survey form manual.* Circle Pines, MN: American Guidance Service.
86. Cole, M., & Cole, S. R. (1996). *The development of children* (3rd ed.). New York: W. H. Freeman.
87. Sroufe, L. A., Cooper, R. G., & DeHart, G. B. (1992). *Child development: Its nature and course* (2nd ed.). Toronto, ON: McGraw-Hill, Inc.
88. Trawick-Smith, J. (2003). *Early childhood development: A multicultural perspective* (3rd ed.). Upper Saddle River, NJ: Prentice Hall.
89. Baltes, P. B. (1997). On the incomplete architecture of human ontogeny: Selection, optimization, and compensation as foundation of developmental theory. *American Psychologist, 52*(4), 366–380.
90. Baltes, P. B., Staudinger, U. M., & Lindenberger, U. (1999). Lifespan psychology: Theory and application to intellectual functioning. *Annual Review of Psychology, 50,* 471–507.
91. Kaufman, S. R. (1986). *The ageless self: Sources of meaning in late life.* Madison: The University of Wisconsin Press.
92. Rutter, M. (1989). Pathways from childhood to adult life. *Journal of Child Psychology and Psychiatry, 30*(1), 23–51.
93. Thomas, J. L. (1992). *Adulthood and aging.* Toronto, ON: Allyn and Bacon.
94. Wheaton, B., & Gotlib, I. H. (1997). Trajectories and turning points over the life course: Concepts and themes. In I. H. Gotlib & B. Wheaton (Eds.), *Stress and adversity over the life course* (pp. 1–25). New York: Cambridge University Press.

Endnotes

[1]Principles that govern development in childhood/adolescence commonly found in the literature are active child, interaction of heredity and environment, behavioral reorganization, continuity/discontinuity, expanding environments, learning/plasticity, and motivation (1, 36, 48, 86–88).

[2]Principles governing development in adulthood/older age commonly found in the literature are continuity, trajectories and transitions, multidirectionality, plasticity, history and context, and multiple causality (11, 12, 14, 16, 37, 38, 58, 59, 78, 89–94).

CHAPTER 7

The Occupational Nature of Social Groups

Charles H. Christiansen and Elizabeth A. Townsend

OBJECTIVES

1. Understand the occupational nature of communities and societies.
2. Describe the relationship between participation in occupation and a sense of connectedness.
3. Appreciate how participation in occupation shapes a social group, both positively and negatively.
4. Provide examples of various social occupations and their role in community building.

KEY WORDS

Adaptation
Allee effect
Altruism
Competition
Connectedness
Cooperation
Diversity
Division of labor
Ecological niche
Exaptation
Free rider problem
Game theory
Exclusion/inclusion
Interdependence
Meme
Memetics
Norms
Prisoner's dilemma
Sense of community
Sociobiology
Social capital
Society
Stigma
Sustainability
Tribe
Virtual community

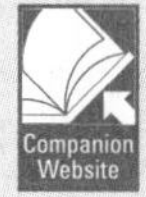

www.prenhall.com/christiansen

The Internet provides an exciting means for interacting with this textbook and for enhancing your understanding of humans' experiences with occupations and the organization of occupations in society. Use the address above to access the interactive Companion Website created specifically to accompany this book. Here you will find an array of self-study material designed to help you gain a richer understanding of the concepts presented in this chapter.

CHAPTER PROFILE

This chapter describes the occupational nature of communities and societies from the standpoint of humans as a group-living species. In doing so, it addresses the factors that contribute to group living and describes the advantages and challenges of occupational engagement in promoting the survival of humans as members of social groups. It proposes that shared or cooperative occupations are a central feature of successful social groups and discusses the role of language in the evolution of group living. Specific biological concepts influencing group living, including altruism, ecological niche, cooperation, and competition within species, are also discussed with reference to the occupational nature of communities. The chapter continues with an examination of socio-cultural environment factors that contribute to the success of social groups, including social values; cultural rituals of exclusion and inclusion; shared history; tribal connections; art, magic, and religion; volunteerism; work; social sanctions; and sustainable, occupational practices. The chapter profiles occupational characteristics of successful communities that build social as well as economic capital and occupational characteristics that fail to support success, such as the absence of trust and the lack of collective occupations for the common good (which together build social capital), as well as the presence of violence and injustices. Throughout the chapter, it is emphasized that people doing things together with a common goal and values, such as compassion, connectedness, and resilience, are central features of fully flourishing social groups.

INTRODUCTION

As a group-living species, humans have evolved occupations that not only contribute to their survival, but also have led to the formation of communities and societies. In this chapter, we consider the occupational nature of social groups by examining the answers to three questions:

1. What makes social groups inherently occupational?
2. How and why did occupations that promote group living develop?
3. How and why do occupations determine a social group's potential to flounder or flourish?

WHAT MAKES SOCIAL GROUPS INHERENTLY OCCUPATIONAL?

Human communities consist of groups of people who do things together and individually. People participate collectively through shared interests and activities (occupational pursuits) in work, sports, hobbies, volunteerism, home life, and civic involvement. Bonds that draw and keep people thinking about each other and occupied together may include shared beliefs, shared geography, shared interests, shared experiences, shared traditions, or shared kinship (1).

Although the terms *social groups, community,* and *society* are closely linked, they represent distinct but interwoven structures and characteristics. Social groups are usually identified by shared characteristics, such as age, gender, social class, or religion. It is useful to think of a community as a bond among people with strongly similar backgrounds and interests and a society as a set of systems that govern connections between those groups. Social groups, communities, and societies can be institutionalized in rules, laws, and shared conventions, but, generally speaking, societal connections are more often formal, whereas community connections tend to be more informal in nature.

Because their connections are more formal, societies can be described according to their economic, socio-cultural and political structures and complexity and include bands, tribes, chiefdoms, and state societies. Societies are also organized according to their means of subsistence, providing clear evidence of the important link between human occupation and society as a structure that formally organizes social groups. The earliest subsistence-based societal category is known as the *hunter-gatherer society,* followed by the *nomadic pastoral,* the *simple farming* or *horticulture society,* and the *intensive agricultural society,* also called *civilizations.* The *industrial* and *postindustrial* societies are new additions to this classification, marking clearly different characteristics from the agricultural societies while again linking these categories to aspects of human occupation that are key to survival. One characteristic of all societies is that they render aid or generate havoc in times of crisis depending on a society's approach to a crisis. They also confer status on their members for specific behaviors that are seen as valuable to the group, and they impose sanctions for behaviors that are considered contrary to the well-being of the group.

Michael Ignatieff, a Canadian historian and politician, describes himself as a citizen of the world. He has written about the deep bonds of "blood and belonging" as the basis for the cultural and religious conflicts that have festered for years in some parts of the world, including the drive for distinct recognition of the (French-speaking) heritage of the founding people of the province of Quebec, Canada (2). His insights emphasize the interdependence and reciprocity of kindness in everyday actions required for people to consider the "needs of strangers" as well as their own needs (3). His recent writings on the Rights Revolution highlight the importance of creating social groups, communities, and societies where bonds are based on both equality and differences. He indirectly points to shared and individual occupations (decorating ourselves, dressing) in the communities through which we

> commit ourselves to a special way of thinking about the relationship between human equality and human difference. . . . What we have in common as human beings is the very way we differentiate ourselves—as peoples, as communities, and as individuals. So it is not the naked body we share in common, but the astoundingly different ways in which we decorate, adorn, perfume, and costume our bodies in order to proclaim our identities as men, women, members of this tribe or that community. (4, p. 41)

The earliest social groups were based on kinship, not unlike the blood relationships of families. Because of their geographic proximity and close bonds, they were also communities. Societies began historically as geographically and genetically defined groups of people who shared the occupations of survival, such as hunting, gathering, and defense against enemies. Today, without restriction to geographic boundaries or genetically linked clans or tribes, there are also societies of shared interests, such as musicians around the world, or societies that form through shared experiences (see Box 7-1). These social groups may be communities or societies, depending on their formal arrangements, that have formed because of bonds related to such diverse experiences as culture, disability, family life, geography, ethnicity, old age, race, religion, rural or urban living, or sexual orientation. Clans and tribes are societies that draw on shared geographic history, heritage, and ancestry. These social groups are now geographically scattered around the world. Many people retain a sense of pride and belonging as members of clans or tribes who may engage in the shared occupations of cultural rituals and artistic expression wherever members may be.

Worldwide virtual groups are now connected in the shared occupations of e-mail correspondence, synchronous or asynchronous web group discussions, online blogs and journals, podcasting, shared videos placed on YouTube, and numerous "wikis." A wiki is a collaborative Website, such as Wikipedia, an online multilingual encyclopedia with over one million entries that has been collaboratively developed by scholars and users all over the world. More and more, the information age is creating networks of people whose shared occupations are the basis for creating virtual communities and societies. These retain many of the characteristics of social groups in physical presence, but have additional features that add value while also creating new challenges. For example, virtual groups make information sharing faster and more convenient, but they also must contend with problems related to factual accuracy, false identity,

BOX 7-1 Clans as Places of Refuge and Barriers to Connectedness

Alistair MacLeod (100), a Scottish-Canadian writer, wrote an award winning novel, *No Great Mischief* about the dilemma of clans being both a source of identity and a trap. His main character, Calum, a member of "clan Chalum Ruaidh" of the MacDonald clan, finds himself both nurtured and stuck in his clannish connectedness with Cape Breton Island in Nova Scotia. Clan and occupation are intricately tied. Calum chances losing his mining job in Ontario to drive for over 30 hours to participate in the clannish occupation that is his grandfather's wake on Cape Breton Island. Within the clan-strong communities and occupations of this island, language is used to search for connections in conversations that inevitably start with "What's your name?" "What's your father's name?" "What's your mother's father's name?" (p. 28), and family remind each other, "Always look after your own blood" in finding each other jobs (p. 204). The grandfather, who enjoyed his occupations of dancing as well as hard work, utters the essence of strong, nurturing, occupation and clan-based communities in his frequently repeated statement that ends the book, "All of us are better when we are loved" (p. 283).

accountability, and potential exploitation. Although these have always been social problems, the global environment of the digital world has made them more visible and more difficult to manage.

There are many kinds of social groups, but they have in common interaction through what they do together, whether sharing interests, beliefs, knowledge, or the completion of functional and creative goal-directed projects.

The defining features of closely knit social groups include respect, connectedness, belonging, reciprocity, mutual aid, care for others, and often an altruism to both help and protect one another (3–7). Consider that the words *community* and *society* are from Latin words with roots in the concepts of friendship and altruism. For example, the words *community* and *communicate* are from the Latin root word "commune," which means to share. Similarly, the word *society* is derived from French and Latin terms meaning companionship, or being in the company of others.

From earlier work, we might say that diverse "ways of knowing" (5) produce diverse ways of doing. In other words, the occupational nature of social groups is characterized by gender, race, and many other differences in the ways people understand, accomplish, and speak about what they do. The struggle for rights to be equal, while also respecting difference, is universal. Equality and difference are actually grounded in the ways people come to know and experience everyday life. That is to say, the occupational nature of social groups is grounded in similarities while also confronting difference. Where there are strong social groups based on shared experience, mutual interest, trust, respect, and common goals, differences may or may not be accommodated. One prevailing view emphasizes the important role of strong social groups in balancing the interests of the individual with the interests of the larger group. Progress occurs because groups adopt the innovations, or new ideas, of individuals who risk thinking about or doing things differently. In fact, tolerance and reasonable accommodations for difference are essential to group harmony and progress (6).

Indeed, Rubin (7) maintains that a community's main function is to act as a go-between—between the individual and larger society. Rubin asserted that individuals relate to their larger societies through both geographic and nongeographic substructures, or communities. Prior to the establishment of modern communication technologies, social groups were, of necessity, primarily geographic and often based on kinship, such as in extended families. But today, technology permits other kinds of groups to develop and serve the purposes of sharing traditions, values and goals. Examples are professional societies, labor unions, or sports clubs that maintain themselves through a membership organization created through shared occupational interests. These groups may meet face-to-face periodically and communicate regularly through non-face-to-face means with their members to establish ethical standards, enable professional communication, and represent the interests of members to the state or internationally.

Rubin developed his beliefs of community from the writings of French sociologist Emile Durkheim (8), who believed that if the state were the only organized structure available to people, the individual would become detached and the larger society would disintegrate. Durkheim wrote: "A nation can be maintained only if, between the State and the individual, there is [introduced] a whole series of secondary groups near enough to the individuals to attract them strongly in their *sphere of action* [emphasis added] and drag them, in this way, into the general torrent of social life (8, p. 28). Furthermore, people need communities to "serve as buffers between the individual and the larger society" (p. 60).

From Durkheim's work, Rubin (7) identified five structural characteristics for a community to mediate between an individual and society. Each characteristic (size, focus, stability, social structure, and participation) makes it possible to experience shared occupations (see Table 7-1 ■).

The implication here is that positive experiences of shared occupation are founded on discovering the just-right-size group, whether it is the result of geographic proximity, kinship, or a common interest. Rubin advocated that a central focus will generate a sense of connectedness through what people are doing. He highlighted the interconnectedness of communities, or the glue that keeps them together, as that sense of shared focus, purpose, mission, or project. One might suppose that groups that fish together, that dance or generate art together, that protect the environment together, or that worship together all share a focus that makes belonging to that group worthwhile. As Rubin noted, communities succeed when there is relative stability. He cited the characteristics of having a shared history (stability over time) or a core nucleus of members (stability of persons) as strength-building features of communities.

The stability of community engagement might also be important in building community strength. Stable community engagement refers to the ability of a group to maintain its focus on particular projects or actions over time, with sufficient attention to completion so that members experience the shared satisfaction of creative expression, work, or play that is done well. Rubin's characteristics of communities also include the need for both structure and participation. In other words, a framework of habits, customs, policies, or regulations makes it possible for people to participate together with congeniality as they go about their shared occupations.

Interdependence is a fundamental experience in shared occupations, such as the traditional "barn raising" that brought families and communities together in a

TABLE 7-1 *Rubin's Structural Characteristics of Communities (7)*

Characteristic	Features
Size	Size should be intermediate—small enough to provide a sense of community and large enough to enable members to feel they are part of a larger social structure.
Focus	Should address some of the important central problems of social life to help members feel connected to the larger society.
Relative stability	Should have a history and core nucleus of members.
Concrete social structure	People should be able to interact and identify with each other.
Participative and congenial social interactions	Interactions should be primary and secondary and allow for social structure.

common occupation (see Figure 7-1 ■). Condeluci describes interdependence as the expression and satisfaction of being and doing with others (9). Alternately, mutual dependence, sometimes referred to as codependence, may negatively draw people into collusion in harmful occupations. Examples are groups who are negatively occupied interdependently, with a mutual dependence that is fraught with violence or codependent families caught in alcohol, drugs, gambling, or other addictions. Positive interdependence, however, can generate mutual aid and reciprocal giving. As Brown noted, interdependence is founded on mutual respect, acknowledgment, accommodation, and cooperation that both connect people and provide them with the independence to develop their communities (10). Interdependence engenders a spirit of social inclusion, mutual aid, moral commitment, and responsibility to recognize and support difference. A common example is the sense of belonging and connectedness generated when groups grow, prepare, and eat food together. Religious groups have long recognized the power of breaking bread or breaking a fast with others when there is a sense of purpose and focus. Health and social programs have a long history of involving people in shared occupations to sustain collective farms, or community mental health programs (11–13). Intentional communities may support "independent living" by people with a disability, or activism against poverty, drugs, or crime (14, 15). Schools may seek to create a culture of inclusion so that students with diverse intellectual or physical abilities can all benefit from educational programs.

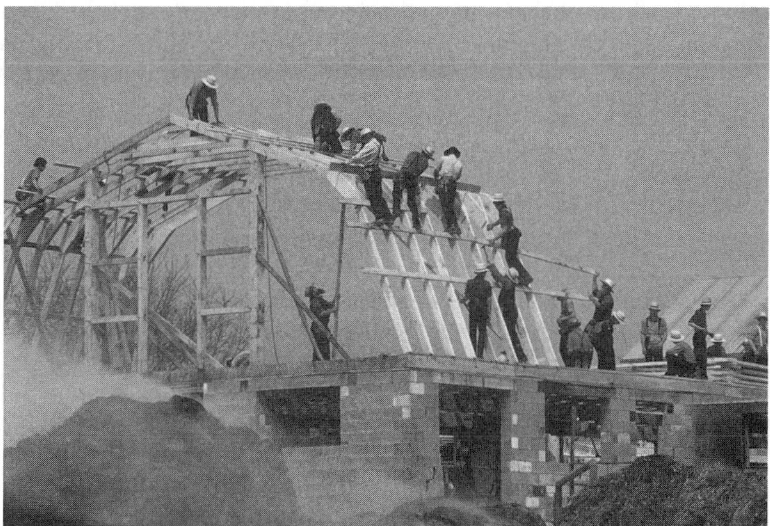

FIGURE 7-1 The concepts of community cooperation and interdependence are clearly exemplified in collective efforts to build a physical structure—either for the community-at-large or for individuals. In this photo, the practice of "barn raising" is shown. In rural areas, it is not uncommon for neighbors to collectively assist with harvesting or building barns, especially when a family or individual is facing misfortune, such as a fire, accident, or health crisis.
(© by Dennis L. Hughes, 6/20/2002. Courtesy of Dennis L. Hughes.)

To participate means to take part, or to share in the doing of something. History-making and documentation are occupations that seem necessary for the continuity of groups, whether communities or societies. Those who participate in recording or documenting historical events or who write stories about their shared experiences create public tools for generating connectedness and a sense of belonging. The making of written histories, group photographs, visual documentaries, films, plaques, cemetery tombstones, logos, plaid tartans, uniforms, or ceremonial clothing are history-generating, shared occupations. These are occupations that often spark a sense of recognition and reconnection within social groups. Such occupations express group values, customs, rules, sanctions, and a shared identity. When we visit a cemetery, we are instantly reminded of the times when we participated together in occupations such as building a house, celebrating an anniversary, or playing games. When we read stories about the development of a shared project, the rebuilding of a town after a fire or flood, or the genealogy of a clan, we remember doing something in particular times and places and with particular people. Historical as well as organizational documentation is fundamental, not only for sentimental reasons, but also in the organization of groups who are able to work together to attain desired aims for collective benefit (16).

Individual identity is irrevocably connected with the occupational nature of social groups. Ironically, the Internet and communication technologies have enabled occupations that create virtual communities at the same time that people around the world are experiencing an erosion of connectedness and moral responsibility in their daily occupations. Many have noted this, such as American sociologist Amatai Etzioni, who has advocated what he refers to as communitarian practices. Like other communitarian advocates, Etzioni proposed that we should more carefully balance individual rights with a community member's responsibilities to the greater good (17). Social groups develop a sense of commitment and emotional support in times of need as members generate shared beliefs, traditions, and goals through shared occupations. Feeling safe and supported by a group engenders feelings of loyalty and attachment. McMillan (18) described four ways in which members generate a psychological "sense of community": Create a sense of belonging, fulfill member needs, provide influence, and offer shared connections.

The occupations that foster individual identity also give rise to shared identity (19). Social groups can support or limit individual development of identity or selfhood. Neither is separate from the other as identity emerges in two fundamental directions, each creating tension with the other (20–22). The first direction is to satisfy individual and shared needs for power, autonomy, status, and excitement. The second is to satisfy individual and shared needs for love, intimacy, acceptance, respect, belonging, connectedness, and interdependence. In his classic work, Bakan (23) described these two directions as agency and communion. Agency refers to mastery, self-assertion, and the capacity of individuals to reason and exert power through thought, language, and action. Communion refers to joining with others to become part of a larger whole. Dan McAdams, a psychologist who studies life stories, has noted that the themes reflected in life stories tend to belong to one of agency (accomplishing significant tasks) or communion (developing strong relationships with others) (24).

Considered together, agency and communion are both necessary to and are the results of participation in shared occupations. Shared occupations are a platform for individual experiences of power, autonomy, status, and excitement, as well as for the development of communal experiences of love, intimacy, respect, belonging, and connectedness. Individual identity and group identity are intertwined. As Page and Czuba highlighted, "the individual and community are fundamentally connected" in a multidimensional journey in which people learn either to dominate and disempower others, or to share power in the empowerment of everyone (25, p. 3).

The collective efficacy of a community appears to generate cohesion among neighborhood residents combined with shared expectations for informal social control of public space. Collective efficacy is a concept that combines the efficient use of resources to achieve what a group defines as important. Collective efficacy builds on the beliefs people have about themselves and the actions they take to address those beliefs. Included in this concept are information and knowledge, skills to do what people need and want done, and the ability to learn and apply new information and skills to develop their communities. Consistent with the experiences of shared occupations already noted, collective efficacy emerges in supportive conditions that foster mutual respect, commitment, informational integration, mediation, compromise, and social cooperation (26, 27). Conditions that do not foster these qualities result in scenarios that have led to the Broken Window Hypothesis that is presented in Box 7-2.

BOX 7-2 The Broken Window Hypothesis

One theory of violence and crime in cities is called the Broken Window Hypothesis (101). This theory suggests that when conditions called "structural disorder" occur in neighborhoods, there is a rise in crime (Figure 7-2 ■). Structural disorder results when neighborhoods are not maintained. Participation declines, and people become less trusting (102). Fear may increase because crime is perceived as more common on the streets. Structural disorder in neighborhoods is said to be caused by poverty and mixed land use—an example being where residential dwellings are combined with businesses and/or places of manufacturing. Structural disorder in one neighborhood prompts residents to migrate to other neighborhoods. The community that is abandoned experiences lower investment, economic decline, and higher rates of robbery as the most prevalent crime. It is important to note that structural disorder does not directly promote crime, although the two are related. Both structural disorder and crime are closely associated with poverty.

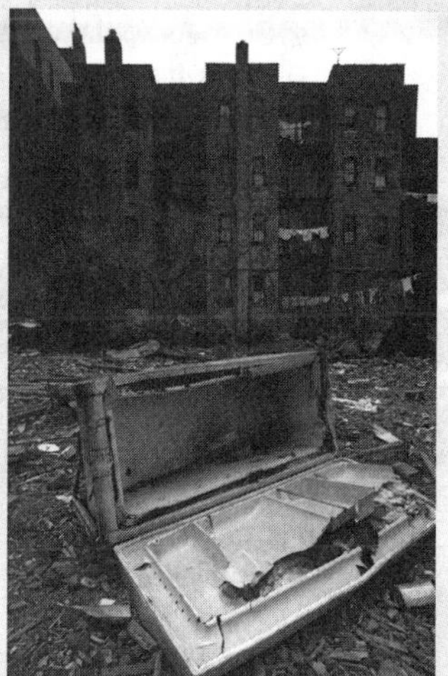

FIGURE 7-2 The broken window hypothesis suggests that when structural disorder occurs in a neighborhood, a rise in crime results.
(S. Meltzer, Photolink/Getty Images.)

HOW AND WHY DID OCCUPATIONS THAT PROMOTE GROUP LIVING DEVELOP?

Humans came to live in groups specifically because we are social and occupational beings who are genetically predisposed to exist and act together (28–30). Mutuality and reciprocity appear to be an evolutionary necessity for humans (31). Although the biological basis for humans living in groups is a complex topic, the field of neuroscience has provided some useful theories regarding why and how group living occurred. A key event in group living was the incredible increase in human brain size over thousands of years. Brain size has been closely related to the development of language.

Language to Communicate Ideas about Occupations

One theory proposes that language evolved as a functional necessity for group living. Interestingly, this theory directly relates language development to group occupations. It seems that language development correlates with the greater amount of time humans spend in social grooming. From observation of primates, it seems that social grooming, a basic occupation of self-care and care of others, enables social relationships to be established. Social grooming requires individuals to be in close, physical proximity to each other for purposes other than procreation. Social and physical proximity enable the development of social relationships, initially for mutual support. Mutual support is necessary to protect one's standing in the larger social group. As social groups develop, social grooming extends to other shared occupations such as food gathering and play within groups and posturing or fighting with other social groups. In other words, the interaction of shared occupations requires language, and language fosters more shared occupation.

A more widely accepted theory suggests that language was a consequence of group hunting or protection, which required that individuals be able to direct others to the location of threats or prey. Pinker and Bloom (32) suggested that language evolved in humans for two reasons. First, early humans cooperated in their endeavors, especially those related to protection and support. Second, they had a need to share knowledge about the local environment and their ways of doing things with their family and group members to sustain the group over time. As humans evolved beyond hunting and gathering to the development of agricultural communities, there was great benefit to dividing labor. For example, cooperation in the division of labor enabled such innovations as the construction of irrigation systems. Communities gain stability and a sense of belonging over time by transmitting customs, rules, and beliefs from one generation to the next. This requires the use of language, which evolved to a point during the history of humankind where written symbols could be used to provide an enduring record.

Compared to other animal species, *homo sapiens* are not large, fast, or strong. Humans, however, have used intellectual capacities to compete with other species and the forces of nature. A key part of this intelligence and survival has been the development and use of language. Social groups are possible because of the ability to communicate, and civilizations have evolved as ideas are transmitted through oral, written, or other expressions of language from one group to another and from one generation to the next.

Ideas, like genes, replicate over time through successive generations. However, ideas also replicate immediately through communication between people. A "meme" refers to an idea, belief, or other bit of information that gets replicated through transmission to others immediately or over time (33). Memetics is the science that studies the process and impact of idea generation and adoption (34). As with the science of genetics, the science of memetics has recognized that memes have benefited from the contrasting forces of cooperation and competition (35). Moreover, idea generation is closely linked to human occupations because ideas typically refer to beliefs and knowledge that emerge from everyday experience and influence ways of living (see Box 7-3). The digital revolution is an interesting case in point. The idea that information can be harnessed electronically has enabled humans to create new industries that drastically change the manner in which people transmit or gain information (such as through the Internet and its extensions of podcasting and vodcasting and smart phones), pursue leisure (such as through electronic gaming) and perform other daily occupations from shopping to writing letters or balancing bank statements and building cars.

BOX 7-3 Memes: The Genes of Language

A central feature of group living is the development and spread of innovations or new ideas. Computer technologies have produced the Internet and created instant communication that assists in diffusing or spreading new ideas. This is an important development for human language and human occupation because the sending and receiving of novel ideas sparks occupations that prompt community growth. During the 1970s, the concept of "memes" emerged to describe the evolution of cultural ideas. Memes and memetics, the study of memes, were first described by Richard Dawkins in *The Selfish Gene* (33). The term refers to ideas that are imitated, extended or otherwise spread through human cultures and across generations. Dawkins argued that human beings are different from other social animals in that they can replicate in ways other than through genes. Because of the ability to think symbolically, humans are able to communicate ideas through stories, music, and concepts. Like genes, memes evolve, are replicated, and are refined over time as they are passed along through generations of communication.

The concept of memes, as an important aspect of human evolution, has gained significant scientific support. Memes appear to be particularly important in the emergence of occupations that express culture through creative thought. Heylighen (35) points out that memes are countergenetic. That is, they serve to propagate themselves under conditions that are directly contrary to genetic means of replication. He uses the contrasting examples of celibate priests and suicide bombers as illustrations of this paradox. In both cases, there is no genetic transmission of the species. However, in each case, the goal of replicating or spreading powerful ideas is accomplished.

The development of language also resulted in something more important than the ability to communicate. It enabled the problem-solving ability and creativity associated with intelligence (36, p. 70). As William Calvin observed, the superior intellect accompanying a larger brain not only enables humans to develop language and symbolic thought, but it also enables the capacity for music, poetry, and humor (36). Early humans were sufficiently advanced that they were able to make and use tools, throw spears, and communicate in a primitive fashion. At some point during the human evolutionary process, for reasons that remain unclear, the human brain increased in volume as well as in problem-solving and creative ability.

Ian Tattersall suggested that the Cro-Magnon humans, who inhabited Northern Europe 40,000 years ago, were significantly more advanced in the complexity of language, occupations, and social relationships than the Neanderthals (37). Tattersall proposed that their inferior tools and poorer problem-solving ability made the Neanderthal highly vulnerable to environmental change. In contrast, the Cro-Magnons, with their larger brains, were able to begin shaping their world rather than becoming victimized by it. Apparently Neanderthal burial sites are devoid of symbolic objects, whereas Cro-Magnon graves provide evidence of a deeply spiritual way of life (37). The ability to think, to communicate, to solve problems, to share experiences and emotions, and importantly, to anticipate the future has enabled humans to develop increasingly complex social groups with increasingly complex variations in everyday occupations. Thus, language has played a key role in fostering the shared occupations that are fundamental to group living in communities.

Biological Forces Prompting Group Living in Communities

Sociobiology has been the traditional field generating much of the theory and research on biological evolution as a basis of group living, although many disciplines are now joining this quest. It appears that humans have taken advantage of several evolutionary strategies to survive and flourish. These include adapting to an ecological niche and finding ways to cooperate in groups to achieve survival advantage. A central process in species evolution is genetic trial and error, which enables a species to adapt to the requirements of a given environment. At the cellular level, trials take the form of successive stages of replication, which can produce advancement quickly because cells divide and multiply rapidly. Cellular changes, or adaptations that succeed are retained. Those replications that fail fade into extinction. Surviving cells then replicate, only to be replaced by cells with characteristics more suited to survival. For this reason, genes are said to be selfish based on their insistence that only cells with strong survival traits continue. Accumulated changes occurring over generations usually result in greater chances of survival according to the environmental conditions in which the cell must exist and reproduce. It is important to note that evolutionary changes occur at three main levels: in cells, in organs, and in the characteristics of multicellular organisms such as humans and other animals, who may be organized into social units, such as communities.

Three concepts that are fundamental to an understanding of the past, present, and future evolution of social animals (and, thus, of communities) are *ecological niche, competition,* and *cooperation. Ecological niche* refers to the environments or environmental conditions to which a particular species can successfully adapt. As noted earlier with cells, species evolve with genetic characteristics that give them the best chance for long-term survival. For humans, it appears that the development of group living in occupational communities has been key to human evolution and survival. *Competition,* in biological terms, refers to the rivalry or struggle between or within species to secure the resources necessary for survival. Humans' symbiotic development of language and survival occupations appears to have been critical in the competition for food and shelter resources with other species and other humans. *Cooperation,* also known technically as the group or *Allee effect,* occurs when members of a species work as a group to ensure reproduction and survival of the species (38). Cooperation is rare in animals because it runs counter to the genetic tendency to be selfish, that is, for genes to compete for evolutionary survival at all cost. Thus, there is little cooperative behavior in most species of insects, fish, lizards, birds, or mammals except occasional demonstrations of cooperation among family groups, parents and offspring. Where cooperation does exist, it never reaches the level of complexity in daily occupations achieved by human societies.

Biological Cooperation and Altruism as Foundations for Shared Occupations

Both language and biological traits of problem solving and creativity have made it possible for humans to develop cooperation and altruism in shared occupations. According to Trivers, the willingness of an organism to cooperate with another for survival requires altruism (39). These two biological traits are actually the building blocks for shared occupations discussed earlier under the question, *What makes social groups inherently occupational?* In biology, altruism means the active donation of resources to one or more individuals at cost to the donor. This definition is strictly resource-based and has no moral connotation. It goes beyond the sharing that occurs among parents and offspring (known as kin selection) to a reciprocal sharing of resources among members of a group who are not related. Beyond humans and other primates, examples of reciprocal altruism have been found only in a few species of animals such as vampire bats, dolphins, elephants, and in some species of monkeys and apes.

Certain conditions must exist for altruistic cooperation to succeed biologically. The biological tendency to compete for advantage and survival results in attempts by some group members to take advantage of the efforts of the group. This is known as the "free rider problem." Biological cooperation succeeds in nature only when there are biological penalties (being eaten or poisoned) or social sanctions against those who cheat or take advantage of the circumstances by not doing their share. The expression "gaming the system" means cheating, or taking advantage of a group's lack of effective safeguards against cheaters. Nonhuman species, such as elephants or wolves, exert social sanctions by ostracizing members who bully the group or by attacking and killing those who interfere with mating or parenting of the young.

Because every group will have rule breakers, effective cooperation requires precautions, often in the form of systems for the detection of cheating and exploitation, and mechanisms to confirm group identification. Debates about the need to enforce immigration laws, which occur in many countries, are examples of how the concepts of trust, social consent, group identification, and systems to prevent cheating and exploitation reveal themselves in public discourse. Systems of social consent or trust develop as a result of long-term group living, where members are able to recognize each other as individuals, recall the history of cooperation by each member, and keep track of help given and help received.

Reciprocal altruism can occur in the absence of close genetic relationships, but only if those who receive aid do so with the understanding that they will reciprocate (39). Moore took the idea of reciprocity to the practical level of everyday occupations in an analysis of the need to synchronize human activity cycles for group cooperation (40).

Adaptation and Exaptation in Shared Occupations

Language and biological evolution underpin theories such as game theory, as well as concepts such as adaptation and exaptation. The word *adaptation* is formed by the combination of the Latin words *ad* + *aptus*, which together mean "toward a particular fit." The adaptation described here refers to the fit between biological organisms and the demands of their environments. Rather than adapting, some species have experienced *exaptations*, a term proposed by Gould and Vrba (41). Exaptations refer to evolved traits that are functional. They have emerged not as the result of genetic changes, but rather as opportunistic consequences of such changes. Gould and Vrba (41) cited as an example the human hand and its ability to write. They noted that humans did not evolve fingers to hold pencils and pens (see Figure 7-3 ■). However, a side effect or consequence of manual dexterity, which was evolved for reasons other than writing, enabled the ability to write. It may be useful to view exaptations as extensions of evolutionary adaptations. The invention of many tools, and their corresponding occupations, are examples of exaptations rather than adaptations. Imagine the disadvantage posed to communities in the modern world if members could not read or write or use banks and accounting systems. Exaptations have thus led to many occupations that are vital to group living and quality of life.

Game Theory and Shared Occupations

Because cooperation is a central feature of group living, there has long been an interest to understand the conditions under which cooperation evolves. One interpretation comes from game theory. Game theory is the mathematical study of games and strategy and represents one of the most important 20th-century developments in the social sciences. The most significant early work in this area was done in the 1940s by John von Neumann and Oskar Morgenstern (42). The purpose of game theory is to determine the most likely strategy to be used by each player from a given set of rules and to find the best strategy. Game theory tries to understand the strategy of a game rather than its elements of chance. Its purpose is to understand how decisions are

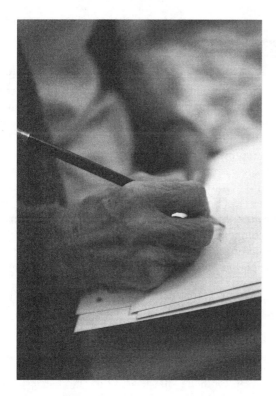

FIGURE 7-3 The ability to hold a pencil or writing tool is an example of an exaptation.
(Photodisc/Getty Images,. Inc.)

made between individuals or groups, based on beliefs that players in any competitive situation have preferences and multiple options, and that they pursue their individual interests logically and to the best of their ability.

Game theory proposes that competing strategies create balance that furthers the survival of the population. This is known as an *evolutionary stable strategy.* Game theory also suggests that social animals learn that cooperation is in their best interest. Game theory emphasizes the importance of communication and symbolic reasoning and suggests that the evolution of these capabilities in humans has helped to create the conditions that enabled cooperation to become a viable strategy in evolution. Game theory provides evidence that the communication of ideas (memes) in modern society may be equally important to the transmission of genes (43). The evolution of community occupations requires reciprocal altruism in the form of cooperation that was made possible by the development of language. Because cooperative strategies place a group at risk for free riders, rules and sanctions are necessary to ensure conformity and maintain the group while also teaching behavioral expectations to younger group members. Box 7-4 describes an exercise called the "prisoner's dilemma" used to study cooperation. Consider the options in this exercise from the perspective of human occupation. Note that one choice will lead to a restriction in a person's actions (in prison), whereas the other will release the person to engage in a wider range of pursuits.

BOX 7-4 Game Theory: The Prisoner's Dilemma

In the social sciences, game theory has focused mostly on non-zero-sum games, particularly those where payoffs are such that players are better off if they select strategies of cooperation, rather than competition. The classic model of this situation is called "prisoner's dilemma" (103). The prisoner's dilemma game (and its variations) is used to illustrate and understand economic, social and political conflict and the coordination that is required for social groups to work. Game theory has been used as a means of demonstrating how cooperative strategies may explain the evolution of social groups and communities. This theory of cooperation contradicts evolutionary theories as explained by genetics. Whereas game theory considers cooperation, evolutionary theories consider competition as a "zero-sum" process. That is to say that competition results in winners and losers, in contrast to cooperation in which everyone can be a winner, or everyone can be a loser. Game theory proposes that people select strategies of cooperation with varying results.

The name of the prisoner's dilemma game is derived from the following situation typically used to exemplify it:

> Suppose that the police have arrested two people whom they know have committed an armed robbery together. Unfortunately, they lack enough admissible evidence to get a jury to convict. They do, however, have enough evidence to send each prisoner away for two years for theft of the getaway car. The chief inspector now makes the following offer to each prisoner: If you will confess to the robbery, implicating your partner, and she does not also confess, then you'll go free, and she'll get ten years. If you both confess, you'll each get 5 years. If neither of you confess, then you'll each get two years for the auto theft.

Most people think that the outcome of the prisoner's dilemma will be that the two prisoners cooperate with each other and each refuses to confess to secure the best outcome for both (2 years in prison). In contrast, the expected outcome of the prisoner's dilemma in game theory is that neither cooperates with the partner to withhold confession. Rather, they both strategize to cooperate with the chief inspector to confess and implicate the partner, thinking that the other partner will not confess. Each strategizes that a confession and implication of the partner will result in personal freedom, while the partner faces 10 years. In other words, under pressure of imprisonment, cooperation with the partner disappears, and cooperation with authority and self-interest prevail. Their shift in cooperation from their partner to the chief inspector results in them both confessing, both implicating the other partner, and both receiving 5 years, rather than the 2 years they would have received if they had retained solidarity with the partner and neither had confessed.

HOW AND WHY DO OCCUPATIONS DETERMINE A SOCIAL GROUP'S POTENTIAL TO FLOUNDER OR FLOURISH?

We now turn to the question of how and why occupations determine a social group's potential to flounder or flourish. A flourishing group appears to offer positive experiences of interdependent participation in occupations (44, 45). Collective achievements are marked by holidays, rituals, and symbols, which may include festivals and commemorative gatherings or parades, often with medals, logos, or other symbols of shared achievement. During these commemorative events, aspects of individual agency (power, excitement) are balanced with communal expressions of mutual respect, love, accommodation, and connectedness (46, 47). The implicit message is that identity and empowerment develop through both individual and shared occupations in a supportive community context (48–50). In today's world, the data used to demonstrate accountability may produce supportive or restrictive contexts. Stein (50) described how a "cult of efficiency" can cloud the judgement of those in communities, such as nursing homes, where concerns for risk management may override staff interests in being supportive caregivers.

In the discussions to follow, a range of occupations and structural features that determine the potential of a group, community, or society to flourish or flounder are considered.

Participation in Occupations

Participation and partnership are two central, interconnected features of flourishing groups, communities, and societies (see Box 7-5). A fundamental principle in community development is that members of groups, communities, and societies are active participants and partners in all action, particularly in decision making (44, 51–53). Participation refers to peoples' intentional involvement in circumstances where doing things together can generate a shared identity. Participatory approaches in health and social services are person-centered, in that they include persons, who may be called "patients" or "clients" of these systems, and who engage with others to shape the service community to support their interests and needs (54–57). As disadvantaged group members participate, rather than accepting their dependence, they develop a common vision and awareness of the changes needed to create a more inclusive community structure and organization (58, 59). An important feature in person-centered, participatory community occupations is their generation of optimism and hope (60). In recent years, participatory research has grown as a means for involving oppressed or disadvantaged people through participation in occupations that change their daily life as well as their communities (59, 61–65).

BOX 7-5 The Antigonish Movement as an Example of Participation and Partnership

Scott MacAulay offers an interesting comparison between two powerful community economic development traditions in Nova Scotia on Canada's East Coast. He analyzes similarities and differences in citizen participation in the Antigonish movement (from 1939 to the present) and the family of community development corporations (starting in the early 1970s), which includes New Dawn Enterprises Limited, the oldest community development corporation in Canada (104). These are examples of changing community practices by engaging in strategic occupations that promote participation, education, and decision making. As he says,

> The innovation of the Antigonish Movement was its combination of a commitment to economic democracy through consumer cooperatives with a program of adult education that was to be brought directly to workers and primary producers (p. 113).
>
> Whereas, the Family of community development corporations is a strategic effort by a small group of people in the community. They volunteer their expertise and scarce time to work on behalf of the whole community (p. 115).

Participation by citizens and partnership with government officials sparked a variety of volunteer and community-oriented initiatives that had as their aim social change as well as economic development. Quoting Jim Lotz, a local commentator on community economic development, MacAulay considers that these participatory initiatives offer lessons for the world.

> The Antigonish Movement flowered here, and the community economic ventures that started with New Dawn have created a history of local achievement through which both local residents and government officials have learned much about working together in mutually beneficial ways. That history, in fact, is a rich and marketable resource. (p. 253)

In discussing "continuities and discontinuities" between these movements, MacAulay points to differences in participation and partnership in educational and decision-making occupations. The Antigonish movement was based on community cooperatives and study clubs that promoted reflective self-awareness and active participation in economic, educational, and social occupations. In contrast, the "Family" of community development corporations was managed by a core group of volunteers who took a business approach with a focus on policy and economic occupations.

Occupations That Express Cultural Rituals and Rules

From their research on Australia's Aboriginal communities, Williams and colleagues (66) proposed that rules or expectations for successful group living have evolved over time. Groups need to ensure health and survival, as well as adequate biological reproduction. However, groups, communities, and societies only flourish when there is a means to socialize children into the group as productive members. Also needed is a means of communicating skills and values to all group members. Of major importance for groups to flourish is a system of sanctions or authority mechanisms to ensure that group members comply with expectations or abide by rules (16, 67). This is a delicate matter of balance. On the one hand, social groups flourish when a society regulates compliance with everyday occupations that create cohesion (driving on the same side of the road, sanctions against violence, etc.). On the other hand, social groups also flourish when regulations and policies protect and encourage individuals and groups to express their diverse ideas and beliefs, and view all persons, regardless of differences, as valued citizens (68).

As the oldest, continuous cultural groups on earth, Australia's Aboriginal communities have been studied extensively for clues regarding societal development. Australian Aboriginal settlement dates back over 50,000 years, and the tools and symbols used in the occupations of this culture are reminiscent of those used by early Europeans. Their language and occupations appear to have been used to define the cultural rituals and rules of their communities. As well, the everyday occupations of sharing living quarters appear to be closely tied to biological and social survival. Lévi-Strauss, one of the early anthropologists who studied Australian Aboriginal people, points out that taboos against incest are made possible through designations of kinship that provide guidance for alliances and residential arrangements (69). Australian Aboriginal people resisted agricultural occupations, possibly because subsistence was provided through plentiful seas and the natural animals and plants of the Australian bush. They also relied on a loosely organized tribal elder system for the occupations of group decision making, rather than developing more formalized institutional systems (69).

We can learn from Australian and other aboriginal groups about the making of successful communities (70, 71). Rituals and rules that encourage voluntary cooperation in the division of labor are extremely important. Also critical is the huge range of decision-making and management occupations that make social governance systems work. Primary resource societies rely on social groups, such as farmers, people who fish, and timber workers. In contrast, industrial and technical communities rely on the occupations of social groups, such as plant workers, scientists, teachers, health professionals, and many others. Collectively, social groups, communities, and societies need to engage in occupations that attend to the cultural rituals and rules required for them to flourish. Communities also need to support diversity and to foster ongoing negotiation among their constituencies. Parents, teachers, and child-care workers help to socialize children into social groups that encourage some uniformity while concurrently encouraging children to give voice to their differences. The balance of uniform and diverse social group occupations will attract interest in the legislative, law enforcement, judicial, and correctional systems where professionals and others strive to develop systems of rules and sanctions for group living.

Occupations That Offer Artistic Expression

Artistic expression has occupied humans almost since the dawn of this species (see Box 7-6). Groups that flourish appear to support occupations that offer artistic expression. These include the pursuit of literature, music, dance, and forms of visual art that enrich the experience of life and contribute to the *soul* of a culture. In the minds of many, occupations that offer artistic expression are a distinguishing feature of thriving versus merely surviving communities. Philosophy, religion, home design, community planning, and the creative use of everyday materials are all expressions that occur through what people think and do each day. Humans understand that life is finite. Within that sense of time and opportunity, groups seem to flourish when members are at liberty, individually and collectively, to explore a sense of self, relationships with and perceptions of other beings, creation, purpose, and place within the universe.

BOX 7-6 Evidence of Artistic Expression by Prehistoric Humans

Approximately 20,000 years ago, humans in Europe lived primarily as hunters. It is likely that questions about the nature of life were occurring to these people, who sought to understand the world about them. Early explanations of existence gave rise to ideas about magic and mythology. The greatest evidence of such ideas is found in prehistoric cave paintings. These mainly depict animals, which, in their primary occupation as hunters, the people believed were their source of life (Figure 7-4 ■).

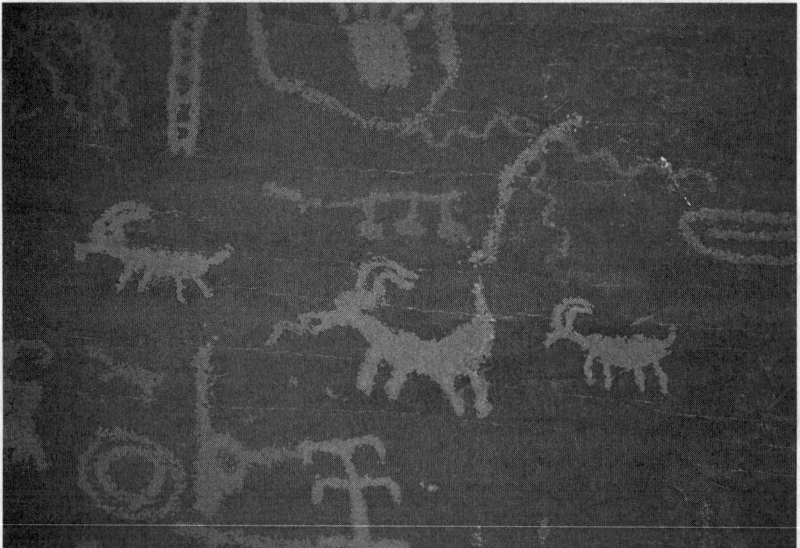

FIGURE 7-4 Prehistoric cave paintings provide clues to early humans' thinking about magic and mythology.
(Albert J. Copley/Getty Images.)

Occupations that Sustain Social Groups

A key concept in modern societal development is *sustainability* (72). The current world emphasis on sustainability gained prominence in a United Nations conference called the Earth Summit held in Rio de Janeiro, Brazil, in 1992. The United Nations defines a sustainable society as one that meets the needs of the present without sacrificing the ability of future generations to meet their own needs (73). It is noteworthy that the idea of conserving natural resources is not new. Indeed, concerns for the environment date back more than two thousand years.

According to Model Principles for Sustainable Communities proposed by the Ontario (Canada) Roundtable on Environment and Economy (Box 7-7), sustainable communities take responsibilities for themselves. They do not compromise the sustainability of other communities or of future generations. The occupations related to sustainability include those that organize, use, and protect energy, those that study natural resources, those that tend the natural environment, and those that

BOX 7-7 Model Principles for Sustainable Communities

A sustainable community is one that:

1. Recognizes that growth occurs within some limits and is ultimately limited by the carrying capacity of the environment
2. Values cultural diversity
3. Has respect for other life forms and supports biodiversity
4. Has shared values among the members of the community (promoted through sustainability education)
5. Employs ecological decision making (e.g., integration of environmental criteria into all municipal government, business, and personal decision-making processes)
6. Makes decisions and plans in a balanced, open, and flexible manner that includes the perspectives from the social, health, economic, and environmental sectors of the community
7. Makes best use of local efforts and resources (nurtures solutions at the local level)
8. Uses renewable and reliable sources of energy
9. Minimizes harm to the natural environment
10. Fosters activities that use materials in continuous cycles.

And, as a result, a sustainable community:

11. Does not compromise the sustainability of other communities (a geographic perspective)
12. Does not compromise the sustainability of future generations by its activities (a temporal perspective).

Source: Ontario Roundtable on Environment and Economy, 1994 (77, pp. 43–47)

address humans' needs for food, shelter, goods, enjoyment, and biological reproduction within the capacity of the environment to regenerate itself. Human occupations that are consistent with sustainability involve the production, purchasing, and selection of energy and environmentally friendly goods, meaning goods that do not deplete finite resources. *Re-use, renovate and recycle* are becoming familiar occupations that now take considerable time in many homes and businesses. Sustainability occupations may also reinforce particular values, such as cultural diversity and respect for life forms other than humans, including plants and animals.

Sociopolitical occupations of sustainability control public and private decision making on policies and regulations (58). A prosperous economy is of little use to a local community if its people are not employed in paid occupations or if the available paid occupations undermine community sustainability. When the only paid occupations are in factories that pollute the air, land, or water of a community, community members may find that their occupations and ideas about a sustainable planet are in conflict with their paid work. An economically vibrant community will not thrive for long if it does so at the expense of people's health or without safeguarding the environment for the future.

The dilemma is that many businesses and occupations that generate economic wealth necessary for communities are reluctant to move to places where workers may be driven by values for environmental sustainability and quality of life, beyond the generation of monetary wealth (74). A debate continues between those who view natural resources as finite and likely to diminish as population growth continues and those who believe that human enterprise and ingenuity will create solutions to problems through technology and resourcefulness (75). Inherent in this debate are difficult occupational choices for individuals and groups if they want sustainable, flourishing communities.

The proximity of people living in communities also enables the shared occupations that promote flourishing. Shared initiatives can be created that enable communities to flourish. New partnerships are springing up that involve participants in occupations as individuals, as members of community environmental groups, as industry and business partners, as representatives of universities and schools, or as representatives of local and national governments.

The Healthy Communities Movement is an example of advocacy for sustainable, healthy communities (see Box 7-8). Shared occupations were proposed to focus on health, with a common purpose of creating stable, ongoing community structures as well as positive experiences of participation in health-producing behaviors. Group empowerment through community movements is both a means and a result of a strategy to involve a total community in health promotion occupations (48, 76–78).

Of particular note is the importance of creating a health-enhancing built environment to encourage health-promoting occupations. An interdependence or compatibility is needed between what society builds and how the built environment influences the overall quality of life of people living there, as measured by health, safety, welfare, transportation, and land development. Frank and Engelke (79) analyzed literature on transportation and land use planning to illustrate the impact on physical activity of the built environment. They concluded that "land development patterns define the arrangement of activities and impact the proximity between trip origins and destinations" (p. 210) in the choices people make about walking, cycling, and using their cars or public transportation.

BOX 7-8 Group Advocacy for Community Improvement: The Healthy Communities Movement

The Healthy Communities movement was started by Trevor Hancock and Len Duhl in 1986 in Toronto, Canada, as part of a World Health Organization initiative (105). Its purpose was to assemble health institutions, businesses, nonprofit organizations, community groups, and individuals to address community well-being using a systems perspective. This approach viewed communities as environments that enable the well-being of their inhabitants. Healthy communities provide the jobs, educational systems, public safety, and health services necessary to support satisfying lifestyles. A key part of a Healthy Community is the involvement of the entire community in problem-solving occupations. Participation in group problem solving is viewed as a group occupation necessary for the community to flourish.

Interestingly, the historical roots of this initiative go back to the Healthy Towns movement in mid-19th-century Britain. Hundreds of communities across the globe are now making efforts that started almost two centuries ago to improve the health of the working poor in growing industrial cities. A Healthy Towns commission looked into the causes of health and saw a direct correlation between poor health and the conditions within towns and cities. The Healthy Towns movement spread beyond Britain and led to major improvements in public health, building, and sanitation, such as the creation of improved water supplies.

The growth of the worldwide Healthy Communities Movement gathered energy from social sentiments that favor local solutions over the bureaucracy required for action at the national level. Concerns about community issues, such as the rise in violence, crime, poverty, and abused and neglected children, have created a sense that communities are disconnected and threatened. These concerns have been used to spearhead community approaches that promote health by tending to a community's root problems.

Most supporters of the Healthy Communities Movement looked for solutions beyond improving the physical health of communities. At its core, this Movement required power sharing among individuals and groups in an effort to improve the quality of life for all. Their efforts are aimed at the development of social capital and the creation or rejuvenation of community spirit. To foster change, groups that were attracted to the Movement became learning communities that were seeking to modify strategies rather than just attain goals. The idea was that community change will not last unless shared approaches to decision making and responsibility, including power sharing, become an established part of community life.

Magic, Religion, and Science

Magic, religion, and science are terms that describe collective thinking aimed at understanding the world and the events that happen in it. These *occupations of understanding* each have creeds, codes, and cultures. That is, they represent certain beliefs, they establish doctrines or expectations for behavior based on those beliefs, and they evolve practices that encourage or enforce the principles of the belief system. Throughout the ages, humans have wanted to know about natural phenomena that occur and cannot be controlled (such as death, lightning, or earthquakes). The ideas of magic and religion, which predated empirical science as ways of understanding the world, have been intertwined over the centuries because they each deal with nonmaterial aspects of life. Humans have developed ideas and actions of magic, witchcraft, or religion as explanations for accidents, chance occurrences, or events that happen in nature (80).

Cultural groups, even those with complex civil structures, have typically developed occupations to divine the meaning of natural or supernatural events. Examples of occupations involved in divination are tarot card reading, palm or tea leaf reading, and the reading of astrological charts. Rituals have either linked humans to gods and goddesses, or granted a select group the occupational status of divine representation. The daily lives of North American peoples and those elsewhere commonly reflect vestiges of concern with the supernatural. Many people wear amulets, or good luck charms, and their occupations are shaped by superstitions, such as avoiding being under a ladder or throwing salt over the shoulder if it is spilled. The rituals and practices of organized religions can be viewed as spiritual occupations that draw groups of people together in action toward mutual goals (81). Whether this involves traditional or new forms of religious or spiritual expression, such occupations foster mutuality, interdependence, and reciprocity within a particular community. Community rituals are sustained in many ways, apart from the supernatural or religious rituals. Weddings are an example of a ritual that, with variations, seems to be part of the everyday occupations to officially recognize partnerships around the world (see Figure 7-5 ■).

Philosophers over the ages, beginning with Aristotle, began to counter supernatural explanations of occurrences with a preference for experimentation and logic (82). The scientific revolution that started in the Middle Ages has not been able to change beliefs in magic or other supernatural forces for many people because they continue to ponder as yet unanswered questions (82). Nevertheless, a new wave of scientific investigation includes empirical work but also values the insights and diverse ways of knowing generated through cooperative, participatory, interpretive, and critical inquiries about people's everyday life experiences (83, 84).

The importance of magic, religion, and science in communities is apparent in the occupations attached to them. As well, groups that flourish also seem to value and preserve buildings, artifacts, symbols, traditions, routines, and rituals. The occupations that express these interests are visible in the horoscopes, worship rituals, and other accepted ways of knowing, understanding, or explaining employed within a community. Flourishing groups seem to tolerate diverse occupations that express

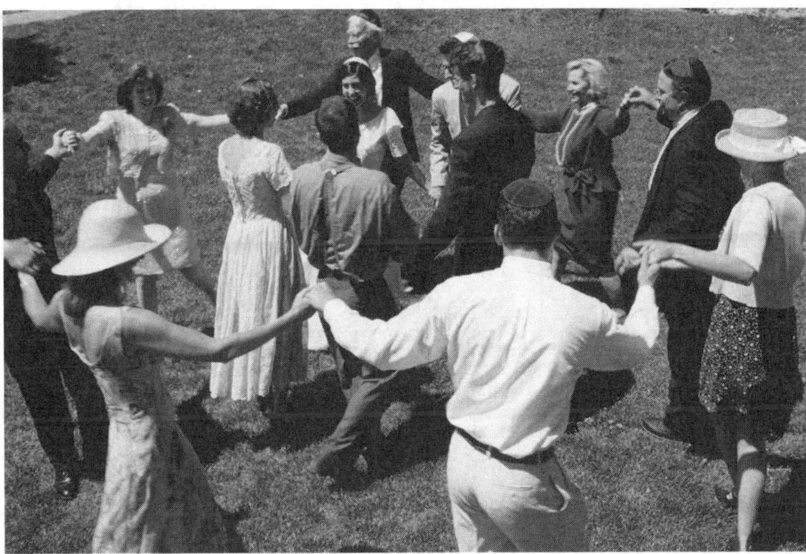

FIGURE 7-5 Weddings as community rituals. Throughout the world, weddings serve as a common and visible reminder of the importance of public ceremonies and rituals in fostering shared beliefs and traditions. Typically, weddings involve symbols, rituals, superstitions, and elements of religion. In this photo, friends and neighbors enjoy a traditional Jewish dance following the wedding ceremony. (Photodisc/Getty Images)

diverse ideas about magic, religion, and science. In groups that are floundering, conflict and violence appear to erupt where ideas and occupations associated with magic, religion, or scientific ideas are restricted. Unequal sanctioning of these important occupations thus divides flourishing from floundering communities.

Volunteer Occupations

Volunteer occupations appear to build cooperation and enhance the social and possibly the economic strength of social groups and communities. Volunteer occupations are those in which people give time, resources, effort, skills, and abilities to serve other people without formal expectation of recognition or reward (85). Ellis and Noyes defined volunteerism as those "acts taken in recognition of a need, with an attitude of social responsibility. . . . To volunteer is to go beyond one's basic obligations" (86, p.4).

Through a tremendous range of volunteer occupations, people help others in almost all aspects of life. Volunteers help to construct homes, provide health services, care for elderly citizens, attend to children, tutor students, welcome newcomers, judge projects at science fairs or Special Olympics, and maintain public areas. Retired workers, persons without employment, and others may also volunteer to support public or nonprofit agencies by publishing newsletters or preparing correspondence.

There are many benefits to volunteerism, both to communities and organizations, as well as to the volunteers themselves (87). Benefits to communities include developing informal support networks that provide assistance otherwise not available and providing meaningful roles for retired individuals and others seeking opportunities to serve. Although businesses are oriented to private interests and governments are oriented to public interests, volunteers focus on the interests of social groups within the society—including disadvantaged groups whose members are poor or living with a disability (88).

Wuthnow noted: "Voluntarism [sic] symbolizes the antithesis of impersonality, bureaucracy, materialism, utilitarianism, and many of the other dominant cultural trends we worry about in our society (89, p. 305). Benefits of volunteerism to individuals include developing a sense of self-satisfaction, learning new skills, developing rewarding social relationships, enhancing career opportunities, and providing affirmation and a sense of completion through doing something that others say is important. Coles (90) suggests that the most successful volunteers are those who enjoy interacting with others, who do not view volunteering as a sacrifice, and who realize that volunteering is a practical occupation that conveys reciprocal benefits.

Work and Employment: Occupations that Generate Economic Capital

Work is the most publicly recognized occupation. In fact, the most typical answer to the question, "What do you do?" is for people to describe their paid work, even though they are actually occupied in many ways, from parenting, maintaining a home, studying, caregiving, sports, games, to other occupations. Most writing about occupation in communities is about work and employment—the interests are primarily in work when researchers examine occupational classifications and the division of labor, occupational health and safety on the job, occupational satisfaction with career choices, occupational training and retraining or retooling, occupational transitions as people change jobs or retire, and related topics.

It is clear throughout this chapter that the occupations of work and employment are only part of the occupational nature of social groups. Work and employment are not even the full source of community economic development when one considers the family, neighbourhood, community-building, bartering and self-sufficiency occupations that sustain an informal, underground economy.

Being employed in work occupations has obvious financial benefits for individuals, their families, and their communities. The income gained through employment provides the means to purchase goods that meet basic survival needs, such as housing, food, and clothing for individuals but also that meet community needs to engage in the reciprocal buying and selling that are fundamental to the economy of a community. The economic profits of paid work also provide people with financial independence and the opportunity to make choices about what they will purchase or do within their community. The quality of employment in one's working life and the income derived from occupational pursuits have consequences for financial independence in retirement when retirees need and want to participate actively in the economy of their community.

Beyond meeting individual and community material needs and desires, employment has many nonfinancial benefits that enable groups as well as individuals to flourish. Having a job provides individuals with a sense of identity and contributes to the common good. As well, employment provides individuals with opportunities to form social associations that foster connectedness outside the family. Paid work involves people in regular physical, intellectual, and social interactions that offer communities the resources of their knowledge, skills, and capacities. Employment also imposes a collective routine or time structure to the day and week within social groups and communities and allows nonwork time to be defined and used in other ways, such as in leisure.

Occupations That Generate Social Capital

The concept of social capital was proposed to counter the emphasis on economic capital as an indicator of a community's well-being. Social capital is defined as the set of values or norms shared among members of a group that permits cooperation among them (91). Social capital is not a static phenomenon; it is actively built and destroyed through human actions and processes. Drawing together the ideas of Putnam and Coleman, social capital has been described as: (1) obligations, expectations, and trustworthiness of structure; (2) information channels or networks; (3) norms and effective sanctions (92, 93). The idea of social capital has grown from the concept of mass society (Box 7-9). In a world with weakening kinship, impersonal neighborhoods and feelings of isolation and alienation, social capital is viewed as an antidote to mass society.

Volunteerism, civic participation, parenting, social and political involvement, and community engagement are the occupations through which trustworthy structures, networks, and norms are founded and facilitated within communities. Occupations that generate social capital facilitate the interdependence, communal experiences, and identity (individual and/or collective depending on the society) that are fundamental to flourishing groups. Although the ideal is for all citizens to contribute to social capital, history tells us that the primary participants in occupations that generate social capital are women, many of whom may be poor with little education (94). The presence of occupations that generate social capital, in effect, is a barometer of cooperation and community success. Cooperation, as has been noted, is a fundamental requirement for the evolution of humans living in groups, and cooperation remains essential if societies are to flourish. Co-operation in the occupations of social capital makes it possible to develop efficiencies and accountability for creating community life beyond economic wealth. An example is the cooperation needed to develop the social capital of offering efficient and accountable care for children whose parents or other caregivers go outside the home to work. It seems reasonable to assume that flourishing social groups generate both social and economic capital, neither one being sufficient for humans without the other.

BOX 7-9 The Concept of Mass Society

The concept of mass society underpins interest in fostering the idea of social capital, including the idea that successful communities develop trust and cooperation. A mass society is viewed as one in which industry and bureaucracy have eroded traditional social ties. The concept of mass society refers to communities and societies that have deteriorated to the point where there is weak kinship, impersonal neighborhoods, and a feeling by individuals that they are isolated and alienated.

The concept of mass society is based on the work of Emile Durkheim (8), Ferdinand Tonnies (106), and Max Weber (107). The major argument is that the scale of modern life has increased in size as a result of industrialization. The result has been an increasing rate of change, an increasing gap between social differences, and a weakening of moral values. Modern communities lack the solidarity required to clearly define and uphold social sanctions. In a mass society, people are known more by their jobs than through kinship, and personal communication has gradually been replaced by mass media. Advocates of the concept of mass society argue that there may be some benefits to changes taking place in communities. However, geographic mobility, mass communications, and tolerance for social diversity in modern communities have eroded traditional values. Furthermore, individual rights and freedom of choice are achieved at the expense of cultural heritage. In such communities, individuals have too many choices and very few boundaries to define what is important to the community. Although individuals have many rights, responsibilities, and freedoms, they also feel isolated, powerless, and materialistic.

Occupational Nature of Social Groups that Flounder

The lack of certain occupations or occupational experiences can undermine social groups. Communities that flounder, in essence, are those without the occupations, the experiences of shared occupation, and the organization and built environment through which social groups flourish. Lacking are experiences of interdependence, shared history, and possibilities for individual identity to grow within a supportive, interconnected, respectful communal environment. Lacking also are occupations that enable social groups to express a diversity of routines, rules, artistry, magic, religion, and science. Volunteer and paid occupations that build only economic capital leave communities without sufficient social capital. Lack of cooperation can undermine the trust, effective communication, and systems required to govern group living. Lack of organizational and physical, environmental support makes it impossible to participate in some communal occupations. Without supportive organization and structures, social groups limit or bar some citizens from participation in some occupations. A concrete example would be a community that lacks sufficient organizational capacity and resources to provide sidewalks and bike trails, thereby preventing inhabitants from gaining the healthful benefits of walking or biking.

In addition, it seems that social groups flounder if some members are deprived of opportunities to engage in occupations that contribute to their social or economic well-being. As Whiteford has shown, social groups from refugees to prisoners and those living in geographically isolated conditions may experience occupational deprivation. This refers to the inability of some groups of people to engage in daily occupations that they define as meaningful for reasons beyond their control (93–95). Communities also flounder when there is a major discrepancy between social groups that have nothing much to do and groups that are overburdened by too much to do. Such a gap is particularly dangerous to communities if those deprived of participation or active engagement in meaningful occupations live in poverty and crime while others without such limitations maintain economic advantages and social privileges. These occupational discrepancies are symptoms of occupational injustice—injustices in everyday occupations that go beyond limitations of legal rights, responsibilities, and freedoms. Occupational injustices occur when some social groups in society are deprived of occupations or alienated from their true occupational selves while others in the same community are not (96).

The poverty inflicted by unemployment has many material and nonmaterial effects, including limiting occupational choices, social participation, and social networks. Moreover, violence is caused by multiple factors, including the disintegration of family life, poverty, social influences such as the availability of weapons, antisocial peer influence, and substance abuse or mental illness (97–99). Floundering communities seem to lose the struggle to address painful occupations resulting from child abuse and neglect, adolescent delinquency, adult criminality, senior abuse, or other forms of violence.

CHAPTER SUMMARY

Three questions have been addressed in considering the occupational nature of social groups: What makes social groups inherently occupational? How and why did occupations that promote group living develop? How and why do occupations determine a social group's potential to flounder or flourish?

A leading premise of the chapter is that occupations are a central feature of successful groups because occupations are essentially social and occur in a social context. Literature and examples have illustrated experiences of shared occupations, biological forces shaping occupations, and various occupations that appear to be necessary for social groups to flourish. It was noted that, conversely, groups that lack the conditions and occupations that promote positive occupational experiences for all citizens seem more likely to flounder. It seems that communities need occupations that generate social as well as economic capital, with a supportive organization and built environment. Individuals need community support for occupational experiences of positive interdependence respect, connectedness, and resource sharing. The occupational nature of social groups is thus central in determining whether individuals and communities will flourish or flounder. This means that communities have the power to use and support occupations to generate both social and economic benefits in areas such as education, parenting, health, employment, retirement, transportation, land use planning, decision making, and policy development. Occupations, it seems, are the foundation for economically productive, socially vibrant, just, and healthy communities, where participation for all in a quality everyday life is paramount.

STUDY GUIDE

Study Guide Author: Kate Barrett

Summary of Main Points

This chapter helps us understand the social nature of participating in occupations. Occupations bring people together in various ways; occupations enable people to develop bonds with one another when they participate in work, leisure, volunteerism, and other occupations. The chapter shows us that this has been true throughout time as well as throughout the world. How people participate in occupations together has the power to shape whether a social group will flourish or flounder.

Application to Occupational Therapy

Occupational therapists work with people on many different levels: one on one, group settings, family settings, and at the systems level with communities, organizations and populations. Working at any level, occupational therapists recognize the occupational nature of social groups. Conversely, occupational therapists also recognize the power of enabling occupation in social groups to promote human doing, being, becoming—and particularly belonging. For example, a baseball player is not just an individual player. He or she is a *member* of a team. Being a member of the team affects the meaning of playing baseball in significant ways. The team is formed around particular values and cultural rituals about playing ball, and around particular practice routines and habits to prepare for ball games. Moreover, being a member of a ball team in the United States may differ greatly from being a member of a ball team in Korea or South America or Northern Canada. Not only are the geographic conditions different for ball playing in each place, but the economics, social values, gender roles, and time use expectations around leisure and sports will determine what kinds of supports are available for ball playing for children, men and women. Players with disabilities or seniors who wish to continue playing ball will find different resources and attitudes toward their participation in ball playing. These differences will all determine how, where, when and with what resources occupational therapists enable participation in ball playing.

When working in a group or policy context, occupational therapists use occupation to positively affect groups and community cohesion. Occupational therapists appreciate the importance of how *doing* brings people together. In addition, occupational therapists have the ability to recognize when *doing* is negatively affecting a social group and can adapt the setting or occupation to promote group cohesiveness. The occupational therapist's skills in enabling participation in group occupations may be to adapt programs or environments, to coach or coordinate participation by diverse social groups, or to consult with and educate those involved in social groups, such as members of a group home or a retirement community. Occupational therapists may also advocate with and for social groups, particularly when they collectively experience occupational deprivation, such as when a lack of reasonable workplace accommodations excludes persons with disabilities or chronic diseases from paid employment.

This chapter explains how participation in occupations influences how a person experiences connectedness to a group of people. Understanding the social aspects of occupation is vital for occupational therapists to gain insight into the multiple and diverse meanings of occupation for different social groups or communities. This is particularly true since the meaning of occupation is socially constructed through time, place, and experience with others. To practice occupational therapy effectively, practitioners consider personal factors (the individual's physical, emotional, and cognitive abilities), as well as the contextual and environmental factors (people, places, objects, etc.) that shape occupations collectively for particular individuals, families, groups, communities, organizations or populations.

Individual Learning Activities

1. Reflect on a group in which you feel belonging. What is it about this community that gives you this sense of belonging? How do you participate with other people in this community, and what do you do with others in this community? Is there a physical space that is meaningful to the community?
2. The chapter introduced the concept of social capital, suggesting that the most effective communities are characterized by participation, trust, and social connectedness among their members. But is it possible that too much connectedness may be counterproductive? In the book *Bowling Alone* (written by Robert Putnam, © 2000 and published by Touchstone/Simon & Schuster), it was pointed out that people in the United States tend to be less active in civic matters than they were 50 years ago. Yet tolerance for difference has improved among younger generations of Americans during that period. How do you explain that relationship?

Group Learning Activity

As a group, watch the movie, *Pleasantville*, a satirical look at community differences in the United States between the 1950s and today. Reflect on how this movie portrays a sense of community. Think about the positive and negative aspects of belonging to a community. (*Pleasantville* was produced in 1998 by Touchstone Pictures and starred William H. Macy and Joan Allen). Or readers outside the United States may wish to choose a movie that portrays a social group from a local cultural context.

Study Questions

1. Rubin identified five structural characteristics for a community to mediate between an individual and society, which do not include:
   a. Sharing
   b. Focus
   c. Social structure
   d. Stability
2. McMillan and Chavis described four ways in which members generate a "psychological sense of community"; they include all of the following EXCEPT:
   a. Creating a sense of belonging
   b. Through fulfillment of member needs
   c. Social skills
   d. Offering shared connections

3. Occupations consistent with sustainable communities participate in:
   a. Composting
   b. Recycling
   c. Using natural resources
   d. All of the above
4. Mutual dependence, mutual aid, moral commitment, and responsibility to recognize and support difference describes which characteristic of community?
   a. Structure
   b. Participation
   c. Interdependence
   d. Independence
5. The environment to which a particular species can successfully adapt is called
   a. Competition
   b. Ecological niche
   c. Cooperation
   d. Evolution

REFERENCES

1. Poplin, D. (1994). Theories of community. In D. Poplin (Ed.), *Communities: A survey of theories and methods of research* (2nd ed., pp. 63–107). New York: Macmillan.
2. Ignatieff, M. (1995). *Blood and belonging.* London: Farrar, Straus, & Giroux.
3. Ignatieff, M. (1984). *The needs of strangers: An essay on privacy, solidarity and the politics of being human.* New York: Penguin Group.
4. Ignatieff, M. (2000). *The rights revolution.* Toronto, ON: House of Anansi.
5. Belensky, M. F., Clinchy, B. M., Goldberger, N. R., & Tarule, J. M. (1986). *Women's ways of knowing: The development of self, voice and mind.* New York: Basic Books.
6. Nemeth, C. J., Nemeth-Brown, B. (200). Better than individuals? The potential benefits of dissent and diversity for group creativity. In P. Paulus & B. Nijstad (Ed.), *Group creativity: Innovation through collaboration* (pp. 63–84). Oxford: Oxford University Press.
7. Rubin, I. (1983). Function and structure of community: Conceptual and theoretical analysis. In R. L. W. L. Lyon (Ed.), *New perspectives on the American community* (pp. 54–64). Homewood, IL: Dorsey Press.
8. Durkheim, E. (1964). *The division of labor in society.* New York: The Free Press.
9. Condeluci, A. (1990). *Interdependence: The route to community.* Orlando, FL: PMD Publishers Group.
10. Brown, K. (1990). Connected independence: A paradox of rural health? *Journal of Rural Community Psychology, 11,* 51–64.
11. Pentland, W., Krupa, T., Lynch, S., & Clark, C. (1992). Community integration for persons with disabilities: Working together to make it happen. *Canadian Journal of Occupational Therapy. 59,* 127–130.
12. Townsend, E. (1997). Inclusiveness: A community dimension of spirituality. *Canadian Journal of Occupational Therapy. 64*(3), 146–155.
13. Townsend, E., Birch, D., Langille, L., & Langley, J. (2000). Participatory research in a mental health clubhouse. *Occupational Therapy Journal of Research. 20,* 18–44.

14. Lord, J. (1987). *Toward independence and community: A qualitative study of independent living centres in Canada.* Canada: Secretary of State.
15. Oakley, P. (1998). Community development in the Third World in the 1990s. Review Article. *Community Development Journal. 33*(4), 365–376.
16. Maton, K. I., & Salem, D. A. (1995, October 23). Organizational characteristics of empowering community settings: A multiple case study approach. *American Journal of Community Psychology 23*(5), 631–656.
17. Etzioni, A. (1993). *The spirit of community: Rights, responsibilities, and the communitarian agenda.* New York: Crown.
18. McMillan, D. W., & Chavis, D. M. (1986). Sense of community: A definition and theory. *Journal of Community Psychology, 14*(1), 6–23.
19. Pretty, G. (1990). Relating psychological sense of community to social climate characteristics. *Journal of Community Psychology, 22,* 346–58.
20. Hogan, R. (1983). A socioanalytic theory of personality. In M. M. Page(Ed.), *Nebraska symposium on motivation* (pp. 55–90). Lincoln: University of Nebraska Press.
21. Adler, A. (1927). *The practice and theory of individual psychology.* New York: Harcourt Brace.
22. Kegan, R. (1982). *The evolving self: Problem and process in human development.* Cambridge, MA: Harvard University Press.
23. Bakan, D. (1966). *The duality of human existence: Isolation and communion in Western man.* Boston: Beacon Press.
24. McAdams, D. P. (1997). *The stories we live by: Personal myths and the making of the self.* New York: Guilford Press.
25. Page, N., & Czuba, C. (1999). Empowerment: What is it? [Electronic Journal]: *Journal of Extension.* Available at: http://www.joe.org
26. Bandura, A. (2000). Exercise of human agency through collective efficacy. *Current Directions in Psychological Science, 9,* 75–78.
27. Peterson, E., Mitchell, T., Thompson, L., & Burr, R. (2000). Collective efficacy and aspects of shared mental models as predictors of performance over time in work groups. *Group Processes and Intergroup Relations, 3*(3), 296–316.
28. Clark, F. (1997). Reflections on the human as an occupational being: Biological need, tempo and temporality. *Journal of Occupational Science: Australia, 4*(3), 86–92.
29. Wilcock, A. A. (1998). Reflections on doing, being and becoming. *Canadian Journal of Occupational Therapy. 65*(5), 248–256.
30. Wilcock, A. A. (1998). *An occupational perspective of health.* Thorofare, NJ: Slack, Inc.
31. Kropotkin, P. (1989). *Mutual aid: A factor of evolution.* Montreal, PQ: Black Rose Books.
32. Pinker, S., & Bloom, P. (1990). Natural language and natural selection. *Behavioral and Brain Sciences. 13,* 707–784.
33. Dawkins, R. (1989). *The selfish gene* (2nd ed.). Oxford: Oxford University Press.
34. Aunger, R. (Ed.). (2000). *Darwinizing culture: The status of memetics as a science.* Oxford: Oxford University Press.
35. Heylighen, F. (1992). Selfish memes and the evolution of cooperation. *Journal of Ideas, 2*(4), 77–84.
36. Calvin, W. H. (1986). *The river that flows uphill: A journey from the big bang to the big brain.* San Francisco: Sierra Club Books.
37. Tattersall, I. (1998). *Becoming human: Evolution and human uniqueness.* New York: Harcourt Brace.
38. Allee, W. C. (1934). *Animal aggregations: A study in general sociology.* Chicago: University of Chicago Press.
39. Trivers, R. L. (1971). The evolution of reciprocal altruism. *Quarterly Review of Biology, 46,* 35–57.

40. Moore, A. (1995). The band community: Synchronizing human activity cycles for group cooperation. In R. Z. F. Clark (Ed.), *Occupational science: The emerging discipline* (pp. 95–106). Philadelphia: F. A. Davis.
41. Gould, S. J., & Vrba, E. S. (1982). Exaptation—a missing term in the science of form. *Paleobiology, 8,* 4–15.
42. von Neumann, J. M., & Morgenstern, O. (1944). *The theory of games and economic behavior.* Princeton, NJ: Princeton University Press.
43. Maynard Smith, J. (1982). *Evolution and the theory of games.* Cambridge, MA: Cambridge University Press.
44. Boyce, W. (1993). Evaluating participation in community programs: An empowerment paradigm. *The Canadian Journal of Program Evaluation, 8,* 89–102.
45. Castelloe, P., & Watson, T. (1999). Participatory education as a community practice method: A case example from a comprehensive Head Start Program. *Journal of Community Practice, 6*(1), 71–89.
46. Gould, R. (1989). Power and social structure in community elites. *Social Forces, 68:2,* 531–552.
47. Ross, L., & Coleman, M. (2000). Urban community action planning inspires teenagers to transform their community and their identity. *Journal of Community Practice, 7*(2), 29–45.
48. Braithwaite, R. L., & Lythcott, N. (1989). Community empowerment as a strategy for health promotion for Black and other minority populations. *Journal of the American Medical Association, 261,* 282–283.
49. Dossa, P. A. (1992). Ethnography as narrative discourse: Community integration of people with developmental disabilities. *Rehabilitation Research, 15,* 1–14.
50. Florin, P., Wandersman, A. (1990). An introduction to citizen participation, voluntary organizations, and community development: Insights for empowerment through research. *American Journal of Community Psychology, 18,* 41–54.
51. Aryeetey, E. B. D. (1998). Consultative processes in community development in Northern Ghana. *Community Development Journal, 33*(4), 301–313.
52. Campbell, M., Copeland, B., & Tate, B. (1998). Taking the standpoint of people with disabilities in research: experiences with participation. *Canadian Journal of Rehabilitation, 12*(2), 95–104.
53. Bird, S. M., Wiles, J. L., Okalik, L., Kilabuk, J., & Egeland, G. M. (2008). Living with diabetes on Baffin Island: Inuit storytellers share their experiences. *Canadian Journal of Public Health, 99(1),* 17–21.
54. Korten, D. (1984). People-centered development: Toward a framework. In D. Korten & R. Klauss (Ed.), *People-centered development: Contributions toward theory and planning frameworks.* West Hartford, CT: Kumarian.
55. Krogh, K. (1998). A conceptual framework of community partnerships: Perspectives of people with disabilities on power, beliefs and values. *Canadian Journal of Rehabilitation, 12(2),* 123–134.
56. Zimmerman, M. A., & Rappaport, J. (1988). Citizen participation, perceived control, and psychological empowerment. *American Journal of Community Psychology, 16,* 725–750.
57. Wallerstein, N., & Berstein, E. (1994). Introduction to community empowerment, participatory education, and health. *Health Education Quarterly, 21,* 141–148.
58. Mulenga, D. C. (1994). Participatory research for a radical community development. *Australian Journal of Adult and Community Education, 34,* 253–261.
59. Stewart, R., & Bhagwanjee, A. (1999). Promoting group empowerment and self-reliance through participatory research: a case study of people with physical disability. *Disability and Rehabilitation, 21*(7), 338–345.

60. Kuyek, J. N. (1990). *Fighting for hope: Organizing to realize our dreams.* Montreal, PQ: Black Rose Books.
61. Davis, S. M., & Reid, R. (1999). Practicing participatory research in American Indian communities. *American Journal of Clinical Nutrition 69*(4 Suppl), 755S–759S.
62. Diaz, M., & Simmons, R. (1999). When is research participatory? Reflections on a reproductive health project in Brazil. *Journal of Women's Health, 8*(2), 175–184.
63. Freire, P. (1970). *Pedagogy of the oppressed: The letters to Guinea-Bissau.* New York: Continuum Books.
64. Freire, P. (1976). *Education: The practice of freedom.* London: Writers and Readers.
65. Freire, P. (1985). *The politics of education: Culture, power and liberation* (D. Macedo, Trans.). South Hadley, MA: Bergin & Garvey Publishers.
66. Williams, R., Swan, P., Reser, J., & Miller, B. (1992). Australian aborigine communities: Changing oppressive social environments. In D. Thomas & A. Veno (Eds.), *Psychology and social change.* Palmerston North, NZ: Dunmore Press.
67. Davies, L., & Shragge, E. E. (1990). *Bureaucracy and community.* Montreal, PQ: Black Rose Books.
68. Belenky, M. F., Bond, L. A., & Weinstock, S. (1997). *A tradition that has no name: Nurturing the development of people, families, and communities.* New York: Basic Books.
69. Lévi-Strauss, C. (1969). *The elementary structures of kinship.* Boston: Beacon Press.
70. Macaulay, A. C., Delormier, T., McComber, A. M., Cross, E. J., Potvin, L. P., Paradis, G., et al. (1998). Participatory research with native community of Kahnawake creates innovative Code of Research Ethics. *Canadian Journal of Public Health, 89*(2), 105–108.
71. Simpson, L. R. (1998). Aboriginal peoples and the environment. *Canadian Journal of Native Education, 22*(2), 223–237.
72. Scandrett, E. (1999). Sustainable development in communities. *Adults Learning England, 10*(5), 12–14.
73. Affairs UNDoEaS. (1992). *Report of the United Nations Conference on Environment and Development.* New York: United Nations. Report No.: A/CONF.151/26 (Vol. I) Contract No.: Document Number.
74. Kemmis, D. (1990). *Community and the politics of place.* Norman: The University of Oklahoma Press.
75. Bailey, R. (Ed.). (1999). *Earth report 2000: Revisiting the true state of the planet.* New York: McGraw-Hill.
76. Flynn, B. C, Ray, D. W, & Rider, M. S. (1994). Empowering communities: Action research through healthy cities. *Health Education Quarterly, 21,* 395–405.
77. Labonte, R. (1989). Community empowerment: The need for political analysis. *Canadian Journal of Public Health, 80,* 87–88.
78. Mildenberger, V., & Rosenfeld, E. (1992). Strengthening community health services: An exercise in knowledge development. *Health Promotion, 31,* 7–14.
79. Frank, L. D., & Engelke, P. O. (2001). The built environment and human activity patterns: Exploring the impacts of urban form on public health. *Journal of Planning Literature, 16*(2), 202–218.
80. Kieckhefer, R. (2000). *Magic in the Middle Ages* (2nd ed.). Cambridge, MA: Cambridge University Press.
81. Staral, J. M. (2000). Building on mutual goals: The intersection of community practice and church-based organizing. *Journal of Community Practice, 7*(3), 85–95.
82. Shapin, S. (1996). *The scientific revolution.* Chicago: University of Chicago Press.
83. Depoy, P., & Gitlin, L. (1998). *Introduction to research: Multiple strategies for health and human services.* New York: Mosby-Year Book.

84. Jackson, W. (1999). *Methods: Doing social research.* Scarborough, ON: Prentice Hall Canada.
85. Rebeiro, K. L, & Allen, J. (1998). Voluntarism as occupation. *Canadian Journal of Occupational Therapy, 65*(5), 279–285.
86. Ellis, S. J., & Noyes, K. J. (1990). *By the people: A history of Americans as volunteers* (Rev. ed.). San Francisco: Jossey-Bass.
87. Fischer, L. R, & Schaffer, K. B. (1993). *Older volunteers.* Newbury Park, CA: Sage.
88. Najam, A. (1996). Understanding the third sector: Revisiting the prince, the merchant, and the citizen. *Nonprofit Management and Leadership,* 7(2), 203–219.
89. Wuthnow, R. (1991). *Acts of compassion: Caring for others and helping ourselves.* Princeton, NJ: Princeton University Press.
90. Coles, R. (1993). *The call of service: A witness to idealism.* Boston: Houghton Mifflin.
91. Fukuyama, F. (1995). *Trust, the social virtues and creation of prosperity.* New York: The Free Press.
92. Coleman, J. S. (1988). Social capital in the creation of human capital. *American Journal of Sociology, 94*(Supplement), S95–S120.
93. Whiteford, G. (1995). A concrete void: Occupational deprivation and the special needs inmate. *Journal of Occupational Science, 2*(2), 80–81.
94. Whiteford, G. (1997). Occupational deprivation and incarceration. *Journal of Occupational Science: Australia, 4*(3), 126–130.
95. Whiteford, G. (2000). Occupational deprivation: Global challenge in the new millennium. *British Journal of Occupational Therapy, 64*(5), 200–210.
96. Wilcock, A., & Townsend, E. (2000). Occupational justice: Occupational terminology interactive dialogue. *Journal of Occupational Science,* 7(2), 84–86.
97. Levine, F. J., & Rosich, K. J. (1996). *Social causes of violence: Crafting a science agenda.* Washington, D C: American Sociological Association.
98. Rae-Grant, N., McConville, B. J., Fleck, S., Kennedy, J. S., Vaughan, W. T., Steiner, H., et al. (1999, March). Violent behavior in children and youth: Preventive intervention from a psychiatric perspective. *Journal of the American Academy of Child and Adolescent Psychiatry, 38*(3), 235–241.
99. Reiss, A. J., Jr., & Roth, J. A. (Eds.). (1993). *Understanding and preventing violence.* Washington, DC: National Academy Press.
100. MacLeod, A. (1999). *No great mischief.* Toronto, ON: MacLennan and Stewart.
101. Wilson, J. Q., & Kelling, G. L. (1982). Broken windows: The police and neighborhood safety. *The Atlantic Monthly,* 29–38.
102. Perkins, D. D., Florin, P., Rich, R. C., Wandersman, A., & Chavis, D. M. (1990). Participation and the social and physical environment of residential blocks: Crime and community context. *American Journal of Community Psychology, 18,* 83–115.
103. Axelrod, R. (1984). *The evolution of cooperation.* New York: Basic Books4.
104. MacAulay, S. (2001). The community economic development tradition in Eastern Nova Scotia, Canada: Ideological continuities and discontinuities between the Antigonish Movement and the Family of community development corporations. *Community Development Journal, 36(2),* 111–121.
105. Duhl, L. J. (1991). *Social entrepreneurship of change.* New York: Pace University Press.
106. Tonnies, F. (1957/1887). *Community and society* (Gemeinschaft und Gesellschaft). Lansing: Michigan State University Press.
107. Weber, M . (1968/1921). *Economy and society.* New York: Bedminster Press.

CHAPTER 8

Occupational Transitions: Work to Retirement

Hans Jonsson

OBJECTIVES

1. Describe characteristics of occupational transitions.
2. Identify positive and negative meanings of work and attitudes toward retirement.
3. Describe three different directions evident in narratives about retirement.
4. Identify common changes in the rhythm of life and meaning of occupations after retirement.
5. Discuss the six characteristics of engaging occupations in retirement.
6. Examine images of retirement in the media.

KEY WORDS

Life transitions
Occupational transitions
Retirement
Engaging occupation
Narrative methodology
Narrative slope
Narrative plot
Freedom
Occupational balance
Occupational rhythm
Meaning

CHAPTER PROFILE

This chapter considers occupational transitions that have a major impact on what people do and how they organize their time. Retirement as an occupational transition is studied as a major transition of ordinary life in the Western world. Phenomena

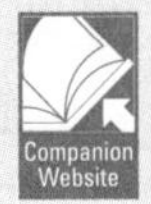

www.prenhall.com/christiansen

The Internet provides an exciting means for interacting with this textbook and for enhancing your understanding of humans' experiences with occupations and the organization of occupations in society. Use the address above to access the interactive Companion Website created specifically to accompany this book. Here you will find an array of self-study material designed to help you gain a richer understanding of the concepts presented in this chapter.

like the meaning of occupations, rhythm of daily life, and the relationship between inner motivation and external expectations/demands are explored through this chapter. The presence or absence of an engaging occupation is analyzed as a key determinant for experiencing satisfying occupational patterns in retirement and is also discussed in more general terms. The chapter ends with a discussion of cultural images of retirement and how they might mirror and shape expectations and attitudes in society.

INTRODUCTION

An occupational transition can be defined as a major change in the occupational repertoire of a person in which one or several occupations change, disappear, and/or are replaced with others. There are many transitions in the life course, and some of them have a major influence on what people do and how they organize their daily living. Transitions can be expected and awaited, such as when a student becomes a worker or a parent leaves work and becomes the caregiver of a newborn child. They can also be unexpected and unplanned, such as unexpectedly becoming unemployed or experiencing a disease or accident resulting in a chronic disability that will heavily influence daily living. A transition can be expected and desired, or it may be unexpected and feared in different combinations. On the one hand, different occupational transitions have characteristics that are unique. On the other hand, significant transitions in people's lives share some common characteristics.

This chapter focuses on one type of major transition: the transition from worker to retiree, and is based on a seven-year longitudinal study in Stockholm, Sweden (1). Thirty-two participants were interviewed when they were 63 to 64 years of age and working at least half time. This was followed with interviews with the same persons at age 66 to 67 ($n = 29$) and at age 70 to 71 ($n = 26$). The participants varied in gender, marital status, blue- or white-collar work, and full- or part-time work, as shown in Table 8-1 ■.

The collected interview data were transcribed and analyzed using narrative (2, 3) and constant comparative methods (4). One study was focused on the anticipation of retirement from the perspective of being a worker (5). Two studies were focused on the experiences and narratives that were told when the participants were newly retired (6, 7). One study analyzed the narratives of the participants when they were established retirees (8).

TABLE 8-1 *Demographic Characteristics of Participants*

Total	Men	Women	Living in Partnership	Living Alone	Workers Blue Collar	Lower White Collar	Higher White Collar	Working Full-time	Working Part-time
32	16	16	19	13	11	15	6	14	18

RETIREMENT AS AN OCCUPATIONAL TRANSITION

From an occupational perspective, retirement can be seen as the exit of a person from one established occupational form (9, 10), paid work, that has been occupying and organizing time and space in that person's life for many years. For the generation on which the studies in this thesis focus (i.e., those born in the late 1920s), paid work had been a part of their lives for about 50 years. Many participants said that they began to work at about 12 to 13 years of age and had worked continuously since then. The end of this occupational form in an individual's life is accompanied by the loss of the personal values and meanings (9, 10), both positive and negative, that each individual finds in paid work. The end of this large occupational form greatly affects the whole organization of the individual's occupational pattern (11); it opens new possibilities for a person to expand performance of other already practiced occupations and to take up new ones. A new pattern will develop (12, 13, 14) in which time and space are organized without the presence of paid work. This is not a sudden change but a process of adaptation over time (15) for individuals who go into new circumstances, anticipating this change in a certain way, then experiencing it, and finding (or not) ways of adapting to the new circumstances.

Attitudes toward Retirement

Studies in Europe and North America show that a great majority of people have a positive attitude toward their retirement and report a basically positive experience (16–19). Given this, it is important to note that some people report difficulties adapting to their life as full-time retirees. A study by Andersson in Sweden showed, for example, that about one-third would have liked to continue to work full or part time if they could have decided for themselves (16). A survey in the United States showed that a large majority wished to have the possibility to work part time (20). Importantly, other factors such as enjoyment, challenge, and social contacts were reported as the most important reasons for this attitude (20, 21). Although most statistical studies show that a majority are positive toward retirement as well as being retired, maybe the most important finding is that attitudes differ greatly. This finding is also confirmed in qualitative studies about retirement. A 70-year-old woman reported her retirement transition in this way:

> Now when I look back to the period of my retirement it was really like a part of me was amputated. (22)

She told how, at work, she was a special person who was treated in a certain way that did not correspond to the way she was treated in the rest of her life. When work no longer was a part of her life, she did not feel like a complete person any longer. This woman told a story of retirement that was connected to losses in life quality. Some people will recognize themselves in such a description, but not all. A person who had been retired for about a year told the following story:

> "Well I had prepared myself for this time, planned what to do and what activities to be engaged in. And everything has worked as I have thought it would be."(1)

This man described retirement as a period in his life where he could increase his engagement in occupations that really interested him.

As negative and positive experiences of retirement exist parallel to each other, it is important that theories and models for working with retirees incorporate such differences. Traditionally, theories in gerontology have been critiqued because they do not readily incorporate big differences between individuals (23, 24, 25) and because they may or may not describe and understand the variety in retirement experiences.

In the following sections we further examine retirement experiences as they were narrated in this author's longitudinal study on retirement (1).

Leaving Work for Retirement—What Are You Leaving?

The first question concerned the values of work as they were expressed while those studied were still working but approaching retirement. In the first part of the study, the participants were 63 years of age, and their retirement was coming in one to two years (5). Retirement was, first and foremost for these participants, defined as being no longer working. Narratives about retirement were invariably stories about "not working." Consequently, to understand retirement, it was important to understand what leaving work meant for the participants by looking at how persons interpreted their work. A number of positive and negative meanings could be seen in the narratives that could be sorted into five different categories regarding the meaning of work: social, doing, organization, material, and productivity (see Figure 8-1 ■).

Regarding values, participants talked about the positive aspects of work life by mentioning the following factors: social contact and fellowship, being part of a larger whole, use of one's knowledge and capacities, having something to do, earning one's income, being productive, freedom and autonomy in work, doing something useful, and having an external structure.

Social contact and fellowship, in the sense of being part of a working team, was the factor mentioned most frequently as a positive value of work. One person characterized this element of work as "*working and toiling together with the others, having fun together.*" Another fondly referred to the teamwork:

> The discussions, the problem solving, the eagerness to find something good, to convince someone of something, balances between different wills . . . to get people to come together for something that produces a result.

When the participants talked about negative aspects of work life, they mentioned the following factors: uninteresting work and boring routines, negative changes affecting the workplace structure and staff, diversion of energy away from preferred activities, stress and the burden of responsibility, and the rigidity of the external structure of working.

The most frequently mentioned negative factor of work was the lack of freedom due to the work routine. Four persons cited undesirable changes in the structure and staff at work (i.e., reorganization and structural changes connected to ownership

POSITIVE MEANINGS	CATEGORIES	NEGATIVE MEANINGS
• Having social contact and fellowship	**Social**	• Having unwanted social contacts
• Making use of your knowledge and capacities • Having something to do	**Doing**	• Experiencing boring routines, uninteresting tasks • Experiencing stressful, unwished for responsibility
• Giving life a preferred external structure • Having freedom and autonomy in work	**Organization**	• Giving life an unpreferred external structure • Experiencing stressful changes in structure and staff • Perceiving external stressors
• Experiencing economic importance	**Material/Economic**	• Experiencing no economic benefit or using scarce resources
• Doing something useful and being needed • Being part of a bigger whole	**Productivity**	• Using energy that one would like to be placed elsewhere

FIGURE 8-1 Meanings of work as expressed by 32 working Swedish persons at the age of 63.

changes) as reasons for work being undesirable overall. As one person noted, *"Thanks to the new owners, . . . I will enjoy leaving."*

These participants had mixed thoughts and feelings about the structure created by work. As noted earlier, lack of freedom was the most commonly mentioned negative aspect of work. Yet, several others found the structure to be valuable. As one person expressed, work is "*something permanent, something time-bound . . . [that] I and people in general need.*" Another person pointed out the importance of having to get up and off to work:

> If I'm at home I feel a little out of sorts . . . I stay in bed until nine, half past nine, maybe ten. And then nothing is really done. . . . So I want to get up.

> I feel now that I have leisure all the time. I guess when one is a retiree this is the only time in life one really owns.

After turning 60, many of the participants described working life as requiring more energy. One did not have the same total capacity as in earlier years. So work took more of a person's total energy, and evenings and weekends were more likely spent in rest and recovery from work. This was put in contrast to earlier years in which the participants had the stamina and energy to do other activities besides work. From that perspective most of the participants were looking forward to retirement. Once one enters retirement the new freedom is appreciated. You own your time. But at the same time there is another side of this freedom in the analysis called the *paradox of freedom.* Everything is up to oneself, and no one expects anything from you. A woman who went from full-time work to full-time retirement expressed the following:

> When I now look backwards at my retirement I really would have liked to stepwise withdraw from work—worked for a couple of hours and then decrease it. For one really misses the actual doing in work. And also the social part with colleagues and all the chats we had. I think I miss that very much.

A man who had a job as a manager felt the need for something more organized:

> I would very, very, very much like to have a small job. Not like in the old company but some small job that I can manage. Like cutting the lawn or a hedge. Or go out with old people for a walk or shopping.

Participants found it difficult to replace the externally created routines that employment generated, when they had to manage new routines themselves. This can be exemplified by a man who started a small consulting business after retirement; he found himself having difficulties in being the ruler of his own time:

> It has been hard to create new work routines. Maybe I should call it life routines. . . . In 25 years I knew what ruled me and what I ruled. And I was very pleased and life rolled on. But now—to find a new life-discipline to do the things I want and have imposed on myself to do takes time and I'm not sure if I'm ready for that yet.

One could look at this paradox of freedom as going from one imbalance in one's occupational life as a worker to another imbalance as a retiree. As a worker, some participants felt an imbalance in which work took too much of their energy and engagement. As a retiree, they felt an imbalance in which too much time was available, requiring decisions to occupy time that were not needed during work. Retirement brought a lack of interaction with other people and institutions that previously created demands and expectations for time and energy. The freedom that the subjects looked forward to in retirement was often not experienced as real freedom. One could say that to experience freedom required having to give away a part of the freedom. One participant, who had chosen to continue to work about 10 hours a week, expressed it in this way:

> . . . still I feel that I have my free-time, it's my own. I can use it—and I do not want to use it for free-time—I want to use it for activity [referring to his job]. That's a very nice feeling, that's fantastic. Yes, that's freedom.

The freedom that subjects had anticipated could—when reached—be experienced in a paradoxical way. A woman expressed that structuring time was very energy demanding, and that everything was up to herself. Every day she had to push herself, telling herself that she should do this, or do that, motivating herself in an inner dialogue. To not have demands and expectations could also be experienced as stressful. It resulted in an imbalance between inner motivation and external demands and expectations.

Gliding into a Slower Rhythm in Life

The participants described how during the first year as a retiree they had adopted a slower rhythm of daily life. Morning was described as the period during the day when this was most apparent. Eating breakfast and reading the paper page by page took almost all morning. The transformation in rhythm was described as a gliding process, an adjustment that they just went into without actually being aware of it, before or during this process. Some participants were surprised when they reflected on the present situation compared with the situation before retirement. These participants asked themselves how they ever had the time to do the things they needed and wanted to do, when they were working. One participant demonstrated her reflection on the change of rhythm and revealed a perplexing experience of the time available:

> When I'm going to do something today it takes a whole day. Before I had the time to do several things.

It seems that a new time structure is created after retirement. This transition was described as a gradual process that led to a slower rhythm of life. Most of the participants described this change in positive terms, as a feeling of ownership of one's day. Expressions like, *"It is calmer now"* and *"It's less stressful"* were used to describe the new rhythm. However some participants experienced their new pace as a slower rhythm that caused emptiness that they didn't know how to fill. A few had hoped to fill time with meaningful occupations, but had found this difficult to realize.

This sheds light on another finding related to temporal adaptation, namely the participants' plans for new occupations in retirement. Most of the participants had anticipated that they would take up new occupations or resume occupations from their younger days, but these were still mostly possible plans, rather than a reality. And there were no evident health problems or economic reasons for not realizing these possible plans. One participant stated: "Yes I have been thinking of it but no action so far." When the participants reflected on this, they expressed surprise about not having the time to realize their plans. The finding that only a few participants took up new occupations can be related to the transformation into a slower rhythm in daily life. When the participants were working, they expected they would have a lot of available time in retirement to perform new occupations. Their slowed rhythm of daily life, however, meant that available time for taking up new occupations also decreased. A slower rhythm meant that more time was now spent on performing each occupation, and thoughts of taking up new occupations remained largely as ideas and intentions.

Change in Meaning

Within the new temporal structure, some participants described a changed meaning of occupations or difficulties in experiencing the same meaning as before retirement. One man who worked full time four days a week before retirement reported a change of meaning in going to his summer cottage:

> It was a real peak to get out to the summer cottage on Thursday evenings after you had worked four days. I had the whole weekend to relax. Now it's not the same any longer. I don't have the same feeling for it. . . . It doesn't matter if it's Sunday now we don't have to go into town. And the differences between weekend and the other days have disappeared.

This describes a change in meaning for an old and well-known occupation when it was performed in another occupational structure. The structure that work had created before retirement influenced the meaning experienced in other occupations—one occupation created important conditions for others. This first became obvious for individuals when the old occupation was carried out in the new daily structure.

The significant meanings given to times and days of the week, provided by an organized, work-structured life were discovered only when work routines were lost. One man who, before retirement, had been longing for the day when he could leave his work said:

> It's a special life one lives when you have this, with work in the morning and the weekends free. And there are Monday mornings and all that. And as all of that has gone I really miss it. Now the days don't matter any longer—if it's Monday morning or Friday evening.

He found himself (to his surprise) missing the routines of working life in retirement.

Two Types of Retirement Narratives—to Get Time or to Kill Time

At the end of the longitudinal project to study retirement, the narratives gathered when people were new retirees were compared to their narratives as established retirees according to basic characteristics of the narratives (8). The basic plot of the narrative was especially in focus in this analysis. Two types of narratives were found as illustrated in Figure 8-2 ■.

One type was basically flat in its unfolding story line, one occupation after another, narrated without larger engagement or intensity. The story of a day, or a week was to get time going, to kill time as the basic plot of the narrative. One participant who told such a narrative said:

> And then I'll go and take a cup of coffee. So I'll walk around in town for a while. Then I'll take the metro home again. That will make this day pass. You can travel around a bit. You've got to find something to make the time pass.

The other type of narrative was fluctuating. One occupation after another was narrated also in this story but with fluctuation in engagement and intensity. Certain

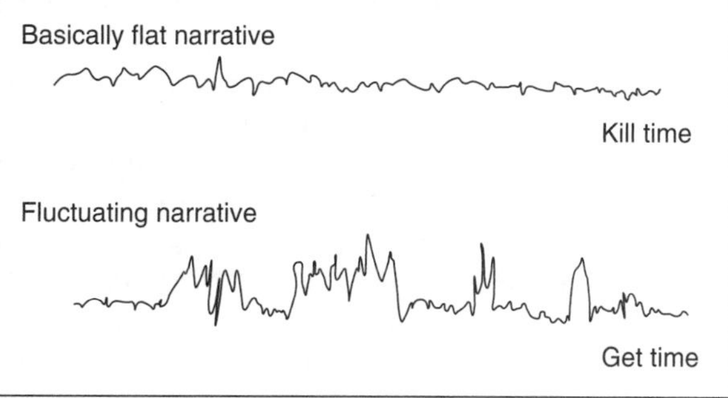

FIGURE 8-2 Two types of narrative with two different plots when describing occupation.

types of occupations were told in an engaging and intensive way. Actually the story was much more organized with these types of occupation in focus. The other occupations were more necessary or complementary occupations. The story line of the narrative was to do the necessary occupations that one had to do, and the plot was to get time for other types of occupations. As one woman said, her important occupations were regularly on Thursdays:

> . . . it's Thursday almost everyday. Thursday, then after only a few days it's Thursday again.

Occupations that went beyond ordinary daily occupations and that evoked a depth of passion or feeling that made them stand out in the participants' narratives were called **engaging occupations.** Engaging occupations were sometimes connected to participants' former work, such as consulting part time in the field where one once worked full time. An engaging occupation could also be a long-term leisure interest that had always been meaningful or exciting for the participant, such as hiking in the mountains. Sometimes engaging occupations were things done with family, such as taking regular care of grandchildren or older relatives.

ENGAGING OCCUPATION FOR A GOOD LIFE AS A RETIREE

The presence or absence of engaging occupations appears to be the main determinant of whether participants were able to achieve positive life experiences as retirees. Those who had difficulty adjusting to retirement had narratives in common: they lacked occupation that was truly engaging. Engaging occupations were done with great commitment, enthusiasm, perseverance, and passion. Participants talked about them in a very emotional way, and discussion of their engaging occupations dominated their narratives. Engaging occupations were a special type of occupation that stood out from the other things a person did. From the participants' stories, we found six constituents common to engaging occupations (8).

Infused with Positive Meaning

An engaging occupation is experienced as highly meaningful and important in several respects. For example, some participants described engaging occupations as especially enjoyable, interesting, and challenging. One participant, who had a full-time pension and who now worked on a variety of minor repair jobs, called this his hobby and said: "*I think it's fun and you meet people and come to talk with them.*" Others stressed how the engaging occupation provided valued social contacts. One, who took care of elderly relatives, highly valued that occupation. Another helped her daughter with her business for the same reasons. A third who engaged in volunteer work for the elderly found that highly meaningful. Engaging occupations sometimes reaffirmed a person's worth or identity. In referring to her consulting and why she found it so engaging, a participant remarked, "*One is quite happy when one is needed.*" In contrast, a participant, who lacked such an occupation in her life, gave one of the most telling descriptions of the meaning of an engaging occupation. She indicated that what she really wanted and did not have was "*something to take a real bite on.*"

Intensity

Engaging occupations involve intense participation. Intensity is a function of two variables: length of involvement and regularity of involvement. Engaging occupations were typically those that the participant did with some sort of regularity over the week. They were not sporadic. Moreover, engaging occupations were also long term in nature, meaning that there was often a long history of involvement that the participant expected to continue on a regular basis in the future.

A Coherent Set of Activities

An engaging occupation consists of a set of activities that cohere or constitute an interrelated whole. The occupation might begin as a single activity, but over time it becomes more intense and involves interrelated activities and projects. For example, one participant belonged to a club for hiking in the mountain area. However, his involvement went well beyond hiking. He attended regular boarding meetings and was assigned responsibility for the club office. He also went out for longer walks in the mountains and took a lot of photographic slides. In the wintertime, he was invited to lecture in club meetings and retiree organizations.

Goes beyond Personal Pleasure

The involvement in an engaging occupation evolves into a commitment or responsibility. Therefore, engaging occupations are often seen as personal duties. The dutiful nature of such occupations was evident in participants' descriptions of how not all aspects of engaging in the occupation were pleasurable. In fact, the very nature of duty seemed to be connected to a willingness to fulfill the required duties, whether or not one actually felt like it. Commitment to one's duty meant taking the bad with the good. One example was one participant's engagement in the activities of a civic club. In the club, he was responsible for planning and organizing a social activity one evening a week. He said that he sometimes felt this assignment was quite "heavy," but at the same time, he accepted it as a responsibility that he highly appreciated, given that it was for the benefit of older and experienced members of the club.

Occupational Community

Engaging occupations ordinarily involve at least some connection to a community of people who shared a common interest in the occupation. Discussions about the occupation, planning future involvement, problem solving related to the occupation, and giving and taking advice from others about how to do the occupation were part and parcel of the sense of community. Even for those occupations, where most of the time was spent alone, this dimension of being involved in a community that shared interest in the occupation was important.

Analogues to Work

Engaging occupations may very well include work for payment. But even without payment, an engaging occupation may take on many of the features of work in the participant's experience, and the person may continue to think and talk about it as work. Although the engaging occupation is ordinarily no longer done as a means of earning a living, it is done with the same kind of seriousness and commitment formerly given to work. One participant, who was formerly a manager, indicated that when his wife (who was still employed) asks him what he has done for the day, he replies: "*I have been at my work. I have been on the golf course. We pros, we are stuck there on the golf course, you know.*" When participants talked about their engaging occupations and tried to explain how complex they were and how they involved several different activities and required ongoing commitment, they often resorted to the analogy or metaphor of work to explain their involvement. Comments that illustrate this analogy were *"One could say that I work at my leisure time"* and *"It's like a sort of work."*

In summary, the analysis drew out six constituents in the narratives of engaging occupations. Not all narratives about engaging occupations had all six constituents, but a majority of them did. In contrast, narratives without engaging occupations were partly about finding meaningful things to do. One participant who lacked engaging occupations told the following story when she went to the local hospital, met a doctor, and watched how occupied and stressed all staff seemed to be:

> . . . then I said can't you find a job for me? I can come down here and take care of the patients until you have time for them, or be of help for the nurses. I'll be happy to work for free. As long as I can have something to do.

One participant who, before retirement, told a narrative about work as his engaging occupation, characterized his experience in retirement as follows:

> You try to prepare yourself, inside your head, for the change. But when it's there, you have a feeling that it's not real. You still feel young, you know, with much left to give. . . . It is a whole new experience. It's like life itself sort of ends! You have worked for 50, 52 years since you were 12, 13 years old.

This participant experienced a larger loss of meaning than expected. His expectation that he would be able to occasionally work for his employer turned out not to be realistic. This disappointed him, and he felt that he "*did not belong anywhere.*" When asked what he did in retirement, he said: "*I don't do anything, not a damn thing.*" In actuality, he had tried some new occupations, but he described them as merely making the time pass.

CULTURAL IMAGES OF RETIREMENT

What types of images exist in society about retirement and, more importantly, about a good life in retirement? Cultural images can be seen as mirroring as well as shaping attitudes and preunderstandings of different phenomena in the society. What types of preunderstanding are put forward in the public arena of retirement? To conclude, the chapter provides some cultural images from different countries in Europe and from the United States. Without comment from the author, readers are encouraged to reflect on them in relation to what has been reported from this longitudinal study of retirement. Where copyright prohibits publication of some of the actual cards/photos, they are described.

The first example is from **Sweden,** where an advertisement can be seen in contemporary media about the importance to start savings for retirement funds.

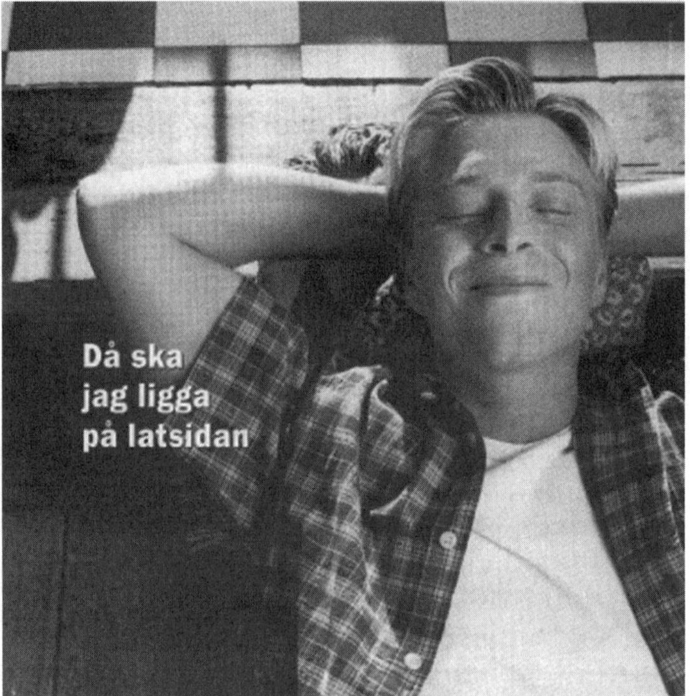

Drömmer du också om ett avspänt pensionärsliv?

Ett pensionssparande hos oss på Folksam kan ge dig både frihet och möjligheter. I drygt 90 år har vi framgångsrikt arbetat med ett enda mål för ögonen – att få våra kunders pengar att växa. Vi kan det här jobbet.

Förutom vår långa erfarenhet har du nytta av att vi ägs av våra kunder. De vinster vi gör kommer våra kunder till del, bland annat i form av låga avgifter på fondsparande.

Hos oss kan du välja bland många olika sparformer. Ring 020-99 10 20 så hjälps vi åt att hitta den bästa lösningen för dig. Du kan också kontakta närmaste Folksamkontor. Välkommen!

www.folksam.se

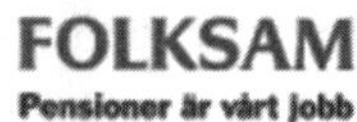

Published with permission from the Swedish Insurance company Folksam. Photographer: Elisabeth Ohlson-Wallin.

The text in the picture says:

"Then I'll really be on the lazy side."

The text below the photo starts with:

"Do you also dream about a relaxed retirement life?"

The second example is from The Netherlands, with a celebration card of retirement:

First page	**Second page**
Text: *Before retirement* Illustration: You see a drawing of a persons sitting behind a computer with tons of paper on the desk almost hiding the person. Some papers are falling down.	Text: *In retirement!* *We wish you luck!* Illustration: You see a man sleeping in a hammock tied to a palm tree and with a drink in the sand below

A third example comes from the United Kingdom, with another celebration card:

First page	**Second page**
Text: *Congratulations on your retirement* Illustration: You see photo of a child standing with a blanket in his/her hand	Text: *... and go to bed without having done it!*

A fourth example is from the United States, with an invitation card to a retirement celebration:

Text:
XXX will now be **GONE FISHIN'!**
Join us in honor of XXX on the occasion of his retirement
[Text continues with date and place of the occasion]

The fifth example is also from the United States, with a celebration card:

First page	**Second page**
Illustration: An abstract drawing with a quote from William Lyon Phelps:	Text:
Text: *"The belief that youth is the happiest time of life is founded upon a fallacy. The happiest person is the person who thinks the most interesting thoughts, and we grow happier as we grow older."*	*Wish you a rich and rewarding retirement*

Finally the sixth example is from Germany, with a celebration card:

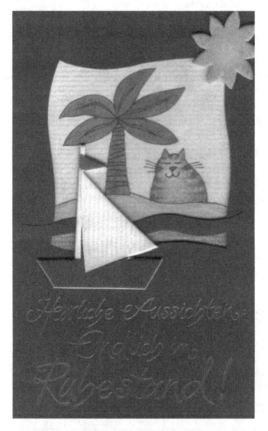

Published with permission from Herlitz PBs Aktiengesellschaft, Berlin, Germany.
The text on the German card reads: *Wonderful future views: Finally in retirement!*

CHAPTER SUMMARY

Studying retirement from an occupational perspective has created knowledge about mechanisms that can occur in any occupational transition. These include changes in the structure of time, changes in the meaning of different occupations or the same occupations, changes in social interaction, and changes in feelings about self worth. The concept of engaging occupation, described as occupational pursuits having several key dimensions including intensity, coherence, socialization, and commitment, was analyzed as an important factor connected to the experience of a good life as a retiree. Research on retirement transitions leads to the conclusion that the concept of engaging occupation not only describes something important about having a good life in retirement; it may also describe a key element of a good life in general.

STUDY GUIDE

Study Guide Author: Julie Bass Haugen

Summary of Main Points

The transition from work to retirement is one of several major life transitions that affects occupational engagement in Western societies. This chapter examined important findings about retirement that emerged from the qualitative narratives in a longitudinal study. One finding from the study is that individuals (and particular social groups) hold various positive and/or negative meanings about work. These perceptions about work life may in turn influence perceptions of retirement. Another finding is that the rhythm and routines of life vary greatly with and without the imposed structure of a work week. Planning for a fulfilling retirement should include development of engaging occupations. Engaging occupations have specific qualities that evoke strong feelings and may be fully described in narratives.

Application to Occupational Therapy

The occupational transition from paid work to retirement is a major area of concern and interest for occupational therapists. Many individuals, groups, or whole communities encountered by occupational therapists may be transitioning from work to retirement; this change may be planned or unexpected due to various medical or social conditions. Retirement will entail new occupations, routines, social networks, and environments. Feelings about the transition will be shaped by the meanings of work for the person and the occupational opportunities available in retirement. Accurate assessment and effective intervention planning will draw on occupational therapists' lifespan perspective on occupational engagement, with an understanding of socio-cultural, political and other environmental conditions, and with understanding and skills in enabling adaptation of lifestyles, educating communities about occupational possibilities in retirement. Occupational therapists may also draw on skills in designing retirement programs and in designing communities, homes, and other spaces to ensure the emotional, cultural and physical inclusion of retired persons. Health promotion is becoming a larger part of occupational therapy practice. Many health-promotion initiatives focus on health and wellness issues for older adults. An understanding of retirement as a major life transition will enable occupational therapy practitioners to develop effective health-promotion programs. Education on the process of retirement may help older adults develop engaging occupations and adapt to the new rhythm of life that is part of retirement.

Individual Learning Activities

1. Identify two to three engaging occupations that you would be interested in during retirement.
   a. Describe the personal meaning of these occupations.
   b. Discuss the six characteristics of engaging occupations as it relates to your selected occupations.
2. Interview a person who is retired and write a paper that includes the following
   a. What were the positive and negative meanings of work for this person?
   b. How did the rhythm of life change for this person after retirement?
   c. What are some engaging occupations that are important to this person?

Group Learning Activity

Form groups of three to four members and investigate evidence and resources for a specific topic related to retirement (You may use the Web links provided in this chapter as a starting point). Share your findings with others in a presentation. Examples include

a. How do the characteristics of retirement vary in different countries and cultures?
b. What factors contribute to improve health and quality of life in older adults? What implications does this have for occupations?
c. What community and Internet resources are available to older adults for retirement planning?
d. What characteristics of the environment support or limit involvement in engaging occupations?

Study Questions

1. Occupational transitions include all of the following EXCEPT:
   a. Minor changes in occupational repertoire of activities
   b. Research questions
   c. Ways of understanding
   d. Intellectual development
2. Retirement was described as a sudden change requiring adaptation.
   a. True
   b. False

3. The factor that was most frequently described as a positive value for work was
   a. Salary
   b. Routine
   c. Social contact and fellowship
   d. Physical activity
4. The paradox of freedom was defined as
   a. Going from an imbalance of too many demands in work to an imbalance of too few demands in retirement
   b. Freedom of time in retirement is used for medical appointments
   c. New people place demands on time in retirement
   d. External demands are fewer in work
5. The meanings associated with times and days were most evident when the work routines were lost
   a. True
   b. False

REFERENCES

1. Jonsson, H. (2000). *Anticipating, experiencing and valuing the transition from worker to retiree: A longitudinal study of retirement as an occupational transition.* Doctoral dissertation, Department of clinical neuroscience, occupational therapy and elderly care research, Division of occupational therapy, Karolinska Institutet, Sweden.
2. Gergen, K. J. (1994). *Realities and relationships: Soundings in social construction.* Cambridge: Harvard University Press.
3. Gergen, K. J., & Gergen, M. M. (1988). Narrative and the self as relationship. In L. Berkowitz (Ed.), *Advances in experimental social psychology,* 17–56. San Diego, CA: Academic Press.
4. Bogdan, R. C., & Bilken, S. K. (1992). *Qualitative research for education—An introduction to theory and methods (2nd ed.).* Needham Heights, MA: Allyn and Bacon.
5. Jonsson, H., Kielhofner, G., & Borell, B. (1997), Anticipating retirement: The formation of narratives concerning an occupational transition. *American Journal of Occupational Therapy 51(1),* 49–56.
6. Jonsson, H., Borell, L., & Sadlo, G. (2000). Retirement: An occupational transition with consequences on temporality, rhythm and balance. *Journal of Occupational Science, 7,* 5–13.
7. Jonsson, H., Josephsson, S., & Kielhofner, G. (2001) Evolving narratives in the course of retirement. *American Journal of Occupational Therapy, 54,* 463–476.
8. Jonsson, H., Josephsson, S., & Kielhofner, G. (2001) Narratives and experience in an occupational transition: A longitudinal study of the retirement process. *American Journal of Occupational Therapy, 55,* 424–432.
9. Nelson, D. L. (1988). Occupation: Form and performance. *American Journal of Occupational Therapy, 42,* 633–641.

10. Nelson, D. L. (1996). Therapeutic occupation: A definition. *American Journal of Occupational Therapy, 50,* 775–782.
11. Kielhofner, G. (1995). *A model of human occupation: Theory and application (2nd ed.).* Baltimore: Williams & Wilkins.
12. Christiansen, C. H. (1996). Three perspectives on balance in occupation. In R. Zemke & F. Clark (Eds.), *Occupational science: The evolving discipline (pp. 431–451).* Philadelphia: F. A. Davis Company.
13. Meyer, A. (1922). The philosophy of occupational therapy. *Archives of Occupational Therapy 1:1. Reprinted: American Journal of Occupational Therapy, 31,* 639–642.
14. Reilly, M. (1966). A psychiatric occupational therapy program as a teaching model. *American Journal of Occupational Therapy, 20,* 61–67.
15. Schultz, S., & Schkade, J. (1997). Adaptation. In C. Christiansen & C. Baum (Eds.), *Occupational therapy: Enabling function and well-being (2nd ed., pp. 459–481).* Thorofare NJ: Slack, Inc.
16. Andersson, L. (1993). *Äldre i Sverige och Europa (Elderly in Sweden and in Europe).* Stockholm: Socialstyrelsen.
17. Floyd, F. J., Haynes, S. N., Doll, E. R., Winemiller, D., Lemsky, C., Burgy, T. M., Werle, M., & Heilman, N. (1992). Assessing retirement satisfaction and perceptions of retirement experiences. *Psychology and Aging, 7,* 609–621.
18. Richardson, V., & Kilty, K. M. (1991). Adjustment to retirement: Continuity vs. discontinuity. *International Journal of Aging and Human Development, 33,* 151–169.
19. SOU, (1985). Statens Offentliga Utredningar, 31: Dagens äldre—fakta kring levnadsförhållanden (Older people today—facts about living conditions). Stockholm: Norstedts Tryckeri.
20. Associated Press. (2000, September 29). *Survey from the Center for Survey Research and Analysis.* Storrs: University of Connecticut.
21. Jonsson, H., Andersson, L. (1999). Attitudes to Work and Retirement—Generalization or Diversity? *Scandinavian Journal of Occupational Therapy, 6,* 29–35.
22. Jonsson, H. (2005). Pensioneringsprocessen i ett aktivitetsperspektiv (The retirement process in an occupational perspective). In H. J. Bendixen, T. Borg, E. F. Pedersen, & U. Altenborg, (Eds.), *Aktivitetsvidenskab i et nordisk perspektiv (Occupational science in a Nordic perspective).* Copenhagen: FADL's forlag.
23. Calasanti, T. M. (1993). Bringing in diversity: Toward an inclusive theory of retirement. *Journal of Aging Studies, 7,* 133–150.
24. Jonsson, H. (1993). The retirement process in an occupational perspective: A review of literature and theories. *Physical & Occupational Therapy in Geriatrics, 11,* 15–34.
25. Light, J. M., Grigsby, J. S., & Bligh, M. C. (1996). Aging and heterogeneity: genetics, social structure, and personality. *Gerontologist, 36,* 165–173.

CHAPTER 9

Occupational Balance and Well-being

Catherine L. Backman

OBJECTIVES

1. Define the concepts of occupational balance, work-life balance, occupational role, role strain, and role balance
2. Summarize the origin and evolution of the concept of occupational balance in contemporary discourse
3. Discuss the relationship of occupational balance to health and well-being

KEY WORDS

Lifestyle balance
Occupational balance
Occupational role
Role balance
Role overload
Role strain
Well-being
Work-life balance
Work-life conflict

CHAPTER PROFILE

The concept of occupational balance is explored in this chapter. People engage in multiple occupations that support different roles in life, and their choices are shaped by the demands of the occupations, the environment, and their personal skills and resources. The extent to which a pattern of occupation is perceived as harmonious, fulfilling, and compatible with one's values is called occupational balance. Related concepts are also discussed, including work-life balance, work-life conflict, and role balance. The relationship between occupational balance, health, and well-being is summarized.

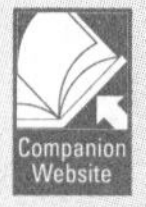

www.prenhall.com/christiansen

The Internet provides an exciting means for interacting with this textbook and for enhancing your understanding of humans' experiences with occupations and the organization of occupations in society. Use the address above to access the interactive Companion Website created specifically to accompany this book. Here you will find an array of self-study material designed to help you gain a richer understanding of the concepts presented in this chapter.

Appreciation is extended to Linda Del Fabro Smith, BSc(OT), MSc(Cand), for assistance updating literature for the initial draft of this chapter.

INTRODUCTION

"Moderation in all things."

Terence, Roman dramatist, c. 185 BC–159 BC

"Moderation in all things" leads to a healthy, happy life. Although this adage captures the fundamental message from the present chapter, it leaves much territory unexplored. Who decides what moderation looks like? And do we really mean *all* things? If not, which things?

People do a lot of different things, or occupations, some of which they value or enjoy more than others. Previous chapters have defined occupation and discussed its scope, from the relatively simple and routine to the more elaborate and carefully planned. Hour-to-hour, day-to-day, and week-to-week, decisions and choices are made to organize tasks and occupations to achieve occupational goals. From time to time people reflect on longer term goals and aspirations and change their pattern of occupational engagement, withdrawing from some occupations and adding others. The extent to which they are able to organize and participate in occupations in a manner congruent with their aspirations and values is referred to as **occupational balance.**

Occupational balance is a perceived state and dynamic process. That is, occupational balance is a subjective, individualized experience that changes over time. People experience occupational balance—we cannot directly observe someone's state of occupational balance, although some behaviors may serve as cues, such as rushing or irritability, suggesting unsatisfactory balance, or an expression of joy or pleasure indicating optimal engagement and balance. Over the life course priorities change, and even within shorter periods of time personal and environmental circumstances dictate priorities. Responding to changing circumstances by making choices about which occupations to do, as well as when, how, and for how long, reflect adjustments made to maintain occupational balance. Sometimes people face competing demands or find themselves doing occupations that misfit their values or beliefs, challenging their ability to effectively plan and manage their lives. When they are able to reorganize these occupations to best match their skills, responsibilities, and priorities, they are more likely to experience a sense of occupational balance. Conversely, an inability to juggle competing demands leads to a state of **occupational imbalance** due to an overabundance of occupations or incompatible occupations. Other people may experience a dearth of occupational opportunity, leading to occupational imbalance of a different sort, arising from lack of participation in meaningful occupation or too much unstructured time. Fluctuations in occupational balance are to be expected in life, reflecting the dynamic nature of occupational engagement. Perceived occupational balance or imbalance influences other perceived states, such as happiness, stress, health, and **well-being.** This chapter discusses the concept of occupational balance and its relationship to well-being.

OCCUPATIONAL BALANCE

Westhorp (1) stated, "This notion of balance in life and in occupations is one that continues to intrigue." Several authors have been similarly intrigued, proposing various theses to describe balance among everyday occupations and its subsequent effect on physical and mental health. The way the balance-related concept is labeled is usually consistent with the underlying assumptions and context for promoting each thesis and may be called occupational balance, life balance, **lifestyle balance**, **work-life balance**, **role balance**, work-family balance, or another term. Selected terms are briefly defined in Table 9-1 ■. The use of so many terms for similar or overlapping concepts has the potential to confuse readers. Consistent with the overall purpose of this book, occupational balance is the predominant concept described in this chapter, with reference to the other terms when drawing on the applicable literature or situating them as contributing to or being distinct from occupational balance. Occupational balance considers a wide range of occupations associated with all aspects of life, including caring for oneself and others, working, playing, learning, socializing, and volunteering, to cite some common categories.

Origins in Occupational Therapy

Although it has been an important tenet underlying the practice of occupational therapy since the beginning of the 20th century, for much of that history occupational balance was more of a philosophical belief than a clearly articulated concept (2). The work-cure prescribed by physicians and followed by early occupational therapists during the mental hygiene movement at the beginning of the 20th century included a balanced regimen of work, play, rest and sleep, and attention to the rhythms of life through activities supervised by pioneering occupational therapists (3, 4). Through

TABLE 9-1 *Occupational Balance and Related Concepts Defined*

Concept	Definition
Occupational balance	Perceived state of satisfactory participation in valued, obligatory, and discretionary activities; occurs when the impact of occupations on one another is harmonious, cohesive, and under control (31, 32).
Lifestyle balance	A consistent pattern of occupations that results in reduced stress and improved health and well-being. Patterns may be viewed on several dimensions, including time allocation, fulfillment of social roles, and meeting psychological needs (4).
Role balance	Satisfactory fulfillment of all valued roles (4).
Work-life balance	Perceived ability to manage individual and family time and perceived conflict in doing so (18).
Occupational imbalance	An individual or group experience in which health and quality of life are compromised because of being overoccupied or underoccupied (8).
Role overload	Having too much to do in the amount of time available; feeling time-crunched (11).
Role strain	Distress or burden arising from excessive demands or insufficient capacity to fulfill the role; capacity includes personal knowledge and skills as well as available resources (financial, educational, social support) (20).
Work-life conflict	Misfit between demands of work and personal/family life. Occurs when the cumulative demands of work and nonwork roles are incompatible such that participation in one role is made more difficult by participation in the other (17). At least three subsets of work-life conflict have been articulated: role overload, interference from family demands to work life, and interference from work demands to family life (11).

the 1980s, emerging theories in occupational therapy reiterated the relationship between occupational balance and health by noting, for example, the fundamental principle that an appropriate balance of self-care, play, work, and rest was necessary to adapt to illness or disability and achieve health. Contemporary occupational therapists continue to refer to a satisfactory balance across the occupational performance areas of self-care, productivity, and leisure as contributing to health (1, 2). However, to some critics, it has become apparent that this view of balance across three categories of occupation is incomplete (1), in part because it reflects a very rudimentary classification of occupation. It also tends to support a simple temporal perspective (time spent in each category) and fails to consider the quality of engagement in occupations, the range of **occupational roles** assumed by individuals, and the relative importance or meaning underlying occupations. Each of these factors influences one's perception of occupational balance. Thus, there is growing curiosity in occupational therapy, extending to occupational science, about the way one's values, culture, and spiritual beliefs shape both the meaning attributed to various occupations (and occupational roles) and occupational choice. However, it is not clear how these factors influence perceptions of occupational balance, other than a general hypothesis that the more meaningful the occupations, the greater likelihood of occupational balance and well-being.

Importantly, Westhorp (1), in her discussion of occupational balance, helps put to rest the myth that "balance" refers to an equal distribution or ideal proportion of time spent in individual occupations or categories of occupation. Instead, occupational balance pertains to a harmonious arrangement of occupations that leads to a sense of well-being. "Harmonious arrangement" is a rather astute metaphor for occupational balance. A satisfying piano composition does not have an equal distribution of key strokes, but rather a harmonious arrangement of high and low notes, some long, short, loud or soft, some in chords, and some alone. The skill of the pianist, quality of the instrument, and presence of an orchestra also influence enjoyment of the piece. So it is with occupational balance. The selection of occupations, quality of experiences when engaged in them, and associated social interactions, as well as time allocated to individual occupations, influence the perception of a harmonious whole or fit with one's goals and values. This view is supported by occupational scientists (5) who purport that occupational balance relates more to qualities than categories of occupation, noting that time use alone is insufficient for explaining and evaluating the construct.

Occupational balance is an individual perception. People are passionate about some occupations and disinterested in others. The combination of occupations that satisfy someone is unique to that person, even if they are shared with others. As people become more skilled, comfortable, and competent with occupations, they will seek new ones as opportunities for personal growth or stepping stones to achieve life goals (1, 6). Just as there is a growing appreciation for eating a balanced diet and ensuring adequate physical activity for good health, an occupational perspective on balance and health recognizes the intrinsic need to "exercise" physical, mental, emotional, and spiritual "muscles" to restore, maintain, or enhance occupational competence. Although some people will consciously plan ways to develop physically, mentally, emotionally, and spiritually, and consequently make choices about which occupations and roles they will pursue, others will not. People's prior occupational experiences and where they are in their life course likely contribute to this consciousness. Even without planning, however, many people will recognize spontaneously occurring moments as influencing their sense of balance, their commitment to certain values, or their enjoyment of a specific role or occupation. An illustration is provided in Box 9-1.

BOX 9-1 Restoring Occupational Balance

A reflective moment contributes to restoration of perceived occupational balance. In this instance, a father and daughter pause on a remote beach during a tropical vacation purposely planned to overcome a period of occupational imbalance (See Figure 9-1 ■). The major contributing factor to occupational imbalance was the father's hip surgery, which resulted in disrupted roles and routines over a prolonged recovery period: a leave from work, changed leisure occupations, and fears about occupational competence.

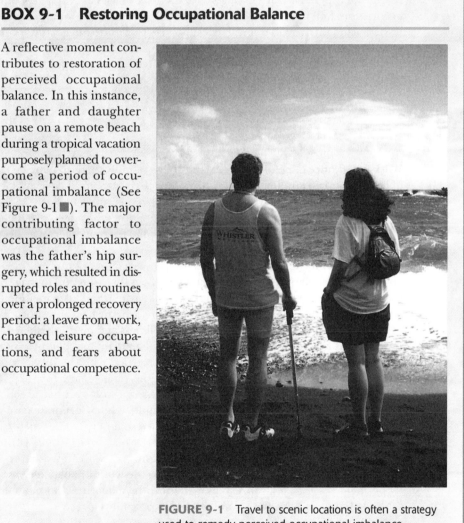

FIGURE 9-1 Travel to scenic locations is often a strategy used to remedy perceived occupational imbalance. (C. Backman)

Occupational Imbalance

The term *occupational imbalance* has been defined as excessive time spent in one area of life at the expense of another (7), or being over- or underoccupied (8). Given the preceding discussion of occupational balance, a broader definition of imbalance is proposed to recognize that occupational imbalance is the lack of congruence across one's occupations, or between occupations and core values. Occupational balance is a relative state and may be visualized on a continuum that is anchored by disharmony and lack of fit (occupational imbalance) at one end, and optimal harmony and congruence at the other (occupational balance), neither of which is a typical experience. Rather, we experience various degrees of occupational balance. Life circumstances and occupational choices result in movement along the continuum, toward greater or lesser balance. Through self-reflection we may recognize our relative position on this hypothetical continuum and seek strategies to resolve occupational imbalance.

Other fields have explored concepts akin to occupational balance and imbalance. The overview that follows demonstrates similarities and differences, beginning with work-life balance and work-life conflict.

WORK-LIFE BALANCE

Work-life balance generally refers to the ability of individuals to manage the demands of both their paid employment and the rest of their lives, most typically, family life (2). Work-life balance differs from occupational balance not only in origin, but also by virtue of its focus on paid employment. Occupational balance considers life's occupations in the broadest sense and therefore applies to all people, regardless of employment, age, roles, or ability.

Throughout the 1980s and 1990s, there was a surge of interest in work-life balance among scholars in organizational psychology, business and managerial sciences, sociology, and vocational counseling. Forces driving this surge included increasing labor force participation by women, declining job satisfaction reported by employees, and the cost associated with stress-related illness and absenteeism (9, 10). Initially perceived as a women's issue, with a focus on balancing paid employment with raising a family (9), work-life balance is now concerned with the broader implications of **work-life conflict** on individuals, corporations, and society (10–12). Responsibilities outside the workplace take on many forms, and role conflict affects all workers, not only women juggling motherhood and employment. Corporate competition and the increasing intensity of a global marketplace that perpetuates the expectation of service 24 hours a day, 7 days a week have increased worker stress (13).

Because the idea of work-life balance resonates with such a large segment of the population (at least, in Western nations), the work-life balance discourse readily permeates the popular press, as evidenced by magazine and newspaper stories, self-help books, Internet sites, and television programs aimed at simplifying life and restoring work-life balance. Consider these newspaper headlines: *A severe case of modern life can make you crazybusy* (14) and *Just 3.5 minutes of eating in lunch "hour"* (15). Both articles describe people overloaded by work and personal demands, with too much to do in the time available to do it. The first headline by Hallowell in the *Vancouver Sun,* based on a psychiatrist's observations, calls this state of being beyond busy "crazybusy." People are distracted, disorganized, overbooked, forgetful, and feeling nothing they do is done well because they are too busy trying to keep up. There is a belief that if they go fast enough, they will create a time when they won't be so busy. As Hallowell noted, this is a "seductive idea, but delusional. The key is to slow down and thrive today" (14). The second headline by Goff also in the *Vancouver Sun* (15) cites time pressures experienced by workers in the United Kingdom (UK), United States (U.S.), and Canada, using their lunch breaks not to eat, but to do "essential" errands (without time to evaluate the extent to which the tasks truly are essential), or to keep up with work demands, reiterating many of the thoughts shared in the crazybusy article. These commentaries are representative of the popular notion of work-life balance, where the problem is perceived as too much to do in too little time and the solution is to simplify, set priorities, and do only those things that are most important.

Being topical in the popular press has the potential to trivialize the seriousness of the problems arising from a state of work-life imbalance. There is ample evidence that imbalance, or work-life conflict, leads to poor health with a subsequent cost to individuals, families, and society. It is estimated that those who experience high work-life conflict are two to three times more likely to experience heart problems, back pain, mental health problems, musculoskeletal injury, infections, and substance abuse than workers who report low work-life conflict (12). These illnesses, in turn, increase the burden on the health-care system. It is, therefore, not surprising that work-life balance "caught the attention of researchers, policy makers, and employers, resulting in the development of a range of employment benefits, legislation and programs aimed at helping people cope" (16, p. 1). Examples of initiatives designed to manage the work-life time bind include flexible work hours, provision of child-care facilities in the workplace, and expansion of workplace occupational health programs to include education on time or stress management. In fact, the governments of many industrialized nations (including the United Kingdom, New Zealand, Australia, Canada, Denmark, Sweden, the Netherlands, France and Belgium) support Web sites with resources for organizations and individuals in support of work-life balance (17). Although some Web sites are largely promotional in nature, aimed at increasing awareness of the need to facilitate work-life balance, others describe legislative changes addressing gender inequities in the labor force, parental leave schemes, sabbaticals, and adjustment of work hours through a statutory workweek.

Interestingly, current work trends suggest a growing polarization of work hours, with increasing proportions of the population working less than 30 hours or more than 40 hours. The standard "full-time" workweek of 35 to 40 hours appears to be declining (5). Additional trends are summarized in Box 9-2.

Based on the assumption that the lack of time to fulfill work and family roles in a satisfactory manner leads to work-life imbalance, several studies have explored whether or not work-life balance improves, predominantly for women, as a result of working part time. Although there is empirical evidence to support part-time work as contributing to more effective time management and greater life satisfaction, the relationships

BOX 9-2 Factors Influencing Initiatives to Address Work-Life Balance and Work-Life Conflict

Researchers have compiled many statistics outlining the changing demographics of the labor force in Western nations. Here is a selection from a 2001 compendium of statistics (9):

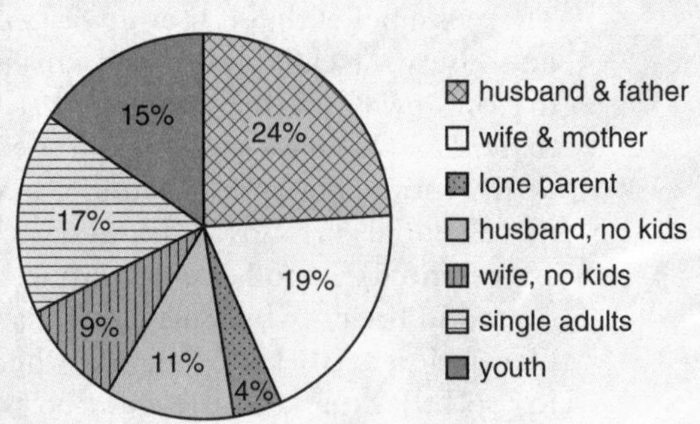

- Representation of women in the workforce has increased steadily over two decades.
- Both men and women in the labor force have child-care demands.
- 15% of employees are engaged in both child care and elder care.
- Many families cite financial pressures: the need for two incomes to keep from losing ground.
- Poverty adds stress to the work-life balance/conflict: high risk groups for poverty are people with disabilities, recent immigrants, and lone parents.

In every 100 participants in the labor force, the distribution relative to family demographics is as depicted in the pie chart and legend above. (See Figure 9-2 ■.)

among amount of work, type of work, family needs, stress, mood, and life satisfaction are quite complex (18). Satisfaction differs depending on the motivation for working part time and the extent to which the work is considered a rewarding career, as just two examples. The nature of the work also contributes to a sense of satisfaction or life balance, possibly more so than a part-time schedule. Women who work in managerial or professional positions report high role overload, regardless of full- or part-time hours, compared to those employed in clerical, retail, or production jobs (18). Aspects of life beyond work and family, including health-maintaining behaviors, financial security, and leisure participation also influence perceived balance. Many part-time jobs are in low-wage sectors. Part-time workers who lack financial security have been shown to be less satisfied with not only their work-life balance, but also their social lives, leisure, and general life satisfaction: therefore, the discourse on work-life balance may be advanced by taking a broader view of how all life domains interact (19).

Work-Life Conflict and Role Overload

A large Canadian study of over 30,000 employees working in public and private companies with 500 or more employees generated considerable data regarding work-life conflict (11). From an occupational perspective, work-life conflict is akin to occupational imbalance, a perceived state of disharmony across occupations.

Sources of work-life conflict were numerous and interrelated, but largely fell into three main categories: **role overload**, work-to-family interference, and family-to-work interference (11). Examples of overload included too many demands for the time available, tight production schedules, and lack of support in the workplace. Escalating technological complexity is an additional cause of work overload (9). Examples of interference are situations where a person feels forced to satisfy the expectations of one role at the expense of another. This occurred in two directions, when work expectations interfered with family activities, and when family role expectations interfered with work responsibilities. To the individual, both work-to-family interference and family-to-work interference contribute to a sense of conflict and, when extreme, have a detrimental impact on health. To employers, work-life conflict has a cost in terms of retaining employees, at-work productivity, and absenteeism. Johnson et al (9) estimated that employees were absent from work for 12 days annually due to family responsibilities.

A content analysis of over 5,000 comments received from respondents to the Canadian national work-life balance study revealed 33 different categories of comments (11). A majority of categories described challenges employees experienced in trying to balance work and family life, many of which stemmed from organizational culture and policies. Other comments indicated the individual struggles and stresses that employees were experiencing. Accounts of these individual struggles are most informative to understanding occupational balance and imbalance. Consider this example of role overload:

> I think most of the stress comes from trying to do everything and still be a good parent, partner, daughter, sister and friend. It's mostly my own fault. Life is simply too fast-paced. The demands to put your children in sports, do well in school, keep entertained, combined with working full-time and a spouse working shift work, make me feel I'm on a high-speed train. (11, p. 27)

This passage offers a glimpse of how competing demands are experienced as **role strain** and internalized as problematic. In this case, competing yet valued roles, together with a need to live up to external expectations, contribute to a perception of imbalance. The quote refers to blaming oneself for not being able to keep up, and the analogy of the high-speed train reflects a pace too fast to perceive life as balanced and rewarding. This experience illustrates how work-life balance and occupational balance are similar constructs.

Edwins et al (20) noted that women tend to experience more role strain than men, but this next comment (from the Canadian national work-life balance study) illustrates that men share similar experiences of work interfering with family life:

> Most days it is a struggle to get through. I do not like bringing my problems home. I don't like getting mad at my wife or kids for things they do which are normal. I'm tired of being angry. My job creates this environment. I wish I could control my life more like the way I envision it. I wish I could have more time with my kids, doing things like other parents do. (11, p. 28)

Not only does this passage describe work-to-family interference (one of the main study findings), but it also points out the consequences of occupational imbalance to emotional health. Karasek and Theorell (21) reported that anger, irritability, and lack of control have been strongly associated with acute and chronic illness, most particularly heart disease. Another participant quote from the national work-life balance study offers an example of how individuals come to recognize the relationship between work-life balance and health:

> I find the area of my life that is impacted the most by the pressures of work and family is my own free time. My family is my first priority, followed by my work responsibilities, which leaves no time for my own physical/spiritual/emotional well-being. I have no time for reading a book, getting some exercise, having a hobby, etc. It makes it difficult to stay healthy when you ignore this. (11, p. 29)

This latter thought—it is difficult to stay healthy when you ignore your own physical, spiritual, and emotional well-being—segues into another construct related to occupational balance: lifestyle balance.

LIFESTYLE BALANCE

Lifestyle balance refers to a pattern of occupations resulting in reduced stress and improved well-being (4). The discourse on lifestyle balance is largely situated in the context of maintaining health or preventing illness, and there is an extraordinary amount of information available to the general public regarding balanced lifestyles, especially on the World Wide Web. A Google search of the term *lifestyle balance* shows top ranking hits are related to health and illness, such as the virtues of adopting a lifestyle that incorporates a healthy diet and regular physical activity. Educational sites on how to make lifestyle changes to prevent and manage diabetes, heart disease, and other chronic illness predominates much of the available information. Materials are available to coach people to adopt a healthy lifestyle and achieve life satisfaction by considering several domains of life: work, family, intimate relationships, friends, leisure, finances, health, spirituality, and self-awareness.

Like many concepts related to health, the notion of lifestyle balance can be linked to early philosophers and medical practitioners. Christiansen and Matuska (4) traced the origins of lifestyle balance to writings from Aristotle (who observed that humans flourish when engaged in activities that are balanced to their interests, goals, and abilities), through to Hippocrates, Galen, and traditional healing practices, all of whom made reference to some aspect of balancing lifestyle choices to achieve health. Lifestyle balance is the outcome of engaging in healthy habits for mind and body, pursuing occupations congruent with one's values, skills, and interests. Lifestyle imbalance occurs when there is difficulty meeting physical, social, and psychological needs in a satisfactory manner, and it is observable when individuals exhibit anxiety, fatigue, or distress coping with life. The environment is an important contributor to lifestyle imbalance, be it social policy, physical demands, or other contextual factors. The consequences of poor lifestyle choices subsequently contribute to the development of chronic illness, further challenging health and well-being. Although there is considerable empirical support that lifestyle factors influence the risk of developing chronic conditions, changing behaviors to adopt a healthy lifestyle remains a challenge.

Amundson (22), in an essay on three-dimensional living, offered an excellent metaphor to help visualize and understand life balance, based on the physical properties of matter. Lives are viewed in the dimensions of length, width, and depth. The length of life is most easily understood: we live in terms of days, months, and years and "need to learn to live with balance: we are given the present and we need to find joy there, while also being aware of both past and future" (p. 116). The second dimension, width of life, reflects our involvement in a wide range of activities. Amundson cautions against wearing "busyness like a badge of honor to reflect our importance" (p. 116) and advises that the point of slowing down is to take time to breathe and remove the excesses of life. "Down time is the lubricant that facilitates movement, and without this lubricant there is going to be friction, and therefore, pain" (p. 116). The third and most significant dimension is depth, which refers to the need to make sense of our lives and live with purpose and meaning. The way we experience purpose and meaning influences the length and width dimensions because it influences choice of occupation and role fulfillment. These three dimensions of life balance comprise an apt metaphor that assists in identifying problematic configurations of balance across the life span, such as overemphasizing width (being too busy to enjoy the important things in life) or sacrificing depth and meaning, which leads to lower life satisfaction. This metaphor may guide an appraisal of lifestyle or occupational balance in terms of considering the length, width, and depth attributed to different domains of life, such as work, leisure, and social relationships, among others.

IS OCCUPATIONAL BALANCE ACHIEVABLE?

Although occupational balance, work-life balance, and lifestyle balance are all generally viewed as desirable states, dissenting opinions have been presented. One example by Beatty and Torbert critiques the premise of the false duality of work and leisure (23), a view that deconstructs the assumption that these two categories of occupation are polar opposites. A second dissenting viewpoint is the observation that creating policies to promote work-life balance may actually undermine people's abilities to lead fulfilling lives (24).

Caproni (24) posits that authors contributing to the work-life discourse in North America are unduly focused on achievement and productivity, applauding the benefits of work-life balance for organizations, individuals, and society and promoting strategies that actually perpetuate the experience of imbalance or role conflict. Reflecting on her own attempt to live a balanced life, she writes,

> I suspected that trying harder, smarter, and faster to balance my life (e.g., learn more time-saving techniques, work harder on my hierarchy of values, make more trade-offs, find a few extra hours in the day) may have been contributing to the problem rather than solving it. Indeed, I considered that I might have been trying to solve the wrong problem. Perhaps the problem—and thus the fix—was not in me but in the conceptualization of work/life balance. I considered that such a

> balance may not be an achievable or even a desirable goal. I realized that the emphasis on work/life balance may be another individualistic, achievement-oriented model based in modern bureaucratic organizational thought, setting us up to strive for one more thing that we cannot achieve and, in doing so, keeping us too focused, busy, and tired to explore the consequences of our thinking and actions. (pp. 49–50)

Any attempt to understand the concept of occupational balance and its potential health-maintaining benefits warrants careful attention to this type of critique. Critical appraisal will encourage the testing of theoretical models pertaining to occupational balance. Caproni's critique supports improved definitions of occupational balance that encompass multiple factors such as the congruence across skills, desires, values, obligations, and the demands of individual occupations and occupational roles. Many of these concepts have been articulated in models of occupational balance put forth by occupational scientists (1, 8, 25).

OCCUPATIONAL BALANCE, HEALTH, AND WELL-BEING

Data from a growing number of studies suggest that pursuing a range of valued, obligatory, and discretionary occupations is associated with health and well-being (2). A long-term qualitative study of a woman with quadriplegia identified a pattern of illness subsequent to periods of too much or too little participation in occupation (26). In a qualitative study of 22 adults with postpolio syndrome, participants declared the health benefits of remaining involved in a range of occupations that matched their abilities and goals (27). Participants with postpolio syndrome also supported the notion that occupational balance is dynamic, because changing symptoms and environmental demands required deliberate decisions to select a satisfying array of occupations. Among people with chronic arthritis, participation in valued occupations has been shown to predict mental health: there is a significant association between loss of valued activities and depression (28). In a cross-sectional study of adults with rheumatoid arthritis, ratings of occupational balance were significantly and positively associated with general health, physical function, and social function and negatively correlated with fatigue and pain (2). One-third of the respondents in this study reported limitations in performing paid and unpaid work as a result of their arthritis, and on average, this group had significantly lower occupational balance than those who did not experience work limitations. This latter finding suggests that engagement in work that matches one's abilities contributes to a sense of occupational balance, a finding that has been confirmed in a study of adolescents and adults from Italy, the United States, and Sweden (5). Ratings of the various dimensions of everyday occupations, such as meaning and stress, have been found predictive of life satisfaction among individuals across three stages of adulthood (college students, mid-career, and retirement) (29).

In research involving working mothers, Erlandsson and Eklund (30) found a lack of control over work and frequent hassles (indicators of lack of occupational balance) to be significant predictors of lower health status and lower quality of life.

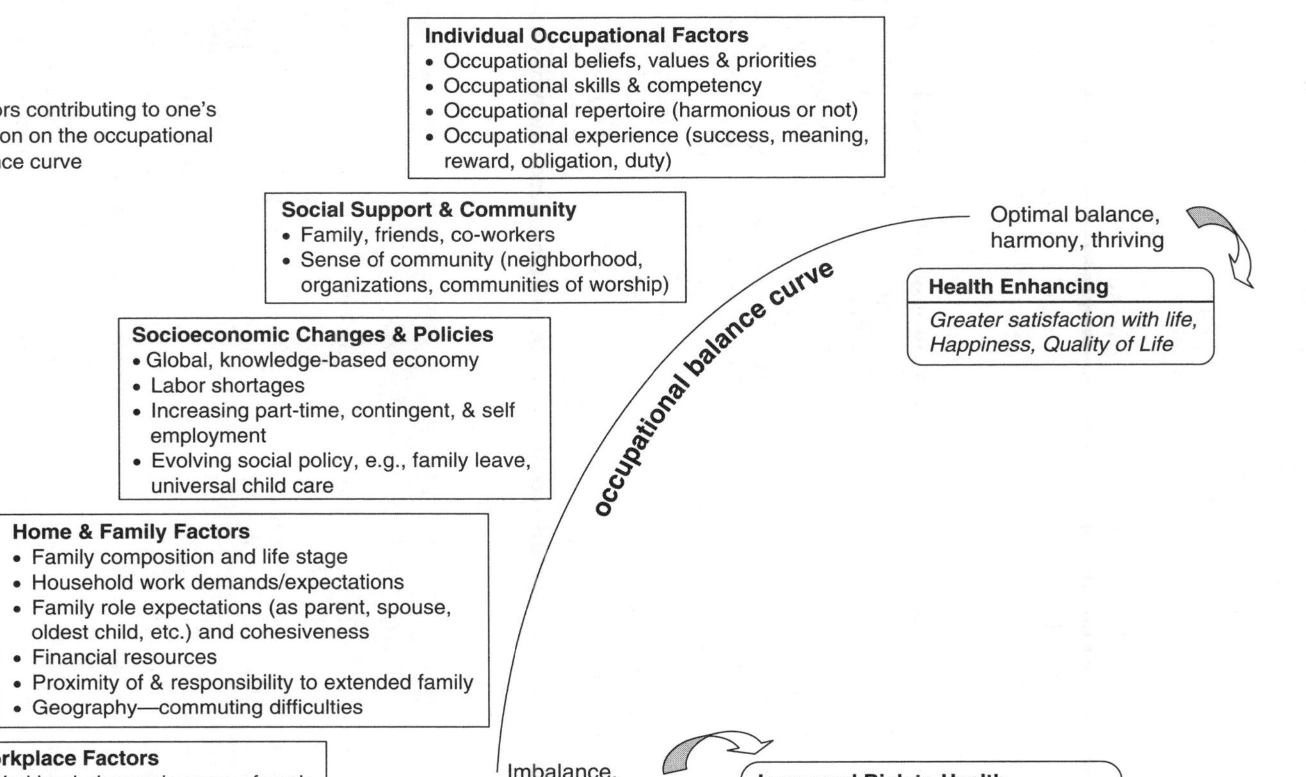

Factors contributing to one's position on the occupational balance curve
Individual Occupational Factors
• Occupational beliefs, values & priorities
• Occupational skills & competency
• Occupational repertoire (harmonious or not)
• Occupational experience (success, meaning, reward, obligation, duty)
Social Support & Community
• Family, friends, co-workers
• Sense of community (neighborhood, organizations, communities of worship)
Socioeconomic Changes & Policies
• Global, knowledge-based economy
• Labor shortages
• Increasing part-time, contingent, & self employment
• Evolving social policy, e.g., family leave, universal child care
Home & Family Factors
• Family composition and life stage
• Household work demands/expectations
• Family role expectations (as parent, spouse, oldest child, etc.) and cohesiveness
• Financial resources
• Proximity of & responsibility to extended family
• Geography—commuting difficulties
Workplace Factors
• Workload, demands, pace of work
• Perceived control, autonomy
• Supervisor, co-worker support
• Organizational culture
occupational balance curve
Optimal balance, harmony, thriving
Health Enhancing
Greater satisfaction with life, Happiness, Quality of Life
Imbalance, role strain, conflict
Increased Risk to Health
Infectious & Cardiovascular Diseases
Anxiety, Depression, Hostility
Substance Abuse

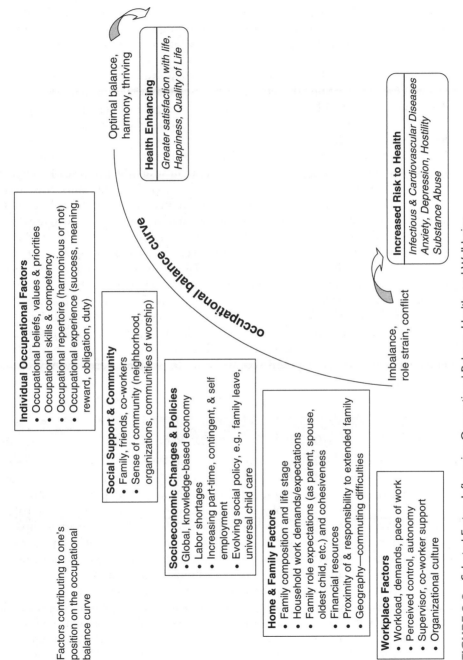

FIGURE 9-3 Selected Factors Influencing Occupational Balance, Health, and Well-being

Increasingly complex patterns of occupation, which generate greater conflict, were associated with lower health status, although the magnitude of the difference was small (30). A focus group study of 19 women recovering from stress-related disorders found that engagement in personally meaningful occupations contributed to a harmonious sense of occupational balance, which in turn contributed to reports of life satisfaction and well-being (25).

These brief examples indicate that a fairly clear association exists between occupational balance and health because it has been consistently found by different researchers working with different populations using different methods. In general, however, the methodological approaches to explore relationships are limited and do not provide empirical evidence of causality; that is, they do not conclusively show that occupational balance leads to good health. Instead, they generate a number of hypotheses worthy of further investigation, and illustrate the promise of such a line of inquiry. Building on emerging theories (1, 4, 5, 17, 25) to advance the study of occupational balance and health, Figure 9-3 ■ summarizes concepts explored in this chapter and makes explicit factors to investigate in future research. The figure depicts numerous individual, occupational, and environmental factors that contribute to occupational balance. It also depicts that the relative state of occupational balance contributes to good health when it is perceived as satisfying, or results in illness when it is perceived as lacking cohesion or creating conflict. Any number of these relationships and their interaction presents a hypothesis for further study to examine what factors lead to occupational balance and in what way occupational balance contributes to health. Individual, economic, social, and environmental circumstances influence the identification of priorities and allocation of time and resources for all segments of society, subsequently contributing to people's perception of occupational balance.

CHAPTER SUMMARY

This chapter opened with an ancient quote: "Moderation in all things." The concept of occupational balance deals tangentially with moderation, in that an overabundance or lack of occupations, or conflict between occupations and personal values, is undesirable. The chapter introduced the concept of occupational balance as a perceived state of harmony across the obligatory and discretionary occupations in which individuals engage on a day-to-day basis. Occupational balance results when occupations are congruent with values and priorities, sufficiently stimulating or challenging, and free from conflict. When occupations or the responsibilities associated with occupational roles are viewed as lacking in importance or meaning, detract from one another, or there is an abundance or dearth of occupational opportunities, occupational imbalance results. Evidence suggests that the consequence of occupational imbalance is an increased risk of ill health. Occupational balance remains an evolving concept that intrigues scholars from a broad range of disciplines. As empirical evidence is accumulated, the extent to which occupational balance influences health and well-being will be clarified.

STUDY GUIDE

Study Guide Author: Kristine Haertl

Summary of Main Points

Throughout our lives, patterns of occupational behavior and engagement change, causing fluctuations in the priorities and time in which we participate in various occupations. This chapter introduces the concepts of occupational balance and lifestyle balance and how they contribute to personal health and well-being. Occupational balance is introduced as an individualized dynamic process, including a harmonious arrangement of occupations that facilitate well-being. Occupational balance is contrasted with occupational imbalance, which refers to a pattern of incompatible or overabundant occupations with an individual's daily life and personal core values. The broader concept of lifestyle balance is reviewed to raise attention to the reflections and critiques of the busy lives of North Americans in particular. The chapter ends with a thoughtful question asking whether occupational balance is achievable.

Application to Occupational Therapy

Occupational therapists consider time use and balance of occupational engagement vital to health, well-being and opportunities for everyone to participate as fully as they wish in society. Role balance and imbalance of occupations (too little or too much) may contribute to mental as well as physical ill health and decreased satisfaction. In engaging people individually or collectively in assessment/evaluation and asking them what they need and want to do to be healthy and engaged in meaningful occupations, the occupational therapist has an excellent opportunity to understand how people use their days, weeks, months and years, and how they participate in occupations in various contexts, from home to community, and depending on circumstances, in the workplace. Goals and objectives for programs with individual, family, group, community, organizational, or population clients can then be developed to address occupational imbalance as perceived by the occupational therapist and the client. Programs can be developed with the client to identify areas of strength and need, occupational patterns, and means to achieve lifestyle, work, and occupational balance. Because values, culture, and spiritual beliefs affect an individual's perception of meaning in occupation, implementation of programs should engage clients in occupations that are both meaningful to them and necessary for realizing their goals and objectives.

Themes of occupational balance have implicitly been part of occupational therapy since the 20th century; however, the author indicates it was more of a philosophical belief than a clearly articulated concept. Several occupational therapy models and frames of references speak to the therapeutic benefit of engaging in meaningful occupations and having a balance of daily occupations, including work, rest, self-care, and leisure/play. Contemporary viewpoints have expanded classifications of occupations to include spiritual, educational, and other occupational areas of meaning. Evaluation of occupational therapy could examine changes in experiences, performance, engagement, or other forms of occupational participation with reference to clients' perceived occupational balance/imbalance before and after occupational therapy. Evaluation might also examine changes in perceived occupational balance with perceptions or measures of overall health and well-being.

A major issue in addressing occupational balance/imbalance in occupational therapy is to understand the socio-cultural context of the client, the therapist and practice to ensure that interpretations of occupational balance/imbalance are culturally sensitive to the context. In contexts where poverty, cultural beliefs, age-based expectations, or inaccessibility for people with disabilities, concepts of occupational balance/imbalance may vary greatly from other contexts where solutions might be based on time management and individualized reallocation of resources.

Individual Learning Activities

1. Conduct a time use diary for three days. Select areas of categorization (i.e., work, leisure/play, rest, activities of daily living (ADL) education, spirituality). Following completion of the time use diary, write a brief two- to three-page reflection. Consider the following questions:
   a. How did you spend your time? Were you satisfied with your time use? What were areas of most satisfaction and perceived competence, what were areas of least satisfaction?
   b. Did you feel as though your time use fit into the categories selected, or did you find yourself with enfolded occupations (i.e., doing things that fit in more than one category at the same time)?
   c. What would you change about your patterns of time use?
   d. Write a personal goal related to your occupational patterns and time use. Include a description of how you plan to achieve this goal.
2. Go to the following Web site and complete the *Headington Institute Self Care and Lifestyle Balance Inventory*. Write a two-page reflection on your results. What areas of strength do you have in self-care and lifestyle balance? What would you change? Did the inventory provide you any interesting insights? Web Site: http://headington-institute.org/Portals/32/Resources/Test_Self_care_inventory.pdf

Group Learning Activity

Form groups of two to four individuals. Each group member should be assigned to an age cohort (i.e., preteen, teenager, college student, working adult, retired adult). Find an individual from this age cohort (for very young children you may need to interview a parent). Interview the individual and ask him/her to describe a typical day/week. As a group, come together and compare and contrast the occupational patterns and balance of the individuals interviewed. How is occupational balance influenced by age and life situation? What contextual factors influence occupational balance (i.e., culture, environment, geographical locale)?

Study Questions

1. Which of the following is true of occupational balance?
   a. Individual perceptions vary related to the state of occupational balance.
   b. The types of balance activities will vary throughout life.
   c. A state of occupational balance is perceived to positively influence health.
   d. All of the above

2. According to the author, current work trends suggest an increasing polarization of work hours with an increased proportion of the population working less than 30 or more than 40 hours
   a. True
   b. False
3. Conceptualizing lifestyle balance in terms of depth would include:
   a. Consideration of how long an individual participates in a certain occupation
   b. Recognizing the number of occupations an individual engages in within a certain time period
   c. The consideration of how an occupation contributes to meaning within the life of an individual
   d. All of the above
4. Leisure and work are considered opposites on the poles of occupation
   a. True
   b. False
5. A state of harmony across the daily occupations in which a person engages
   a. Lifestyle balance
   b. Role balance
   c. Work-life balance
   d. Occupational balance

REFERENCES

1. Westhorp, P. (2003). Exploring balance as a concept in occupational science. *Journal of Occupational Science, 10,* 99–106.
2. Backman, C. L. (2004). Occupational balance: Exploring the relationships among daily occupations and their influence on well-being. *Canadian Journal of Occupational Therapy, 71,* 202–209.
3. Bryden, P., & McColl, M. A. (2003). The concept of occupation: 1900 to 1974. In M. A. McColl, M. Law, D. Stewart, L. Doubt, N. Pollack, & T. Krupa (Eds.), *Theoretical basis of occupational therapy* (2nd ed., pp. 27–37). Thorofare, NJ: Slack, Inc.
4. Christiansen, C. H., & Matuska, K. M. (2006). Lifestyle balance: A review of concepts and research. *Journal of Occupational Science, 13,* 49–61.
5. Jonsson, H., & Persson, D. (2006). Towards an experiential model of occupational balance: An alternative perspective on flow theory analysis. *Journal of Occupational Science, 13,* 63–73.
6. Wilcock, A. A. (1998). *An occupational perspective of health.* Thorofare, NJ: Slack, Inc.
7. Hanson, C., & Jones, D. (2002). Restoring competence in leisure pursuits. In C. A. Trombly & M. V. Radomski (Eds.), *Occupational therapy for physical dysfunction* (5th ed., pp. 745–759). Philadelphia: Lippincott Williams & Wilkins.
8. Townsend, E., & Wilcock, A. (2004). Occupational justice. In C. H. Christiansen & E. A. Townsend (Eds.), *Introduction to occupation. The art and science of living* (pp. 243–273). Upper Saddle River, NJ: Prentice Hall.

9. Johnson, K. L., Lero, D. S., & Rooney, J. A. (2001). *Work-life compendium 2001: 150 Canadian statistics on work, family and well-being.* Guelph, ON: Centre for Families, Work & Well-being, University of Guelph, and Human Resources Development Canada.
10. Chaykowski, R. P. (2006). Toward squaring the circle: Work-life balance and the implications for individuals, firms and public policy. *IRPP Choices, 12*(3), 2–26.
11. Duxbury, L., Higgins, C., & Coghill, D. (2003). *Voices of Canadians: Seeking work-life balance.* Catalog No. RH54-12/2003. Hull, Quebec: Human Resources Development Canada.
12. Health Canada. (2000). *Best advice on stress risk management in the workplace.* Accessed April 30, 2006 at http://www.hc-sc.gc.ca/ewh-semt/pubs/occup-travail/work-travail/stress-part-2/index_e.html
13. Perrons, D. (2003). The new economy and the work-life balance: Conceptual explorations and a case study of new media. *Gender, Work and Organization, 10,* 65–93.
14. Hallowell, E. M. (2006). A severe case of modern life can make you "crazybusy." *Vancouver Sun,* April 8, 2006.
15. Goff, K. (2006). Just 3.5 minutes of eating in lunch "hour." *Vancouver Sun,* May 23, 2006.
16. Kerka, S. (2001). *The balancing act of adult life.* ERIC Digest No. 229, Article EDO-CE-01-229. Retrieved June 1, 2004 from http://www.ericfacility.net/ericdigests/ed459323.html
17. Todd, S. (2004). *Improving work-life balance: What are other countries doing?* Ottawa, ON: Human Resources and Skill Development Canada.
18. Higgins, C., Duxbury, L., & Johnson, K. L. (2000). Part-time work for women: Does it really help balance work and family? *Human Resource Management, 39,* 17–32.
19. Warren, T. (2004). Working part-time: Achieving a successful "work-life" balance? *British Journal of Sociology, 55,* 99–122.
20. Erdwins, C. J., Buffardi, L. C., Casper, W. J., & O'Brien, A. S. (2001). The relationship of women's role strain to social support, role satisfaction and self efficacy. *Family Relations, 50,* 230–238.
21. Karasek, R., & Theorell, T. (1990). *Healthy work. stress, productivity, and the reconstruction of working life.* New York: Basic Books.
22. Amundson, N. E. (2001). Three-dimensional living. *Journal of Employment Counseling, 38,* 114–127.
23. Beatty, J. E., & Torbert, W. R. (2003). The false duality of work and leisure. *Journal of Management Inquiry, 12,* 239–252.
24. Caproni, P. (1997). Work/life balance: You can't get there from here. *Journal of Applied Behavioral Science, 33,* 46–56.
25. Håkansson, C., Dahlin-Ivanoff, S., & Sonn, U. (2006). Achieving balance in everyday life. *Journal of Occupational Science, 13,* 74–82.
26. Spencer, E. A. (1989). Toward a balance of work and play: Promotion of health and wellness. *Occupational Therapy in Health Care, 5,* 87–99.
27. Jönsson, A.-L., Möller, A., & Grimby, G. (1999). Managing occupations in everyday life to achieve adaptation. *American Journal of Occupational Therapy, 53,* 353–362.
28. Katz, P. P., & Yelin, E. H. (2001). Activity loss and the onset of depressive symptoms: Do some activities matter more than others? *Arthritis & Rheumatism, 44,* 1194–1202.

29. Christiansen, C. H., Backman, C., Little, B. R., & Nguyen, A. (1999). Occupations and well-being: A study of personal projects. *American Journal of Occupational Therapy, 53,* 91–100.
30. Erlandsson, L.-K., & Eklund, M. (2006). Levels of complexity in patterns of daily occupations: Relationship to women's well-being. *Journal of Occupational Science, 13,* 27–36.
31. Backman, C. (2005). Occupational balance: Measuring time use and satisfaction across occupational performance areas. In M. Law, C. Baum, & W. Dunn (Eds.), *Measuring occupational performance: Supporting best practice in occupational therapy* (pp. 287–300). Thorofare, NJ: Slack, Inc.
32. Christiansen, C. H. (1996). Three perspectives on balance in occupation. In R. Zemke & F. Clark (Eds.), *Occupational science: The evolving discipline* (pp. 431–451). Philadelphia: F. A. Davis.

CHAPTER 10

Occupations and Places

Toby Ballou Hamilton

OBJECTIVES

1. Appreciate the complex, reciprocal relationship between place and occupation.
2. Understand how environmental affordances and presses shape occupations in place.
3. Understand how the meaning of place is created and experienced.
4. Appreciate how culture influences the ways in which physical space is experienced.
5. Provide examples of how symbols and signs provide both meaning and direction to place.

KEY WORDS

Affordance
Archetypal spaces
Archetype
Avatar
Community
Displacement
Environmental press
Habitus
Life-world
Places
Semiotics
Sense of place
Social geography
Socially constructed meaning
Tele-immersion
Temporal
Virtual places

CHAPTER PROFILE

The study of geography extends well beyond a consideration of the physical features of the planet to consider the interaction of places, cultures, and living things. This chapter focuses on how the cultural and physical features of places influence and are

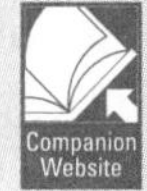

www.prenhall.com/christiansen
The Internet provides an exciting means for interacting with this textbook and for enhancing your understanding of humans' experiences with occupations and the organization of occupations in society. Use the address above to access the interactive Companion Website created specifically to accompany this book. Here you will find an array of self-study material designed to help you gain a richer understanding of the concepts presented in this chapter.

influenced by the occupations that take place there. Topics to be explored include the idea of places with universal meaning and purpose (archetypal places), the various dimensions or characteristics that are used to describe locations and how these influence occupations, how places create meaning, and how movement between places influences lifestyles from a temporal perspective. Other topics considered include the concepts of home and community and the creation of virtual places through modern technology. The chapter concludes with a discussion of the contribution of places to well-being, followed by brief discussions of the consequences of displacement and homelessness.

INTRODUCTION

When people engage in everyday pursuits that capture their time and attention, they must do so in places. The places in which people find themselves strongly influence what they do and the meaning of their time spent there. In fact, the contribution of place is an important and necessary element of occupation. This is because all occupational situations have three components: places, people (with their attributes, thoughts, feelings, and memories), and the occupations in which the people are engaged. Thus, the link between person, place, and occupation is so strong that one cannot consider occupations without considering that they involve people in places.

In this chapter, the term **place** refers to physical surroundings or environments that are either natural or built (produced through human labor). To a great extent, places influence how people work, play, and care for others and themselves. This located or *where* dimension also partly influences the *what,* the *why,* the *how,* and the *how well* of occupations.

Each day, individuals must meet basic human needs, such as eating, grooming, and sleeping, to support their survival and quality of life. Daily life revolves around the places associated with meeting fundamental needs. When surroundings include places that meet these needs, the results benefit individuals as well as their social groups. However, when places do not provide full satisfaction of basic needs, people's engagement in everyday occupations becomes difficult and can have negative consequences that extend beyond the immediate family or living group.

Places influence the occupations that are engaged within them. These influences can be subtle clues based on traditions and social expectations, or they can be more obvious, based on the physical characteristics of a place. Groups of people often establish relationships with places, translating their collective values and personalities into a type of cultural landscape. When people have known and occupied a place that carries such a special relationship, the symbolic meaning that is conveyed is called a **sense of place**.

Similarly, places have a spatial dimension, in that they represent distances from other places. In daily life, distance equates with travel, which requires time. People gain familiarity with regions, cities, and neighborhoods because of their proximity. This familiarity contributes to safety and security, which forms the basis for the ideas of shelter and territoriality.

This chapter will also explore aspects of place and the relationships between places, people, and their occupations. Many of the ideas presented in this chapter are fundamental to the study of social and cultural geography, sociology, and psychology.

UNDERSTANDING PLACE

The word *place* has many meanings, revealing the fact that the meanings of places are "socially constructed." That is, places are given different meanings by different people for different purposes, often as the result of shared experiences. Thus, meanings are attributed to places largely as a result of what happens in them and how people interpret those experiences over time. This multidimensional nature of place is conveyed well by Harvey (1, p. 4), who noted that many terms, such as *region, territory, location,* and *neighborhood,* are used to describe general qualities of places, as well as terms for particular kinds of places, such as *city, village,* and *state.* We also use words such as *home, turf, community,* and *nation* to evoke particular meanings. In addition, we designate places by the kinds of occupational pursuits that take place within them, such as *school, shopping center, football stadium, factory, amusement park, kitchen,* and *bedroom.*

Places as Archetypes

The first experienced environment for all humans is the uterus, and the experiences of the physical properties of the womb influence behavior for a lifetime. The rhythmic sounds of amniotic fluid created by the mother's movement and the muted sensory impressions of vision, hearing, and touch serve to stimulate growth and development of the fetus while providing protection and security. The small dimensions of the womb help explain why swaddling, or tight wrapping in blankets, calms newborn babies. The desire to re-create the pleasure of infantile security and comfort remains in adulthood. Most people enjoy the physical expression of love created by embracing and hugging.

When problems and challenges arise for individuals and groups, they usually seek places of quiet and relaxation to inspire the courage, creativity, and resourcefulness necessary for solving problems. The implicit message behind this adaptive strategy is one of seeking protection and support to meet threats and challenges. All humans possess these basic needs for security and protection.

Just as nature has provided the womb to serve as the primeval shelter, humankind has learned to construct places that serve a fundamental requirement of meeting basic needs. Spivak (2) identified 13 types of places that evoke and support behaviors that meet basic needs. He called these **archetypal places**. An **archetype** is any object that is deeply rooted in human history and serves as a symbol or model for other objects. Hence, Spivak proposed that archetypal places represent the basic settings necessary to sustain human existence. According to Spivak, archetypal places meet humankind's needs for shelter, territory, and the routes that link places for sleeping, mating, grooming, feeding, excreting, playing, competing, working, storing possessions, and meeting with others to fulfill spiritual, educational, and communication needs (2). Spivak's list of archetypal places provides a standardizing approach for classifying places by type.

Although archetypal places are found universally, their forms differ by geographic region and their use varies by the person's age and life stage. As "containers of culture" (2, p. 46), archetypal places necessarily vary from one place to another. Geographic aspects of place support or hinder travel and communication. Despite its small land mass, geographic barriers contributed to Europe's language and cultural differences until technology overcame the barriers. Therefore, differences in archetypal form reflect the geographic, climatic, and natural divisions of the places in which people live. The meanings associated with archetypal places differ by culture and custom across the life span according to the behaviors associated with age and stages of development. For example, the meaning of places for preparing and eating food differs not only by culture but also as one matures from childhood to adulthood. Similar changes influence the perception and use of sleeping areas.

Archetypal places are necessarily associated with the everyday occupations of life that secure our survival and quality of life. Just as certain places evoke particular occupations, occupations dictate design features of the built environments. People typically store, prepare, and clean up from preparing meals in the kitchen. The bedroom is the archetypal sleeping room and often the place for the occupation of sexual expression. We tend to do personal care tasks, such as grooming, hygiene, and dressing, in the bathroom and bedroom. Although such personal care occupations are usually performed as habitual routines, a change in place can offer either a refreshing change from routine or disrupt important and essential habits and routines that support daily life. Generally, unexpected and permanent changes of place represent stressful situations because of their importance in supporting the routine occupations of personal care, work, and leisure.

Dimensions of Place

Every place consists of different aspects or layers, each influenced by the other (3). The most obvious aspect of place concerns its physical attributes, location, objects, and furnishings associated with it. People experience physical space through their senses because of physical properties such as temperature, lighting, color, and noise. Many places have natural attributes or characteristics, such as proximity to mountains, water, trees, or open spaces that make them unique, undesirable, or appealing. It is important to note that the design of urban landscapes and open spaces constitute an aspect of the built environment. Thwaits (4) has proposed a conceptual model for landscape design that emphasizes many of the concepts in this chapter to enable the creation of neighborhood spaces that facilitate movement and the identification of location while also enabling the creation of place related meaning.

In addition to their location, the distance between places is an important dimension as distance influences daily routines. Distances are based on natural geography as well as human planning. London and New York are separated by 3,488 nautical miles of the North Atlantic Ocean—a geographical reality that cannot be changed. Yet, the distance from any office to the nearest staircase or toilet facilities is a function of architectural design. Some places provide locations for sharing commonsense knowledge and contesting social norms; others enable quiet, solitude, and privacy by providing distance or shelter from noise and large numbers of people.

Architects and designers use their awareness of affordance to design objects and places that signify their uses. Perceptual psychologist J. J. Gibson (5) coined the term **affordance** to refer to the particular arrangement of objects in the environment and to estimate the actions allowed by an object. Affordance is an interaction between an object and a person; the object's design suggests its purpose, function, and usability, and the user determines the object's affordance.

Affordances do not have to be visible, known, or even desirable to affect behavior. For example, begin noticing the affordance of doors. Doors with flat horizontal bars in the middle of the door afford the movement of pushing; those with vertical bars on one side afford us to pull (5); those with round knobs afford us to twist and open. We are usually unaware of a door's affordance until a particular door varies from typical designs. Chairs offer another example of affordance through design features such as the height of the seat from the floor, the size and flatness of the seating surface, and weight-bearing capacity. Such properties would not afford effortless use of a chair as a writing surface. Although a particular chair's affordance seems a simple decision, multiple factors go into judgments of the sitability of a chair. We judge a chair's affordance based on properties of the chair and personal physical capacities. Judgment of the chair includes the design features mentioned earlier. Personal or intrinsic capacities include the relationship of eye height, leg length, hip joint mobility, and center of gravity that must be raised above the height of the chair's sitting surface (6, 7). Each person determines affordance by both extrinsic properties of the object in the environment and intrinsic capacities to do the actions that the object affords. For example, adults find chairs designed for preschool children to be too low and small and may express concern that the chair may not support their weight. Young children usually resort to climbing strategies to sit on adult-sized furniture. We test affordance when shopping for chairs, defining comfort to some extent by the ratio of the length of the femur (upper leg bone from buttock to knee) and the length of the seating surface. Airline travelers in economy class certainly notice changes in the affordance of airline seats. The design of airline seats not only considers multiple dimensions of comfort (6, 7) for a range of a population's body dimensions, that in many countries is increasing in size, but also safety factors for emergency evacuation and health issues such as the prevention of deep vein thrombosis (blood clot) due to prolonged sitting (8). Take time to notice how design affordances of buildings and objects affect your experience of the dimensions of place and behavior.

The relationship between person and place can be used to influence behavior. Thus, subtle cues in the design of spaces can facilitate access and movement within a place (Figure 10-1 ■). Similarly, designs may facilitate privacy or social interaction. Objects help to define a place's meaning and shape its physical characteristics. Examples include memorial objects such as gravestones at cemeteries, ancient artifacts displayed at museums, and works of art at galleries.

A second and perhaps more important aspect of place relates to its **socially constructed meaning**. Through experiences, places become associated with events and action that give them both individual and collective meaning. Thrift (9) identified that the social nature of places provides structure for daily routines and life paths by providing opportunities and constraints that influence economic and social life. Places provide an

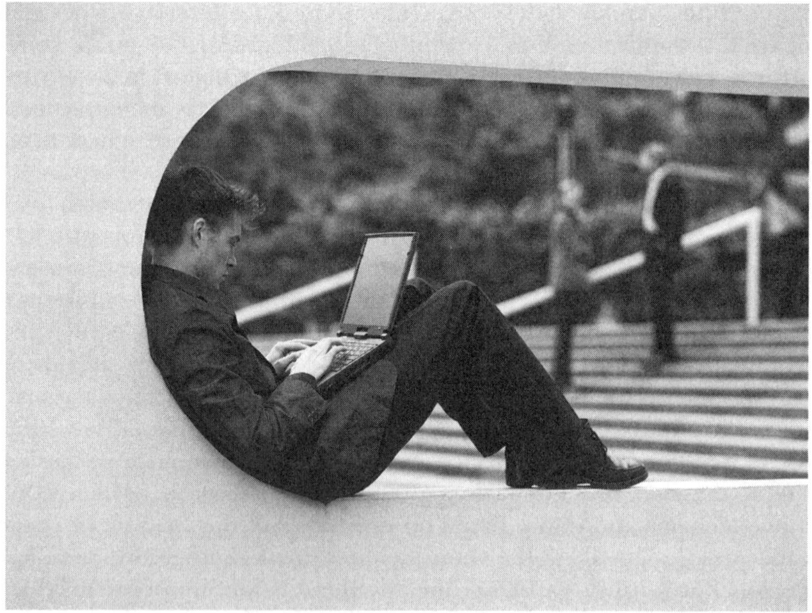

FIGURE 10-1 This campus architectural design has created an affordance for sitting and study. (Photodisc/Getty Images)

arena for social gatherings that are necessary for the development of language, culture, and values and the education to convey them to others. As places become associated with purposes and events over time, they acquire symbolic meanings that influence what goes on within them. These meanings then contribute to a shared identity associated with places through direct experience or stories told over time. The wonders of the world represent places with significant meanings associated with their actual and mythical histories, passed on through generations in a manner that makes them larger than life. On a smaller scale, each region and town has places that convey special meaning to the persons living in that area. These meanings develop over time through shared understanding of the people associated with them. Thus, places hold socially constructed meaning.

Place and Meaning

The meaning attributed to a place is influenced by its familiarity, which is in turn influenced largely by the amount of time a person spends there. People who are familiar with places and locations are *insiders*. The insider's view commonly holds these familiar places to be safe, secure, and nonthreatening (10). Humans are territorial, and safety and security are important dimensions of territoriality. Territoriality makes spaces and places instruments of power, inclusion, and exclusion (11). Places have meaning in direct proportion to the degree of "insideness" that people feel toward them, which relates directly to the time people spend there.

In his book, *The Experience of Place,* Tony Hiss (12) wrote: "The places where we spend our time affect the people we are and can become. Whatever we experience in a place is both a serious environmental issue and a deeply personal one" (p. xi). This personal or experienced part of places is called a *sense of place* (13, 14). Sociologist David Hummon (13) connected sense of place with feelings of community related to satisfaction, attachment, and identity. People clearly have feelings and thoughts about environments that include a subjective assessment of their level of comfort with being there. Taken together, these thoughts, feelings, and evaluations create a sense of meaning associated with place (15). Recent research supports the idea that meanings associated with place are laden with value and are highly dependent on the environment, experience with others, and a person's sense of self or identity (16).

Another aspect of meaning in place comes from semiotics, or the study of signs or symbols and their interpretation (17). Semiotics encompasses words, signs, nonverbal behaviors, gestures, objects, and building designs. We use semiotics to understand how people derive meaning from places and the feelings they experience there.

The concept of human communication through signs dates back to ancient Greece and medieval Europe. Modern semiotics began in the mid-1800s when Frenchman Ferdinand de Saussure and American Charles Sanders Peirce (pronounced "purse") proposed similar triadic relationships between physical signs, the objects to which they refer, and human interpreters. Saussure theorized that a *sign* consists of a *signifier,* or sensory pattern, and a *signified,* the concept that the signifier elicits in one's mind. The signifier becomes a *sign* when interpreted (18, pp. 21–24).

Semiotics involves the collective attributes of a place, its location, objects, memories, and emotions it evokes as symbols. Meanings are apparent when a group of people engage in collective actions and experience emotions evoked by place. Think of groups of people sharing feelings of pride when singing a national anthem while gazing at the collective symbol of a national flag or feelings of grief when gathered at a graveside funeral service.

We constantly encounter signs in place. Simple signs, such as "eat here" or "open" guide our behavior. Other signs offer semiotic challenges. A commonly encountered semiotic puzzle involves selecting the culturally correct public restroom designated for females and males. Typically, the only difference between identical doors is a signifier of stylized figures or words in letters and Braille. Figures and words may be generic or suited to the place. Consider the reading levels and interpretations required when we encounter words or pictures of "ladies," "gentlemen," "men," "women," "guys," "dames," or "señoras" and "señors," as well as the relatively recent "family" restroom. Adults who do not read the language or recognize its culture's symbols and children are often confused about restroom signs that exceed their reading, symbolic, or interpretive levels.

Maps offer another example of semiotics. Harry Beck was a London Underground electrical draughtsman who drew circuit diagrams at work and designed the world-famous stylized London tube (subway) map in 1933 in his spare time. Basing his map on electrical circuit diagrams, Beck ingeniously reduced the complexity of the London Underground system to its bare basics by disregarding geographic detail and distance. Because passengers traveled underground, they could not compare actual geographic features such as the River Thames or streets to the simplified map.

An immediate success, the original tube map generated a variety of similar public transit maps around the world (19). Clearly, the study of semiotics provides a key dimension for understanding occupations in places.

Time and Place

Not only are many places archetypal, but the routes that link them are also an archetype (3). When people commute to work or school or run errands, they are simply connecting archetypal places. Daily occupations link archetypal places into patterns. Just as a piece of cloth consists of vertical and horizontal strands woven together as warp and weft, so too are daily occupations woven into patterns that are influenced by locations and distances.

In a larger sense, the idea of life as a journey is an archetype (20) that has been frequently reflected in the motifs of the world's mythology and folktales (21, 22). The journeys of cultural heroes follow a particular pattern, regardless of the time and cultures that produced them (21). Hundreds of myths and folktales tell of journeys to other worlds, including the upper and lower worlds (21, 22).

For example, the ancient Greeks explained the cycle of seasonal change by the story of Demeter and her daughter, Persephone. After Hades, ruler of the underworld, seized Perspehone, Demeter allowed crops to fail. To restore order to the world, Persephone spent part of the year with her mother and part of the year with Hades. Winter occurred when Persephone was in the underworld with Hades, and her return to earth explained spring and summer.

There is a temporality of place that influences the duration and timing of everyday events. Places often display a rhythm of occupations that is influenced by their geographic location and purpose (23). A farm is an excellent example of a place where daily and seasonal rhythms influence the occupations that are done there. The rising sun brings early morning chores, and the seasons dictate the planting and harvesting of crops. Archaeologists have determined that the position of the sun during the day and during the year influenced the location of various work tasks among the indigenous peoples who inhabited the cavelike pueblos in the southwestern United States (24). The movement of occupations was an example of seasonal adaptation related to the changes in temperature and light as the sun moved through daily and yearly cycles.

Clearly, places are also associated with rituals that mark life events. The cathedral, which towered above other structures in the medieval villages of Europe, was a commanding reminder of religion and the social power of the church. As such, it greatly influenced daily life through the tolling of its bells, its location as a place for regular worship and social meeting, and as a place for baptisms, weddings, funerals, and other ceremonies that signified important points along the life course of villagers.

The locations of places in neighborhoods can also create informal rituals. In many small towns in North America on Saturday nights, young people gather or cruise Main Street to see and be seen by others. Here, place and time acting together create a social ritual. Similarly, if a bakery is located between the workplace and home, a person may develop a personal ritual of stopping on the way home to buy bread or pastry. Families develop personal rituals surrounding locations within the

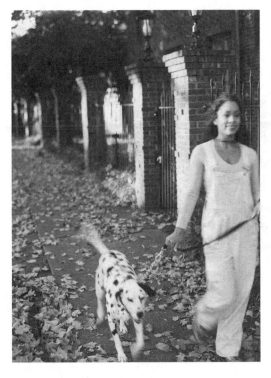

FIGURE 10-2 Occupational rituals are often linked to time and place. Many people have a set time and route for walking their dogs.
(Steve Cole/Getty Images/Digital Vision)

home. These rituals may be related to gatherings around certain parts of the house, such as the fireplace or stove, or to locations such as summer cottages or other favorite locations for regular family reunions or weekend getaways. Many people develop rituals around neighborhood itineraries where they take their daily strolls to exercise or walk the dog (Figure 10-2 ■).

Movement from Place to Place as Occupation

Transportation provides human access to other people and places. Similarly, lack of transportation options can limit access to occupational engagement, including work, school, and various social activities. This lack of access can undermine well-being by limiting earning potential and social participation. As urban areas grow and distances between places become greater, the importance of transportation increases.

In the industrialized world, the growth of urban areas has changed daily life. Many people no longer live and work in their homes or in the same neighborhood. Instead, they commute between home and work, often traveling long distances in cars or public transportation. Commuting has a negative effect on the traveler's psychological state by increasing stress and contributing to insomnia (25). Lengthy commuting times also adversely affect family and social life by reducing the time available for socialization (26). For example, on a typical weekday, the average Canadian commuter spends 48 minutes going to and from work. Significant proportions of workers spend an hour or more each day in travel (27).

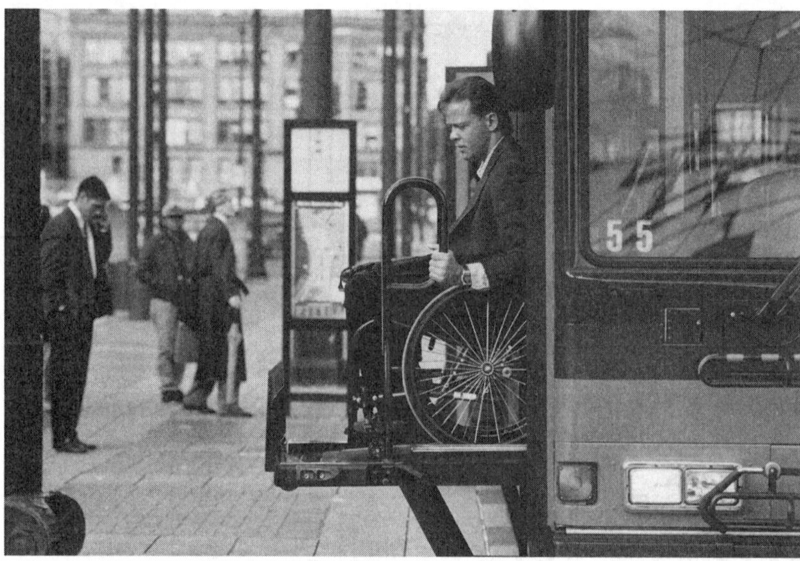

FIGURE 10-3 Movement from place to place is often a key element of participation in necessary and chosen daily endeavors. The significance of available public transportation to quality of life is often overlooked.
(John Photodisc/Getty Images)

The stress of commuting varies by mode of transport as well as the nature of the commute. Traveling on a busy multilane road is not as pleasant an experience as driving along a tree-lined residential street. Some scenic neighborhoods offer drivers many of the visual experiences that make walking or cycling in greenways appealing. Attractive scenery changes the perception of time associated with a commute and reduces stress. Drivers perceive the time spent driving on a suburban arterial road to be 23% more than the actual time elapsed. In contrast, the perceived time spent driving along a traditional tree-lined residential street is experienced as 16% less than the actual time (28).

The cost of transportation is also a consideration, especially for economically disadvantaged people, that can limit access to shopping, education, and recreation. In some parts of the world, money for work-related commuting is given first priority for poor families, often leaving inadequate resources for transportation for other purposes. In many urban environments, the working poor reside in the inner city, with little opportunity to visit suburban areas, which often have limited access by public transportation. This characteristic of place and transportation can have economic consequences that result in pervasive threats to quality of life (29; Figure 10-3 ■).

OCCUPATIONS AS EXPERIENCES IN PLACES

A term frequently used in sociology to communicate daily experiences is **life-world**. A life-world can be defined as the routine patterns and interactions of everyday life. The concept of life-world is experience-based and emphasizes the meanings that people give to the spaces they occupy. Because it is familiar, routine, and recurring, the life-world is seldom given conscious thought. This contributes to its enduring nature, creating a sense of secure, continuous reality as life is lived on a daily basis (30).

When people interact with other people or objects within their life-worlds, their experiences can be described as embodied. Within the embodied experience, individuals employ their own characteristics, dispositions, and attributes to shape and interpret the places they occupy. The sociologist Pierre Bourdieu used the term **habitus** to describe the unconscious patterns of doing, thinking, speaking, and perceiving that people exhibit in these circumstances. These characteristics are basic to the creation of shared meaning within places (31).

In the life-world, a person's doing, thinking, speaking, and perceiving most often take place in the context of daily occupations, which occur in places. Thus, occupations always occur within a context of place and time. Since ancient times, people all over the world have engaged in productive, personal care, and recreational occupations, and they have needed shelter for sleep. In a more restricted sense, occupation happens in a particular place that has observable physical properties that happen within the rhythms of natural, cultural, and personal routines.

Because of the dynamic nature of people, their occupations, and the places in which occupations are done, no element can be understood in isolation. So enmeshed are the person, the place, and the performance of occupation that their respective influences must be considered. In short, a complete understanding of occupations can only occur with careful consideration of the settings and people who are engaging in them. In the sections to follow, these influences are described in greater detail.

HOW PLACES INFLUENCE OCCUPATION

Places invite certain types of occupations and prohibit or restrict others (4). When people go into a store, they look at items and may purchase some of them, but most people would not steal anything. People invite others to talk while eating lunch but expect silence while visiting the cinema. Given the outdoor setting of a playground, children find it easy to run and play but difficult to complete lessons. The elements and rules inherent to a place may combine and build on each other (4). When students enter a classroom, they typically sit in chairs that are placed to face the front of the room where they expect the instructor to stand. Only under special circumstances that alter the rules of the classroom space would students or faculty rearrange the seating.

These behaviors are a consequence of social expectations associated with places. Some customs and rules of social behavior are learned and generalized from one place to another. People learn to be quiet and reverent in spiritual places. Obvious spiritual places, such as mosques, churches, synagogues, temples, cathedrals, or other houses of worship, commonly elicit such behaviors. Behaviors in spiritual places known only to insiders will be less obvious to visitors, and inappropriate behaviors in these places will elicit sanctions by those more familiar with customs.

The traditions associated with behavioral expectations in places have been called **environmental press** and were theorized by psychologist Henry Murray in the

1930s (32). More recent work on behavioral influences has recognized that press is a phenomenon associated with social experiences and the presence (imagined or real) of other people within places. Lewin's field theory (33) and Latane's social impact theory (34) form the basis for more recent research confirming the influence of social expectations on behavior within settings or places. Their frameworks support the basic proposition advanced here—namely, that occupations are influenced by the nature of the individuals and the settings in which people find themselves.

Physical Influences

The physical characteristics of places also influence the performance of occupations—how frequently, efficiently, or effectively people are able to achieve their purposes there. Psychological and emotional factors, simple design and logistical issues related to the demands of given tasks, abilities of people, and environments influence occupational performance and mastery. The science of human factors, or *ergonomics,* evolved as a means of determining how the psychological, physical, and social characteristics of people and environments influence task performance in work settings. A goal of ergonomics is to improve the fit between people and their working conditions while improving safety, productivity, comfort, and efficiency (35). To accomplish these goals, human factors engineers must take the various aspects of place into account. Human factors specialists recognize that psychological issues, particularly those related to the perception and meaning of places to their inhabitants, have important influences on task performance and safety in the home and workplace.

Just as the person brings abilities, capacities, and desire for mastery and competence in a setting, the place [environment] makes demands on an individual's occupational performance which can change within the same setting during the course of a day. The demands that a place makes will have different effects on everyday occupations according to the difficulty, complexity, familiarity, intricacy, speed, effort, integration, exertion, responsiveness, timing, span, and scope of the occupations.

For example, consider the demands that school places on children's occupations. During recess breaks, the physical aspects of the outdoors and the playground equipment challenge children by offering opportunities for swinging, climbing, running, or playing competitive or cooperative games. Back in the classroom, the children must interact in socially appropriate ways with others to complete projects, wait in line, eat lunch or snacks, sit in their seats, and participate in class discussions. Rules regulate their behaviors whenever they move in the classrooms and halls, work or play alone or with others, and even determine when they can meet biological needs to eat or drink. Teachers expect students to be prepared for class, use unstructured school time to meet educational objectives, avoid disruption of others' work, and independently complete assignments and projects at school and at home.

Schools are good examples of places where exploration and experience lead to enhanced abilities. This may explain why school experiences often hold such special meaning for people. In addressing this point, Platt (36) wrote that:

> Places capture experience and store it symbolically. Its collective meanings are extractable and readable by its later inhabitants. This symbolic housing of meaning

> and memory gives place temporal depth. But not only do places of experience store meaning about the past; they also are platforms for visions and plans about the future. Places of experience provide us with identity to venture forth out of this place into less certain or orderly spaces. Places of experience provide categories for managing new adventures and new cycles of old adventures. Places of experience connect the past to the future, memory to expectation, in an invigorating way. Places of experience give us a sense of continuity and energy. (p. 112)

Geographical Variations in Occupation

Part of the continuity of place is related to the traditions and customs that are practiced there. People in different places often do things differently, based on experience and teachings passed down through generations. Often, these ways of living are influenced by natural resources and physical characteristics of the places. A comparison of child-care practices serves as a useful example to illustrate the diversity and similarity of occupations as they vary by geographic places.

Universal child-care includes carrying, bathing, diapering, and feeding babies as well as comforting them when crying and getting them to sleep. Parents protect their infants from weather and the invisible world that consists of either evil spirits or germs, depending on the culture's beliefs (37). Parents find methods of meeting their children's needs by using the physical features of a place and the materials at hand.

A place's climate and available materials influence how mothers carry their babies. Babies may be carried either close or far away from the parent's body, and the infants may be free to move or be tightly swaddled into virtual immobility.

Babies around the globe are carried in slings, hammocks, pouches, nets, or baskets supported on the mother's (and father's in some cultures) front, back, neck, hip, or forehead. For example, mothers in the Amazon rain forests carry their babies from a strap over the mother's forehead so her hands are free to gather food. The manner of transporting the infant determines how much of the world the baby can see and hear. Today, mothers and fathers may carry their babies in front or back pouches or slings for convenience and to provide closeness between baby and parent. Infants carried in a horizontal sleeping position see and hear very little, whereas babies carried upright on the parent's back or hip experience a great deal more of life. In places in which the infant is strapped to the mother's body as she goes about her daily work, the infant not only has rich sensory experiences but also "serves as a witness" to the work occupations in that place (37, p. 17).

Bathing is a part of the personal care routine carried out to remove dirt and germs from the baby's body. People around the world bathe babies in sinks, conventional bathtubs, or small child-sized tubs. In some societies, bathing fulfills the need to cleanse the infant both literally and ritually. Tribal mothers in South America, Africa, Indonesia, and Oceania fill their mouths with water, warm it, and spray the water over the infant for a literal "spit bath." The baby may then be covered with oils, spices, herbs, juices, paints, powders, pastes, or even dung for protection from the elements, disease, and vectors. Tribal babies in Australia, Africa, and India may be cleansed by being held in the smoke of a fire fueled by plant materials and animal

Play in Neighborhoods

Researchers who studied the physical features of four California neighborhoods found that place dictated the play patterns of 11- and 12-year-olds (46). The neighborhood, defined by the distance from home to school, comprised the children's "social universe" (p. 320). In each neighborhood, constraints on children's play patterns included the terrain, the number of and access to other children, ages of the children, the relationship of major streets to designated play areas, and availability of undeveloped, unstructured play space. Children living in hilly, sparsely populated neighborhoods spent more time planning social interactions than other children. Children living in flat neighborhoods with many children spent more time in spontaneous social interactions. In neighborhoods with a higher density of children, friendships tended to be more casual, less structured, and inclusive of a variety of children of different ages.

The importance of this research lies in the fact that the children in all neighborhoods adapted to the assets and constraints that the physical place of their neighborhoods presented. The children's "energy, imagination, and perseverance make it possible for them to define an acceptable play environment" (46, p. 320), despite the physical limitations of the places in which they lived and played.

Variable Notions of Home

What people think of as *home* is a single place that allows them to meet their archetypal needs for shelter, storage, and territory to enable the tasks and occupations of sleeping, mating, grooming, feeding, and excreting (2). Home is itself an archetypal place that ideally offers the security to meet those needs, the opportunity to interact with loved ones, and the freedom to be ourselves. The ideal of such a place as home permeates a society's culture. Dorothy's desire to return home with the magic phrase "There's no place like home" was the basis of the L. Frank Baum's series of books about the mythical land of Oz (47). Because of his intense desire to return to his home planet, the most quotable line in Steven Spielberg's movie, *E. T., The Extraterrestrial* (48), is "E.T. phone home." Advertisers use the archetype of the idealized home to promote products designed to enrich home as place, express our feelings of love and caring, and promote our desire to return home. Many holidays evoke idealized images of home that are reinforced by art, books, food, magazines, movies, theater, and advertisements. Clever real estate agents bake cookies during the showing of a house to evoke a sense of feeling "right at home."

However, not all ideal images of home are actually realized. Domestic or family violence and maltreatment (neglect and abuse) of children and elders represent violations of the idea of home as an archetypal place. Instead of meeting basic needs in an environment of safety and caring, domestic violence and maltreatment are crimes that disrupt personal boundaries and the privacy of homes in ways that negatively alter its archetypal meaning as a place of safety, nurturance, and love. Family violence, defined as violence committed by an offender who is related biologically, legally by marriage, adoption, or co-habitation typifies this violation of home. In the United States, family offenders committed 3.5 million violent crimes, accounting for 11% of

Despite the limitations sometimes imposed by aging as shown by Czaja et al (50), Graham Rowles, a social geographer (51) showed that a lifetime of familiarity with the physical place of one's home can facilitate continued functioning despite limitations or impairments associated with aging. Rowles found that one's house, community, and the habits of neighbors helped the residents of a small Appalachian town to overcome the losses caused by normal aging and poor health. Residents made simple modifications such as moving furniture to aid mobility and enlarging windows to increase the visibility of the outdoors and their neighbors. Some timed their necessary everyday occupations to occur at the same time that certain neighbors walked by their windows. They created elaborate systems of checking on each other through regular patterns of community activity and extensive telephone communication. By skillful use of the features of the place in which they lived, the older Appalachian adults in this study reduced the mismatches in person and place that could have required a move to safer, more structured places, such as their children's homes or nursing homes.

For about four decades, people in the United States and other countries have witnessed a trend to move people with physical disabilities, mental illnesses, or developmental disabilities out of large institutions into independent living places or group residences in community settings. The premise underlying this movement is that if people live and work in more normalized settings, the experiences and opportunities available for them will be more typical, and their lifestyles will be enhanced. Unfortunately, the residences occupied by persons with disabilities in community settings often have retained a character more like institutions than homes (52). These characteristics of place have, in turn, influenced the lifestyles and behaviors of their occupants.

In a study of the relationship of architecture and the behavior of residents in 20 group homes for adults with developmental disabilities, Shinn and Weitzman found that residents living in homelike places behaved more normally and engaged in more typical occupations than residents living in places that were more institutionlike. The residents of homelike buildings were more likely to do household chores independently, help with meal preparation, and pursue individual leisure interests. Residents of less homelike places were observed to be less active and more disengaged. The study found that the design features and furniture of the dining room were the best predictors of resident behavior. The most influential dining room factor was the number of seats at the dining room table. Settings with dining seating exceeding 12 places at a table tended to be associated with more institutionlike characteristics in general and the observation of less normalized behaviors among residents. The researchers found that the physical arrangements of the group homes also affected the behavior of staff, so that all three factors—design of dining room and furniture, dining room seating, and physical arrangements—influenced the behavior of residents (52).

Loss of Place (Displacement)

Changes in place can interfere with the performance of even the most routine occupations. Anyone who travels becomes familiar with the challenges of changing personal

reported and unreported crime from 1998 to 2002. With simple assault as the m frequent type, 40% of family violence resulted in injury. Forty-nine percent of fa ily violence was directed against spouses, and 11% were children victimized by th parents. About 75% of all family violence occurs in or near the home (49).

HOW OCCUPATIONS INFLUENCE PLACES

Places can be classified according to certain fundamental occupations necessary daily life. These archetypal places present important influences of everyday occu tions on places. Examples of occupation influencing place can be seen in hom People who enjoy preparing elaborate meals and entertaining often select hor that feature well-equipped gourmet kitchens. On the other hand, others may m their cooking needs with a single-burner stove and toaster or microwave oven. Exp tant parents often redecorate the baby's room and continue to change its des according to the growing child's interests and hobbies. Families with adult child who have long since left the home often convert the extra living space into ho offices, craft rooms, or storage areas. From these examples, one can see that peo modify places to meet individual occupational needs.

Place as Community

When people consider places that encourage them to engage in public places as p of the life of a **community**, they usually think of two aspects of place. First are the n urally occurring geographic features, such as mountains or ocean beaches. The s ond aspect is the constructed or built place, such as entertainment centers, hik paths, museums, performing arts stages, and parks. When companies search for a n site in which to locate or relocate a business, they consider the geographical locat and available resources and people, as well as the entertainment, cultural, and e cational aspects of place.

However, people can consider community life on a smaller scale, as discussed The Occupational Nature of Social Groups in Chapter 7 . Older persons living in th homes often face challenges in personal care and homemaking occupations. Th challenges result not only from age-related changes in their physical capacities, also from the physical characteristics of the places in which they live. Both demands of daily occupations and physical features of place influence the ability older persons to function inter/independently at home. Daily life requires bendi reaching, carrying, and lifting. These pose the most difficulties for older pers (50). Limitations in any of these performance components influence the occu tions and lifestyles of seniors both in the home and in the community.

Czaja et al (50) found that older persons reported more frequent shopping tr to food stores because they experienced difficulty lifting and carrying their p chases. They also found that meal preparation was affected when weak grasp ma it difficult to open refrigerator and cabinet doors or operate sink faucets. As an alt native to meal preparation, seniors in many countries eat meals at a community c ter or have meals delivered to their homes.

care routines of hygiene, grooming, and dressing. A forgotten toothbrush, the maintenance of clothes, and the inability to easily locate clothing and grooming items from luggage or travel bags create significant disruption that influences the performance of these routines at the moment and also changes the **temporal** pattern of everyday occupations. Mealtimes must be adjusted to the schedules of restaurants, and diets must accommodate to the vagaries of available menu items and the accommodations of waitstaff and cooks. In addition, one must accommodate the difficulties of local travel in an unfamiliar environment. Changes in routines and locations can also upset biological rhythms, making sleep more difficult. Because these consequences are expected even in first-class travel, we can easily appreciate how changes in place can have undesired consequences for people who must move involuntarily. Involuntary displacement from a living environment can occur as the result of hospitalization, progressive aging, or illness that requires supervision or care in attended settings, disasters that necessitate displacement such as fires or floods, and economic situations, such as unemployment or chronic poverty. Because of its growing prevalence in North America, homelessness presents a poignant case study of the consequences of **displacement**.

Homelessness violates the concept of home as a secure, permanent, private place where one meets a variety of archetypal needs. Homelessness is an outcome of complex societal issues for those who may experience domestic violence, mental illness, addiction disorders, low wages, lack of affordable housing, decline in public assistance, and poverty. Families with children comprise the fastest-growing segment of the homeless population, accounting for 40% (53).

Homelessness disrupts the most basic everyday occupations. Without a single place that meets the most basic needs, the everyday occupations of people who are homeless center around efforts to find sufficient food, clothing, and shelter to survive on a day-to-day basis. The inability to meet such basic needs in one place fragments sleeping, eating, and grooming occupations, resulting in a daily routine of traveling to several places to meet basic needs.

People who are homeless have more health problems than the general population, experience social problems that may be exacerbated by their lack of shelter, and are more likely to become involved in criminal activity than the general public (54). Health consequences of homelessness occur because people in these circumstances are exposed to more infectious and communicable diseases and experience more stressors, thus resulting in lowered resistance (55). These circumstances also place homeless people at greater risk for drug addiction, suicide, and other mental health problems (56–58). At the same time, homeless people are often displaced from stable housing because of unemployment, low income, and family difficulties such as spousal or child abuse (59). Of young people on the streets, it is estimated that 70% have experienced physical and sexual abuse (60).

Evidence suggests that people who are homeless may be involved in criminal activity more than youths in the general population (54). Some observers speculate that because of their lack of access to private spaces, the crimes of homeless people are more visible and therefore more apparent. Statistics indicate that the criminal behavior involves crimes against property, such as theft and fraud, prostitution, and minor infractions, such as failure to pay fines and loitering (60). These victimless crimes seem to arise more out of the circumstances of homelessness than serious criminal intent (54). Taken together, the effects of homelessness would seem to underscore the important role that a stable and consistent shelter plays in everyday existence and the consequences of diminished social support that results when living environments are disrupted or substandard.

The thought of not knowing where the next meal will come from or where one will sleep for the night is foreign to many people. The struggle to meet the most basic needs taxes the person–environment interaction in ways that are hard to imagine. A person may be able to sleep in a shelter for the night, but must stay alert to safeguard possessions because of the lack of secure storage of belongings. Staple foodstuffs may be available from food banks and pantries but go unused without the utensils and means of preparing food. A given shelter may offer only one meal a day, necessitating travel between several shelters to eat more than once a day. The place where one gets a meal may be some distance from the place where one sleeps. Although people who are homeless are sometimes eligible for government assistance, no one can receive mail without a permanent address. Meeting archetypal needs through such fragmented occupational performance strains the person—environment interaction when the search for a means of survival dominates one's daily routine (Figure 10-4 ■). Instead of meeting archtypical needs efficiently, safely, and

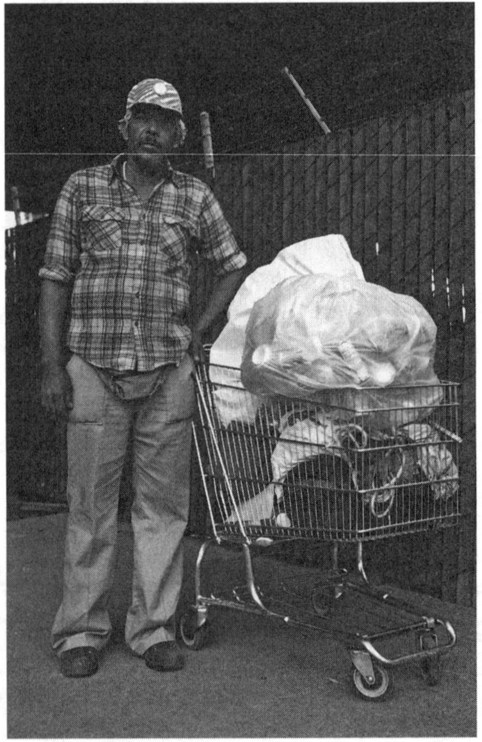

FIGURE 10-4 In the United States, one prevalent symbol of homelessness is a grocery cart filled with personal belongings. (Photodisc/Getty Images)

supportively in a single place called "home", the primary patterns of daily occupation for homeless people to partially meet archetypical needs is to navigate street routes that link various places. The street routes that link various places only partially meet archetypal needs through their primary patterns of daily occupation.

Virtual Places

No one can doubt that computer technology and the Internet have profoundly changed the lifestyles of many people. Using a computer to interact, shop, discover, learn, play games, and even do paid work has become commonplace. As computers have become more advanced, improved processing speeds and data memory have enabled the creation of digital experiences that hold great potential for changing the way life is lived for millions of people throughout the world. The Internet and digital communications create the sense that physical distances are no longer a barrier to social interactions. The ability to instantly engage in everyday occupations across vast distances and to visit **virtual places** can reconfigure the time, place, and pattern of everyday experiences.

Occupations that once required travel to another physical place can now be conducted without leaving the room. Instead of going to a store, we can browse, shop, and purchase goods and services from our computers. We can electronically send and receive mail instantaneously, whereas people used to compose and write a letter on paper, mail it from the nearest post office or letter collection box, and hope our correspondent would receive our letter in a few days. Instead of going to a university campus, students can enroll in and complete courses emanating from a digital campus.

Because it is digital, every Web site can be construed as a virtual place. As technology has matured, Web experiences have become more sophisticated. Using broadband connections capable of transmitting or streaming huge amounts of digital images and sound, computers can display images of real-time events from across the globe. The term *virtual reality* refers to any simulation of a real or imaginary environment in which it is possible for a user to interact with objects and people within that environment. Immersion refers to the sense that users are interacting within an environment represented digitally (61).

The digital representation of environments, or immersive virtual places, is becoming more sophisticated as the environments are rendered in three-dimensional form. Here, the user can move within the virtual environment and experience visual, auditory, and tactile sensations through devices known as haptic interfaces (Figure 10-5 ■). As these technologies mature, the potential for re-creating places and simulating real-world experiences using virtual reality is perhaps inestimable. The term **avatar** refers to a representation of the self that can be used in virtual environments. Avatars can be similar to the self or can be imagined representations. In effect, the use of imagined avatars in virtual places enables people to gain experiences and to experiment with identities that transcend those possible in the physical world.

More recently, scientists interested in interactive virtual reality technology used over distances have used the term **tele-immersion** to describe networked applications of virtual reality that enable immersive three-dimensional interactions from multiple sites (61). The immediate goal of current research on tele-immersion is to

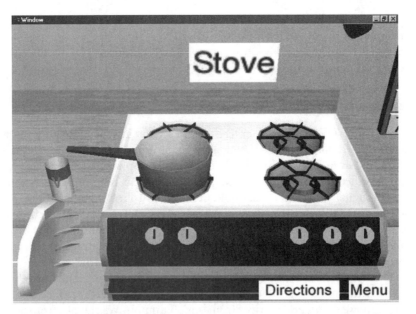

FIGURE 10-5 Virtual environments can vary from entire buildings to specific rooms. This virtual kitchen enables the user to perform many tasks necessary for food preparation, including opening cans, running water, and heating food on an electric range.
(Courtesy of the University of Texas Medical Branch and the Transitional Learning Center of Galveston.)

create work environments that facilitate scientific collaborations in networked-based virtual reality. The potential significance of this and other technological developments on cultures, people, and daily occupations is difficult to estimate.

PLACE, OCCUPATIONS, AND WELL-BEING

Research on the relationship between place, occupations, and well-being has crossed many disciplines and focused on a variety of variables. Much of the current research in **social geography** and cultural geography has occurred in naturalistic settings through ethnographic approaches. *Ethnography* refers to research in which an investigator observes behaviors and places to provide a written description of a social group focusing on cultural characteristics based on concrete experiences (62).

Ecological psychology research has been concerned with specific environmental, physical, and social characteristics and their influence on task performance, perception, or emotions. Studies have repeatedly shown that place influences the type, frequency, duration, and style of behavior, and that it can have both positive and negative influences on lifestyle and well-being. For example, an ethnographic study conducted at six low-rise apartment communities supported the premise that having natural settings in the view from the window contributes substantially to residents' satisfaction with their neighborhood and with various aspects of their sense of well-being (63). Another study of students' favorite places found that natural settings were a high priority and that these settings had perceived characteristics that facilitated relaxation and personal restoration (64). Also linking place, occupation and well-being, a study of the effects of physical environment on the behavior of preschool children showed that ceiling height and wall color in classrooms can influence cooperative behaviors (65).

Although physical characteristics of environments have an influence on performance and emotions, the most important characteristics of places that influence occupations are their social dimensions and the meanings associated with those dimensions, as illustrated in a study by psychologist Ellen Langer (66). In her 1979 study, men aged 75 to 80 years old were asked to either assume or recall their state of mind at age 55. The men were divided into two groups. Men in the experimental group were asked to be the person they were 20 years ago. Men in this group were asked to live as if it was actually 1959, and the men and researchers used the present tense to refer to that year. Langer's team suggested that the men might even feel as well as they did in 1959. Men in the other group also focused on conditions 20 years earlier, but their temporal context was the present. That is, they discussed life as it was in 1959 using the past tense. Before and after a separate 5-day country retreat, researchers measured the men's physical strength, taste, hearing, vision, gait, perception cognition, values, and behavior. The men's faces were photographed and their gait and posture was videotaped. At the retreat, the researchers videotaped the men eating meals to record how much food and with how much vigor they ate and their independence in serving themselves and cleaning up after meals. The men in both groups engaged in the same daily routines with the only difference being the focus on 1959 as if it were the present (experimental group) or past (control group). The experimental group experienced news, music, movies, magazines, television, and sports as if it was 1959, and the other group used media to reminisce about 1959.

The results showed changes in both groups. Both groups showed improvements in hearing and hand strength and all looked younger as judged by the facial photos. Their memories improved. They ate heartily and gained a little weight, were less dependent on others, and were more involved in serving and cleaning up from meals. In fact, all the men in both groups were functioning independently from the first days of the retreat, despite the fact that they had all been dependent on the help of others before the retreat. The differences between the two groups that were apparent in 5 days included gains for the experimental group and losses for the reminiscence group. The experimental group showed changes in their physical condition, including improvements in cognitive skill (IQ and problem solving), vision, flexibility, and overall fitness. The control group showed improvement only in the measures for friendliness and emotional expressiveness.

Langer's study showed that when researchers changed the time context, this dramatically altered the men's experience of where they were. By controlling that aspect alone, Langer found that the men in the experimental group had reversed what had always been considered "irreversible" measures of the aging process (66, p. 112). The interaction of the men and place was altered by time-improved measures of health, perceived well-being, and everyday occupations of the experimental group. Perhaps in the process of depicting an earlier time in their lives, men in the experimental group lived out the everyday occupations of a time when they were presumably healthier.

In another study of place, occupation, and well-being (67), Wallenius examined whether the perceived supportiveness of an environment in connection with an individual's personal projects was related to psychological well-being. Well-being was defined as a person's overall satisfaction with life and the presence of depression as measured by psychological scales. Personal projects referred to the goal-directed pursuits that were currently being undertaken by the study's participants. Wallenius was also interested in determining those specific characteristics of personal projects and everyday places that were associated with the level of perceived supportiveness of the environment.

Wallenius found that approximately one-third of the participants' personal projects were connected to a specifiable place, most often home, the workplace, or sports facilities. Perceived supportiveness of the environment in connection with personal projects predicted life satisfaction but was not related to depression. Highly supportive environments were associated with projects that were accomplishable, socially supported, and difficult to complete successfully. Study participants who showed evidence of depression tended to have projects that were more abstract, more stressful, and more self-related. Each aspect of the environment was perceived to have supportive functions. Informal action by friends and associates was perceived to support personal projects more often than more formal structures in a setting. Wallenius' study provided a detailed understanding of how places supported goal-directed occupational pursuits.

Clearly, the health and well-being of people depend to a great extent on the places in which they work, rest, sleep, play, and care for themselves and others. Although it is important for places to have natural and physical resources, it is the influence of place on social interaction and the social dimensions of places that seem most to affect the quality of life and overall well-being in everyday occupations.

CHAPTER SUMMARY

This chapter has provided an overview of the relationship between places and everyday occupations. Multiple dimensions of places were identified, including their physical and geographic dimensions and their socially constructed meanings. Archetypal places were identified as those that fulfill basic needs in everyday life, many of which serve as focal points for specific daily occupations. The reciprocal influences of occupations on places and places on occupations were described, and geographic differences in occupation by place were illustrated, with examples of how the displacement of homelessness deprives individuals of the basic support provided by the place we call "home." The importance of the time–space dimension related to the location of places and the distances between them was described. Technological developments and the creation of virtual places were identified as a significant development for the new millennium. The chapter concluded with descriptions of research showing how dimensions of place can influence health and well-being.

STUDY GUIDE

Study Guide Author: Kate Barrett

Summary of Main Points

Understanding how the meaning of place develops is vital in understanding how a person experiences occupation. The place in which an occupation is performed may influence when, how, why, and with whom the occupation is performed. Culture and geographic location are significant factors shaping how places are experienced and used. Conversely, occupations affect how a place is constructed. The objects and space required of an occupation as well as the abilities of a person and/or community influence how place is designed for specific occupations, and participation in occupations affects how places are built or culturally organized.

Application to Occupational Therapy

Understanding the concept of place is vital for occupational therapists. Occupational therapists consistently encounter people who are experiencing displacement and/or are in need of re-creating meaning in a new space. Even when the geographic place is unchanged, occupational therapists encounter people who are redefining their use of space to promote their health, build greater community connectedness, or otherwise change their lifestyle. The meaning of place changes as people's abilities to perform occupations, habits, routines, and rituals in those places are affected by illness, injury, disease, or other life-altering experiences.

Occupational therapists frequently work with clients to change or adapt their places to maximize occupational function. To do this in an effective manner, occupational therapists would include attention to place in starting with clients, assessing occupational issues, planning programs, implementing and evaluating the effects of place on occupational engagement. Alternately, rather than coaching and educating people to adapt their lives in place, occupational therapists may collaborate with them to prompt changes in place. In some situations, occupational therapists may advocate for universal design or employment support for persons with mental disorders. In other situations, they may enable people to transform their occupational experiences where they are members of social groups who experience occupational injustice.

The concept of place draws from several disciplines. The understanding of place that is being articulated in occupational science can be used to inform occupational therapy practice. Occupational scientists are concerned with how place is created and experienced, and how occupational engagement can transform places to be more universally accessible or supportive. Occupational therapists may use the concept of place to address issues of survival and participation as well as the meanings of occupations in particular places.

Individual Learning Activities

1. Think back to your childhood and a memory that you have of "being in place," in other words, a memory you have of being somewhere. It may be a place that you only visited once, perhaps on a vacation. It may be a place where you spent a lot of time (kitchen table, bedroom, classroom, etc.). Describe what you remember about that

place. Who was there with you? What do you remember about the physical properties of the place (color, objects, size, smells, sounds, etc.). How did the place shape the activities you did there? What makes the place memorable to you? Was it the people there with you? The experience(s) that occurred there? What emotion is attached to that place? What did you DO there—what were your occupations?

2. Think about an occupation that you participate in at a community level (sport league, church activities, volunteerism, etc.). Describe how the place in which this occupation is performed shapes the performance of the occupation. Does the place shape temporal aspects of the occupation (seasonal, duration, frequency)? Does it shape physical behaviors? What are the affordances in this place?

Group Learning Activity

In a small group, identify a place to visit in the community (park, church, restaurant, store, etc.). Observe people participating in occupation in the chosen community site. What affordances and presses exist in this place that shape occupational performance? How do you think the meaning of the occupation may be shaped by the place?

Study Questions

1. Which of the following is NOT true?
   a. Place shapes how occupation is performed.
   b. Occupations shape the meaning of a place.
   c. Occupations performed in different places always have the same meaning.
   d. Place influences why occupations are performed.
2. Any object that is deeply rooted in human history and serves as a symbol or model for other objects is a(n)
   a. Antique
   b. Archetype
   c. Habitus
   d. Semiotic
3. When people change places all of the following may occur EXCEPT:
   a. A reinforcement of habits
   b. A sense of a refreshing change
   c. A disruption in habits and routines
   d. A sense of stress
4. The social construction of the meaning of place may be built through:
   a. Historical meaning passed on from generation to generation
   b. Shared experiences in place
   c. Acquired symbolic representation
   d. All of the above

5. Habitus, as described by the sociologist, Bourdieu, describes
   a. The place in which one resides
   b. The place in which one experiences community
   c. Conscious patterns of doing, thinking, speaking, and perceiving
   d. Unconscious patterns of doing, thinking, speaking, and perceiving

REFERENCES

1. Harvey, D. W. (1993). From space to place and back again: Reflections on the condition of post-modernity. In J. Bird, et al. (Eds.), *Mapping the futures: Local cultures, global change.* London: Routledge.
2. Spivak, M. (1973, October). Archetypal places. *The Architectural Forum,* pp. 44–49.
3. Barker, R. G. (1963). On the nature of the environment. *Journal of Social Issues, 19,* 17–38.
4. Thwaits, K. (2001). Experiential landscape place: An exploration of space and experience in neighbourhood landscape architecture. *Landscape Research, 26*(3), 245–255.
5. Gibson, J. J. (1979). *The ecological approach to vision perception.* Boston: Houghton Mifflin.
6. Dumur, E., Barnard, Y., & Boy, G. (2004). Designing for comfort. In D. de Waard, K. A. Brookhuis, & C. M. Weikert (Eds.), *Human factors in design* (pp. 111–127). Maastricht, Netherlands: Shaker Publishing.
7. Mark, L. S., Balliett, J. A., Craver, K. D., Douglas, S. D., & Fox, T. (1990). What an actor must do in order to perceive the affordance for sitting. *Ecological Psychology, 2,* 325–366.
8. Quigley, C., Southall, D., Freer, M., Moody, A., & Porter, M. (2001). *Anthropometric study to update minimum aircraft seating standards.* Retrieved August 20, 2006, from https://magpie.lboro.ac.uk/dspace/handle/2134/701?mode=full
9. Thrift, N. (1985). Flies and germs: A geography of knowledge. In D. Gregory & J. Urry (Eds.), *Social relations and spatial structures.* Basingstoke: Macmillan.
10. Ralph, E. (1976). *Place and placelessness.* London: Pion.
11. Sack, R. (1992). *Place, modernity and the consumer's world.* Baltimore: Johns Hopkins University Press.
12. Hiss, T. (1996). *The experience of place.* New York: Vintage Books.
13. Hummon, D. (1990). *Commonplaces: Community ideology and identity in American culture.* Albany: State University of New York Press.
14. Steele, F. (1981). *The sense of place.* Boston: CBI Publishing.
15. Hummon, D. (1992). Community attachment: Local sentiment and a sense of place. In S. Altman (Ed.), *Place attachment* (pp. 253–278). New York: Plenum.
16. Gustafson, P. (2001). Meanings of place: Everyday experiences and theoretical conceptualizations. *Journal of Environmental Psychology, 21*(1), 5–16.
17. Danesi, M. (1994). *Messages and meanings: An introduction to semiotics.* Toronto: Canadian Scholars Press.
18. Cobley, P., & Jantz, L. (1998). *Introducing semiotics.* Lanham, MD: Totem Books.
19. Transport for London. (2006). *History of the tube map.* Retrieved October 2, 2006, from http://www.tfl.gov.uk/tube/company/history/tube-map.asp
20. Stevens, A. (1990). *On Jung.* London: Penguin.

21. Campbell, J. (1973). *The hero with a thousand faces.* Princeton, NJ: Princeton University Press.
22. MacDonald, M. R. (1982). *The storyteller's sourcebook: A subject, title and motif index to folklore collections for children.* Detroit: Neal-Schuman Publishers.
23. Knowles, R. L. (1992). Rhythms of perception. *Places, 8*(2), 72–81.
24. Calvin, W. H. (1986). *The river that flows uphill: A journey from the big bang to the big brain.* San Francisco: Sierra Club Books.
25. James, L., & Nahl, D. (2000). *Road rage and aggressive driving: Steering clear of highway warfare.* Amherst, NY: Prometheus Books.
26. Federation, E. (1984). *Improvement of living and working conditions.* Dublin, Ireland: European Foundation for the Improvement of Living and Working Conditions.
27. Marshall, K. (1994). *Getting there* (Report 75-001E). Ottawa: Statistics Canada.
28. Kulash, W. (1990). Traditional neighbourhood development: Will the traffic work? In *Eleventh Annual Pedestrian Conference* (pp. 4-1–4-2). Bellevue, WA.
29. World Bank (IRBD). (1986). *Urban transport* (Report PB86-194321). Washington, DC: Author.
30. Ley, D. (1983). *A social geography of the city.* New York: Harper and Row.
31. Bourdieu, P. (1990). *In other words: Essays towards a reflexive sociology.* Stanford, CA: Stanford University Press.
32. Murray, H. A., Barrett, W. G., & Hamburger, E. (1938). *Explorations in personality.* New York: Oxford University Press.
33. Lewin, K. (1997). *Field theory in social science.* Washington, DC: American Psychological Association.
34. Latane, B. (1981). The psychology of social impact. *American Psychologist,* 36, 343–356.
35. Wickens, C. D., Gordon, S. E., & Liu, Y. (Eds.). (1998). *An introduction to human factors engineering.* New York: Addison-Wesley.
36. Platt, K. (1996). Places of experience and the experience of place. In L. Rouner (Ed.), *The longing for home* (pp. 112–127). Notre Dame, IN: University of Notre Dame Press.
37. Fontanel, C. (1998). *Babies celebrated.* New York: Harry Abrams.
38. Valentine, G. (2001). *Social geographies, space, and society.* Harlow, England: Pearson Education, Ltd.
39. Christiansen, C. H. (1999). Defining lives: Occupation as identity: An essay on competence, coherence, and the creation of meaning, 1999 Eleanor Clarke Slagle lecture. *American Journal of Occupational Therapy, 53,* 547–558.
40. Sacks, O. (1998). *A leg to stand on.* New York: Touchstone. (First printing: 1984)
41. Hall, E. T. (1981). *Beyond culture.* New York: Anchor Books. (First printing: 1976)
42. Mehrabian, A. (1981). *Silent messages: Implicit communication of emotions and attitudes* (2nd ed.). Belmont, CA: Wadsworth Publishing.
43. Rand, M. L. (2001). Boundaries and the body. *Annals of the American Psychotherapy Association, 4,* 27.
44. Senft, G. (1997). *Space: Studies in Austronesian and Papuan languages.* Oxford: Clarendon Press.
45. Mahler, M. (1975). *Psychological birth of the human infant: Symbiosis and individuation.* New York: Basic Books.
46. Berg., M, & Medrich, E. A. (1980). Children in four neighborhoods: The physical environment and its effect on play and play patterns. *Environment and Behavior, 12,* 320–348.

47. Carpenter, J. L. (1991). *Frank Baum: Royal historian of Oz.* Minneapolis: Lerner Publications Co.
48. Spielberg, S. (Producer & Director), & Kennedy, K. (Producer) (1982). *E. T. The Extra-Terrestrial* [Motion Picture], United States: Universal City Studios.
49. U.S. Department of Justice Office of Justice Programs. (2005). Family violence statistics. Washington, DC: Author. Retrieved November 8, 2006 from http://www.ojp.usdoj.gov/bjs/pub/pdf/fvs07.pdf
50. Czaja, S. J., Weber, R. A., & Nair, S. N. (1993). A human factor analysis of ADL activities: A capability demand approach. *Journal of Gerontology, 48,* 44–48.
51. Rowles, G. (1999). Beyond performance: Being in place as a component of occupational therapy. *American Journal of Occupational Therapy, 45*(3), 265–271.
52. Robinson, T. (1999). Stigma and architecture. In G. S. Steinfeld (Ed.), *Enabling environments: Measuring the impact of environment on disability and rehabilitation* (pp. 251–270). Norwell, MA: Kluwer Academic/Plenum Publishers.
53. Shinn, M., & Weitzman, B. (1998). Predictors of homelessness among families in New York City. *American Journal of Public Health, 88,* 1651–1657.
54. Fischer, P. J. (1992). Criminal behavior and victimization among homeless people. In R. I. Jaheil (Ed.), *Homelessness: A prevention-oriented approach.* Baltimore: The Johns Hopkins University Press.
55. Steiner, L. P., Looney, S. W., Hall, L. R., & Wright, K. M. (1995). Quality of life and functional status among homeless men attending a day shelter in Louisville, Kentucky. *Journal of the Kentucky Medical Association, 93*(5), 188–195.
56. Rosenbeck, C. (1998). Homelessness, health service use and related costs. *Medical Care, 36*(8), 1256–1264.
57. Weinbreb, L., Goldberg, R., & Perloff, J. (1998). Health characteristics and medical service use patterns of sheltered homeless and low income housed mothers. *Journal of General Internal Medicine, 13,* 389–397.
58. Gelberg, L., Linn, L. S., & Leake, B. (1998). Mental health, alcohol and drug use, and criminal history among homeless adults. *American Journal of Psychiatry, 145*(2), 191–196.
59. Williams, J. C. (1998). Domestic violence and poverty: The narratives of homeless women. *Frontiers, 19*(2), 143–165.
60. Davey, T. L. (1998). Homeless children and stress: An empirical study. *Journal of Social Distress and the Homeless, 7*(1), 29–41.
61. Lanier, J. (2001). Virtually there. *Scientific American, 284*(4), 64–65.
62. Marshall, G. (Ed). (1994). *The concise Oxford dictionary of sociology.* Oxford: Oxford University Press.
63. Kaplan, R. (2001). The nature of the view from home. *Psychological Benefits, 33*(4), 507–542.
64. Korpela, K. M., Hartig, T., Kaiser, F. G., & Fuhrer, U. (2001). Restorative experience and self regulation in favorite places. *Environment and Behavior, 33*(4), 572–589.
65. Read, M. A., Sugawara, A. I., & Brandt, J. A. (1999). Impact of space and color in the physical environment on preschool cooperative behavior. *Environment and Behavior, 31*(3), 413–428.
66. Langer, E. (1989). *Mindfulness.* Reading, MA: Addison-Wesley.
67. Wallenius, M. (1999). Personal projects in everyday places: Perceived supportiveness of the environment and psychological well-being. *Journal of Environmental Psychology, 19*(2), 131–143.

CHAPTER 11

Work, Occupation, and Leisure

Jiri Zuzanek

OBJECTIVES

1. Describe the relationships between work, occupation, and leisure and their effects on well-being.
2. Define and discuss concepts of spillover, compensation, and compartmentalization.
3. Examine the leisure effects of occupational culture.
4. Explore the relationship of stress, work hours, feelings of pressure, and the effects on overall health and well-being.

KEY WORDS

Compartmentalization
Compensation
Life satisfaction
Occupational culture
Spillover
Stress
Time pressure
Well-being
Work-leisure relationship

CHAPTER PROFILE

This chapter examines relationships between work, occupation, and leisure and their effects on workers' and employees' well-being. Three major conceptualizations of work-leisure relationship identified in the literature, namely spillover, compensation, and compartmentalization, are examined in greater detail. Additionally, the chapter examines lifestyle and leisure effects of occupational culture, defined as a set of technical, social, and cultural characteristics and attributes associated with one's

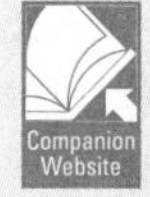

www.prenhall.com/christiansen

The Internet provides an exciting means for interacting with this textbook and for enhancing your understanding of humans' experiences with occupations and the organization of occupations in society. Use the address above to access the interactive Companion Website created specifically to accompany this book. Here you will find an array of self-study material designed to help you gain a richer understanding of the concepts presented in this chapter.

place in the social division of labor. Finally the chapter examines the effects of prolonged hours of work and subjective feelings of time pressure on workers' and employees' health and emotional well-being.

INTRODUCTION

Relationships between work, occupation, and leisure have long attracted the interest of social scientists. In the 1930s, George Lundberg (1) drew attention to the effects of the changes in the labor market on the relations between leisure and occupation. In Europe, effects of industrial work on leisure were examined systematically in the 1950s by Georges Friedmann (2). Sebastian de Grazia pointed out that the connection between work and leisure can be traced back to ancient Greece and Rome where (unlike modern times) work was defined as the opposite of leisure. The Greek as well as the Latin word for work, or being occupied, was *un-leisure.* English has no word to ground leisure more positively than work (3).

The assumption that the character of one's work has a strong impact on one's leisure was shared by most authors in the 1960s. According to Greenberg (4), leisure—even for those who do not work, is at bottom a function of work, flows from work, and changes as the nature of work changes. The same message rings loud in Bennett Berger's classical article, *The Sociology of Leisure.* According to Berger, we must contrast work and leisure, since they have sociological meaning vis-à-vis each other (5). Joffre Dumazedier, a disciple of Friedmann, attempted to redefine the relationship between work and leisure. By emphasizing that in postindustrial societies leisure will increasingly affect the choices and the nature of work, he defined the relationship between work and leisure as reciprocal rather than one directional (6).

The debate about the relationship between work and leisure in the 1950s and the 1960s focused on their respective roles in the advanced industrial and postindustrial societies. Riesman's (7) analysis of the shift from the "inner-directed" to the "other-directed" personality in *The Lonely Crowd* signaled a growing role of interpersonal contacts and leisure (at the expense of work) in the lives of Americans. Dubin (8) and Orzack (9) in the United States and Goldthorpe (10) in Britain suggested that work as central life interest lost ground in most occupations and retained its prominence only among professionals, self-employed persons, and those in higher levels of management. According to John Kenneth Galbraith, by the mid 1960s the notion of a "new era of greatly expanded leisure" had become a "conventional conversation piece" (11). Fourastié (12), in France, predicted that in 1985 men would work only one-third of their life, the length of the workweek would not exceed 30 hours, and 12 weeks of vacation would be guaranteed. Arguing from an economist's perspective, Samuelson (13) suggested that after achieving a comfortable margin over what they conventionally consider to be necessary, people would not seek additional work, even if the wages were to go up, but rather would opt for more leisure. Dumazedier, in the trend-setting book *Towards a Society of Leisure,* suggested that growing amounts and greater role of leisure in modern societies were destined to trigger a "humanistic mutation" of the industrial civilization.

However, not everybody agreed. For economists the relationships between work and leisure always involved a conscious or implicit trade-off between a desire for more free time and foregone earnings (income). Examining historical data, Kreps and Spengler (14) and Owen (15) established that whereas in the 1930s up to 30% of the total societal gain in productivity was transformed into free time, in the 1960s only 8% of it was channeled toward increased leisure. Productivity gains were invested increasingly into consumption rather than free time. This argument was brought to its logical conclusion in the early 1970s by Stefan Linder in his provocative book *The Harried Leisure Class* (16). According to Linder, people in modern industrial societies lead more hectic rather than more leisurely lives because any gains in shorter working hours are compensated by growing demands of consumption. More recently, this thesis has been restated by Juliet Schor in *The Overworked American: The Unexpected Decline of Leisure* (17). Historic preferences of employers for longer working hours, gender inequalities, and the addictive nature of consumption have contributed, according to Schor, to the vicious "work-and-spend" cycle, resulting in a "time squeeze" for both men and women.

Authors in Europe and the United States (18) drew attention to the fact that "flexibilization" of working hours and standards, fostered by globalization and increased international competition, poses a threat to many workers' long-established leisure privileges and has profound lifestyle implications in the rapidly changing work environment.

Apart from the general debate over the future of work and leisure and their interrelation in postindustrial societies, sociologists and psychologists have paid considerable attention to a number of more specific issues of the relationships between work, occupation, and leisure. Four of these issues are particularly interesting and will be discussed in greater detail in this chapter. They are

1. Theoretical conceptualizations of work-leisure relationships
2. Empirical support for the alternative scenarios of work-leisure relationships
3. Effects of social-occupational status on leisure behavior and preferences
4. Effects of long hours of work and "time crunch" on leisure and emotional well-being of employees

WORK-LEISURE RELATIONSHIP: "SPILLOVER," COMPENSATION, OR COMPARTMENTALIZATION?

In a pioneering attempt to define the effects of work on leisure behavior and experience, Harold Wilensky coined the notions of *spillover* and *compensatory* relationships. According to the spillover hypothesis, alienation from work becomes alienation from life, and "mental stultification produced by labor permeates leisure." In the compensatory relationship, the routine of leisure produces "an explosive compensation for the deadening rhythms of factory life" (19).

Reinhard Wippler summarized this issue a decade later:

> A rich terminology has evolved in designating different kinds of connections between work and leisure such as compensatory, complementary, spillover, or continuative. Critical analysis of leisure studies from Western Europe and the United States indicates, however, that all hypotheses can be subsumed under two main hypotheses. When leisure-time behavior differs markedly from that during working time, or when the setting of leisure activities contrasts strongly with the work setting, reference may be made to the *contrast hypothesis.* On the other hand, resemblances between leisure behavior and work behavior and between the physical and social circumstances of work and leisure may be indicated by the term *congruence hypothesis.* (20, p. 58)

Stanley Parker, in *Leisure and Work* (21), pursued a similar line of argument contrasting *extension* or *congruence* work-leisure relationships with *compensation* and *contrast* ones, as well as adding an "in-between" *compartmentalized* relationship.

Historical and ideological roots of these approaches are anchored in the 19th-century critique of industrial work and its impact on workers' lives. Although this critique is usually associated with the Marxian analysis of alienated labor in the *Economic and Philosophical Manuscripts* (22), it can be found already a decade earlier in Alexis de Tocqueville's *Democracy in America.* According to Tocqueville, when a workman is unceasingly and exclusively engaged in the fabrication of one thing, the work is ultimately done with singular dexterity, but at the same time the worker loses the general faculty of thinking about the direction of the work. Workers become more adroit, less industrious, and with improvement are actually *degraded.* The question that this raises is about expectations of workers who spend "twenty years making heads for pins?" (23).

The *spillover* hypothesis stipulates that because work is, for the majority of people, the most important life occupation, it decisively affects the quality of one's self-concept, lifestyle, and leisure. Increasingly fragmented industrial and clerical work does not allow workers to see the final product of their effort, to identify with work, and to control the rhythm and direction of their actions. Assembly-line production turns work into an alienating and mindless toil rather than a meaningful experience. Mindless work produces passive and mindless leisure. Irving Howe believed that the quality of leisure time activity cannot vary too sharply from that of the work. In essence, leisure time must be related to working time since they may appear to be different yet are actually the same. Leisure complements work by providing relief from work monotony so that the return to work is bearable (24). Meissner (25), in a study of Canadian factory workers, observed that lack of discretionary potential on the job resulted in reduced participation in organized and voluntary activities. Workers isolated from their workmates on the job spent less time in social leisure activities away from work, whereas active social interaction on the job resulted in greater participation in voluntary organizations in the after-work hours.

The *compensatory* relationship between work and leisure has been also often associated with negative outcomes. Wilensky's 1964 description of an autoworker using dramatic phrases, such as "gripped bodily for eight hours to repetitive, low-skilled, machine-paced work," "hells down the superhighway," "stops for a beer," "starts a bar-room brawl," "goes home and beats his wife," and lo and behold, "throws a rock at a Negro moving into the neighbourhood" illustrates well this scenario (26). In short, the worker compensates for the lack of excitement at work by outbursts of uncontrolled spontaneity, which often take antisocial and deviant forms (heavy drinking, brawls of soccer fans, drugs, racial harassment). A comment is, however, due here: Most of the evidence in support of this "downgrading" scenario came from journalistic accounts rather than systematic sociological inquiry.

A much more positive interpretation of the compensatory relationship between work and leisure was articulated by Friedmann. According to Friedmann, leisure can provide the worker not only with an escape from the drudgery of the job, but also with a positive compensation for the dissatisfaction with monotonous work. Leisure can be, in Friedmann's opinion, more readily humanized than work. The worker tries to use leisure time to regain the initiative, responsibility, and sense of achievement that is absent from work. Compensation for work is growing with a "fantastic mushrooming" of leisure options, such as hobbies, arts and crafts, photography, pottery, and electronics. On a scale unknown in previous history, there are now "amateurs" on almost everything in the United States (27). Leisure, viewed from this perspective, provides the individual with an independent source of satisfaction, personal involvement, and cultural development. This positive effect is achieved, however, according to Friedmann, at the high cost of dissatisfaction with work.

It is not only the *compensatory* relationship, however, that can assume positive forms. A number of authors have argued that a *spillover* relationship between work and leisure can also produce positive outcomes as a result of technological change. Most of these authors rested their hopes on automation (Theobald; McLuhan) and organizational reforms of industrial work (Karasek & Theorell) (28).

Automation, in the opinion of Theobald and McLuhan, reverses a long trend toward the fragmentation of human work. It represents a different organization of work than mechanization or assembly-line production. Assembly-line technology and Taylor's (29) management practices of work reduced the worker to a cog in the chain of machine operations, subordinating him to the process over which he had little control and which he did not understand. Automation supposedly reverses this trend. In the automated plant, the worker steps out of the production line to assume a supervisory and management role. This is accompanied by a quest for skills, knowledge, and better understanding of the entire work process. In other words, technology, rather than enslaving the individual, will liberate us.

Marshall McLuhan wrote about how automation makes liberal education mandatory because the electric age of "servomechanisms" removes the need for mechanical and specialist servitude, as was necessary in the preceding machine age. McLuhan uses the analogy that, just as the motorcar released human needs for the horse and turned horses over to the world of entertainment, automation is releasing the need for human servitude to machines. The result is that humans are now threatened with the liberation of self-employment and the unknown opportunities yet to be discovered for participation in society (30).

Karasek and Theorell, in a seminal study of Swedish workers, demonstrated that greater decision latitude and psychological demands at work correlated positively

TABLE 11-1 *Theoretical Conceptualizations of the Work-Leisure Relationship*

Type of work -leisure relationship	Scenarios of work's future	
	Pessimistic	**Optimistic**
Spillover/congruence	Spillover—optimistic	Spillover—pessimistic
Compensation/contrast	Compensation—upgrading	Compensation—downgrading
Segmentation/compartmentalization	No relationship	

with workers' health and overall well-being. According to these authors, an active job situation with high psychological demands and high decision latitude is linked to high rates of participation in leisure and political activities (31). According to an Australian study by Kabanoff and O'Brien (32), workers with greater variety and skill use demonstrated higher levels of these attributes in their leisure.

In real life, the effects of automation proved, however, to be less pronounced and clear than expected, and the changes in the organization of work advocated by reformers were implemented only to a limited extent.

In addition to the spillover and compensatory hypotheses of the work-leisure relationship, the *segmentation* or *compartmentalization* hypotheses should also to be mentioned here. According to this hypothesis, first spelled out by Parker, there is virtually no relationship between the worlds of work and leisure. They both exist in different and unrelated universes. According to Parker, segmentalists believe that life is split into different areas of activity and interest, with each social segment lived out more or less independently of the rest. Work is separated from leisure. The production of goods and services is separated from their consumption. The workplace is separated from one's residence, education is not connected to religion, and politics are different from recreation (33). According to Bacon, modern industrial societies are characterized by a more segmented relationship between work and leisure than was commonly assumed. Bacon proposed that work is no long the central focus of life for most people and for many work is a marginal experience (34, 35).

The typology of possible work-leisure relationships just discussed is summarized in Table 11-1 ■.[1]

EMPIRICAL SUPPORT FOR THE WORK-LEISURE RELATIONSHIP SCENARIOS

After outlining major theoretical hypotheses of work-leisure relationships, it is appropriate to ask whether these hypotheses are supported by empirical data, and if so, to what extent? In general, the evidence in support of various conceptualizations of work-leisure relationships is inconclusive. According to Kabanoff, none of the three major work/leisure hypotheses can be fully supported (36). Pennings formulated a similar conclusion even more resolutely, suggesting that the evidence for the three hypotheses resembles an outcome of a hung jury (37). In a recent review of the analyses of work-leisure relationships, A. J. Veal concluded that all three traditions, although still relevant for the understanding of current concerns in the domain of work and leisure, have largely disappeared in the 1980s and 1990s from leisure studies. Today's studies have turned to new approaches and concerns (38).

The reasons for the lower interest in the early concepts of work-leisure relationships can be attributed to three major factors: (a) methodological problems, (b) underestimation of the role of intervening factors, and (c) changes in the labor market and economy.

Several authors (39) pointed out that some of the difficulties in establishing clearer relationships between work and leisure stem from definitional and measurement problems, such as rather general or inconsistent definitions of work and leisure and lack of clarity with regard to the hypothesized associations between different types of work and their leisure outcomes. According to Kando and Summers, literature about the relationship between work and nonwork has a tendency to overlook the complexity of possible relationships between work and leisure and the experiences and interpretations of those who participate in them (40).

A number of authors (41) emphasized the need to pay greater attention to the moderating effects of intervening psychological and social factors and processes. Wippler, whose study is generally supportive of the spillover relationship between work and leisure, observed that, contrary to the expectations advanced in theoretical discussions, variables representing work and career explain only a small part of the variations in leisure in comparison to other predictors (42).

Kabanoff and O'Brien and Iso-Ahola stressed that the effects of work on leisure participation are usually mediated by cognitive processes or personality traits. Iso-Ahola, determined the effects of work (W) on leisure (L) and vice versa by taking into account cognitive variables (O) in a paradigm represented by W-O-L (43). According to these authors, personal dispositions and situational context such as locus of external or internal control, independence, alienation, or affiliation determine to a large extent whether the relationships between work and leisure will take spillover, compensation, or segmented forms. According to Mannell and Iso-Ahola (44), individuals in modern societies enter the workforce with relatively well-formed personality dispositions, which affect choices and structuring of their work and leisure options.

Research has also shown that the work-leisure relationship may vary for different sociooccupational groups. According to Parker (45), the work-leisure relationship could be characterized as mostly *spillover* among successful businesspeople, *neutral* among minor professionals, and *contrasting* among unskilled manual workers and assembly-line workers. Pennings's study reported a spillover relationship between work and leisure among full-time employees in the American Midwest, but observed that this relationship was strongest for employees who deeply identified with their work (46).

The strongest factor that contributed to the fading of interest in the conceptualizations of work-leisure relationship was, however, the change in the labor market that took place in the 1980s and 1990s. The manufacturing jobs that were at the root of the initial conceptualizations of work-leisure relationship were disappearing and so were well-definable lifelong careers. Unwaged groups attracted greater policy interest. It is, therefore, not surprising that Veal was not in support of Parker's bipolar work/leisure approach which neglected and marginalized manufacturing groups in research on leisure studies policy (47).

LEISURE AND OCCUPATION

The relationship between work and leisure has been also examined from a sociooccupational perspective of work. Studies using this approach do not focus on the effects of technical and organizational features of work on leisure, but rather on the lifestyle effects of belonging to a specific sociooccupational group or class.

There is a difference between studies examining how leisure is affected by *social class* and studies examining relationships between leisure and a more narrowly defined *sociooccupational status.* The former studies focus on social and class inequalities and implicitly pose the question of how to reduce or eliminate these inequalities. In a way, these studies are *prescriptive* as well as descriptive. Ultimately they foresee a society with few, if any, marked differences in the population's access to and use of leisure. The studies of the relationship between leisure and *sociooccupational status,* on the other hand, assume that occupational differences are horizontal as well as vertical and will remain present in any society, even the most egalitarian one. This second type of studies usually aims at a better understanding as well as a forecasting of social, leisure, and cultural needs or requirements associated with the changing occupational structure of modern societies. It is these studies that will be commented on next.

Studies of occupational differences in leisure behavior and attitudes may focus on leisure patterns of individual occupational groups, such as blue-collar workers, as was done, for example, by Hoggart or Shostak and Gromberg (48) or they can compare lifestyle and leisure patterns of different occupational groups deemed important in modern societies. Lundberg, in *Leisure: A Suburban Study* (49), examined and compared time use and leisure activities of blue-collar workers, white-collar employees, professionals and executives, the unemployed, housewives, and high school and college students.

Lundberg's classification of occupations was upheld and modified in a number of follow-up surveys of time use and leisure participation. Alexander Szalai and associates (50) examined time use differences between professionals and high and low white-collar employees, skilled and semiskilled labor, and unskilled labor. The United States Bureau of Outdoor Recreation (51) distinguished between outdoor participation of professionals, managers and executives, clerical and sales workers, kindred workers, laborers, service workers, and farmers. Katz and Gurevitch, in *The Secularization of Leisure* (52), examined time use and leisure patterns of Israeli farmers, craftsmen and factory workers, service personnel, professionals, managers and executives, entrepreneurs, and the unemployed.

The 1992 Canadian General Social Survey (53) distinguished between unskilled manual labor, semiskilled clerical and sales personnel, middle management, high-level management, and self-employed professionals. Table 11-2 ■ shows that unskilled

TABLE 11-2 *Time Use and Leisure Participation of Employed Men Aged 24 to 65 by Sociooccupational Status: 1992 GSS, Canada (Minutes per day; Mean Score)*

Activity	Unskilled labor	Semiskilled clerical & sales	Middle management	Higher-level management	Self-employed professionals
Paid work, incl. travel to work	437	452	461	409	527
Domestic work	122	119	131	163	115
Education, study	2	0	2	2	3
Personal needs	559	560	552	545	521
Sleep/naps	462	476	458	439	439
Meals at home	58	49	50	60	43
Personal care	39	35	44	46	38
Religion and voluntary activities	9	7	10	16	13
Free time	311	302	285	305	261
Watching television/video	141	142	103	95	87
Social leisure	93	81	82	117	86
Physically active leisure	29	27	34	28	28
Reading	15	19	34	26	40
Games (incl. computer and video)	10	3	7	7	0
Resting/relaxing	10	11	7	14	5
Other free time	13	19	17	18	15
Total day	1440	1440	1440	1440	1440
Index of leisure participation (1–100)	17.9	21.7	28.4	32.2	36.9

labor and higher-level management, perhaps somewhat unexpectedly, reported shorter hours of paid work than semiskilled clerical/sales personnel or middle management. The longest hours of paid work and the shortest amounts of free time were reported by self-employed professionals. Not surprisingly, self-employed professionals experienced the highest levels of perceived time pressure. The relative shortage of free time did not stop them, however, from participating in a greater variety of leisure pursuits than other occupational groups.

In general, it is surprising how little attention researchers have paid since the 1960s to the impact of occupational differences on leisure. One has to agree with Veal that the study of leisure behavior of different occupational communities has been neglected in the past decades (54).

One of the possible reasons for this lack of interest is the absence of a standardized classification of occupational categories that can be easily applied to the study of daily life and leisure. Statistical agencies often build their occupational classifications around industries or prestige levels, rather than distinct *occupational cultures.* One finds in the 1998 Canadian General Social Survey *six* versions of the Standard Industrial Classification as well as Blishen's and Pineo's socioeconomic indices (55). Categories such as *utilities, construction, manufacturing,* or *trade* are, however, of little help in ascertaining lifestyle profiles of these occupational groups. Likewise, the collapsing (in the same survey) of *skilled workers, employees,* and *farmers* into a single *medium status* category does not do justice to the lifestyle differences between these groups.

Standard industrial classifications of occupations do not reflect respondents' perceptions of their belonging to a distinct and readily identifiable occupational and lifestyle group or culture. From the leisure perspective, it is important, according to Salaman, that "occupational communities" understand and identify with their occupational roles, such as printers, policemen, and army officers, and that the specific qualities, interests, and abilities of occupational communities be carried into their non-work life (56).

It has been suggested by this author in an earlier study of work-leisure relationship (coauthored with Roger Mannell) that future research on the work-leisure relationship may benefit from greater attention to the *occupational culture,* defined as a set of technical, social and cultural characteristics and attributes that are associated with people's place in the social division of labour and with people's perceptions of themselves in the system (57). The implementation of this suggestion has been hampered, however, by the increased fluidity of the labor market. Paid employment in traditional assembly-line production has been replaced, according to Critcher and Bramham, by increasingly differentiated niche markets (58). According to Rojek, unlike the Fordist economies, workers in the new economies have to be flexible and possess a variety of skills that enable them to switch operations according to the market challenges. Globalization and deregulation propagate migratory, nomadic work-leisure experiences (59). For most employees, these changes undermined the notion of a stable *occupational career* spanning most of the life course. The workforce became increasingly unstable and fragmented, making the relationship between work and leisure situational rather than systemic (60). Therefore, it should not be a surprise that the interest in relationships between work and leisure has, in the 1980s and particularly the 1990s, shifted from the effects of jobs and occupations on leisure to the effects on leisure of *long hours of work,* accompanied by the feelings of *time crunch* and *stress.* These topics are politically more urgent and methodologically more accessible.

LONG HOURS OF WORK, TIME CRUNCH, AND LEISURE

The focus of the intellectual debate in the 1980s and 1990s shifted from the work-leisure relationship and the *promise of leisure* to the *problem of time* and *time scarcity.* Wilensky, who pioneered the early hypotheses of work-leisure relationship, was among the first to draw attention to the phenomenon of the *life-cycle squeeze* and time pressure (61). Schor's *The Overworked American* (62), questioned the widely shared belief in the forthcoming abundance of leisure. Perhaps more important than publications by academics was the shift in public opinion. Numerous polls conducted in the

United States and other industrialized nations indicated that people felt more pressed for time in the 1980s and 1990s than they did in the previous decades. Bond, Galinsky, and Swanberg reported that the proportion of Americans who felt that they "never had enough time to get everything done on the job" increased from 40% in 1977 to 60% in 1997 (63). Canadian General Social Survey data demonstrate that the percentage of Canadians who felt "more rushed than five years ago" has risen from 47% in 1992 to 50% in 1998 (64).

There is no unanimity about the extent of and underlying reasons for this trend. Robinson and Godbey, in their book *Time for Life: The Surprising Ways Americans Use Their Time,* acknowledged high levels of time anxiety in Americans but disputed Schor's conclusion about the decline of leisure. The authors argued that from the mid 1960s to the mid 1970s, Americans experienced a substantial reduction in both paid and, particularly, domestic work, and the amount of weekly free time available to Americans in the 18 to 64 age category increased from 34.8 hours per week in 1965 to 38.7 hours in 1975, and 39.6 hours in 1985 (65).

Can the positions of Schor and Robinson and Godbey be reconciled? The answer to this question may rest with the uneven distribution of workloads among different life cycle and occupational groups. Analyses of Canadian time use data show, for example, that although the amount of free time for the entire surveyed population (including adolescents and retirees) has increased between 1986 and 1998, the amount of free time available to the employed part of the population has declined. Tremblay and Villeneuve (66), using official labor statistics, showed that the average length of the workweek in Canada did not change much from 1976 to 1995, but the proportionate share of both long-hour workers (41 hours per week or more) and short-hour workers (35 hours per week or less) has increased. In other words, the two poles of the workload spectrum have expanded at the expense of the middle ground.

Zuzanek and Smale (67) argued in 1997 that the labor force became increasingly polarized along workload lines during the 1980s and 1990s. Time pressure did not affect everybody in the same way. Some population groups (unionized labor) have gained free time, whereas occupational and life cycle groups operating under combined pressures of multiple work and family roles (self-employed, professionals, employed parents with small children, single parents) did not gain additional free time, were pressed for time, and experienced time pressure and stress. It is telling, for example, that in 1992 over 68% of employed mothers and 67% of employed divorced and separated women in Canada reported feeling rushed "every day."

The preceding observations have, of course, serious methodological and policy implications. The process of polarization implies that time use of different population groups evolves along divergent rather than common paths. Under these circumstances, statistical averages of time use for the *entire* population can obscure a widening time use gap between the *haves* and *have nots* and may be inappropriate for the study of time use trends.

The phenomenon of polarization also has important social implications and revives earlier concerns about the nature of the work-leisure relationship. Employees who work long hours usually have financial means to access desirable leisure and recreational resources but do not have the time to take advantage of this opportunity. They often come home tired, spend little time in physically active leisure and, by trying to compress more leisure activities into shorter periods of time, invoke time pressure and stress.

The effects of work overload and time pressure on emotional well-being and health have been examined extensively in the literature. A study of Type A behavior by Friedman and Rosenman (68) concluded that elevated competitiveness and a sense of time urgency typical of Type A personalities exposed individuals to a heightened risk of cardiovascular disease. A 1997 Finnish Quality of Working Life Survey showed that 69% of employees in Finland who reported *high* levels of time pressure frequently experienced fatigue, 50% complained about exhaustion, 45% had sleeping problems, and 19% felt depressed (69). In Japan, concerns about negative effects of work overload resulted in a public debate over the phenomenon of "karoshi," an expression denoting "sudden death from overwork" (70).

Yet, according to some authors, existing research failed to produce carefully specified and measurable proof of the ill effects of long hours of work (71). Long hours of work were associated by some researchers with positive psychological outcomes (72). Analyses of Canadian General Social Survey (GSS) and National Population Health Survey (73) data illustrate difficulties in interpreting the effects of long hours of work on well-being and health. According to GSS, *subjective feelings of time pressure* are associated with negative emotional and health effects, whereas *long hours of work* are associated with average to above average levels of self-assessed health (Table 11-3 ■). The difference between the effects of *perceived time pressure,* as opposed to *long hours of work,* on health has a substantive as well as methodological explanation. Paid workloads in excess of 50 hours per week can hardly contribute to better health. The direction of causality between long hours of work and health is in all likelihood the reverse—healthier people are more willing and more likely to work longer hours.

There is a point, however, beyond which—to use the colloquial metaphor—the straw breaks the camel's back. Even the healthiest people are able to absorb only so much work strain. The negative effects of prolonged hours of work *kick in* when *transformed* into an acute feeling of time pressure and stress. Prolonged hours of work are not only physically exhaustive, but also create tensions in the family that produce negative emotional and well-being outcomes. In the 1998 GSS, the correlation between the length of the paid workload and satisfaction with one's work-family balance was –0.17, and between the length of paid work and satisfaction with one's use of nonworking time –0.07. Job and marital satisfaction have been identified by researchers as some of the strongest predictors of longevity (74).

One should also keep in mind that it is not only the length of work, but also the control over it that affects employees' well-being and health. Feelings of time crunch and stress are associated with the lack of control over one's use of time, lack of interest in one's work, and an excessively fragmented use of time (75). People can work long hours without feeling time crunched or stressed, if they freely choose their work and are interested in it. People working shorter hours, on the contrary, often feel time

TABLE 11-3 *Time Pressure, Stress, Leisure Participation, Emotional Well-Being, and Health by the Length of Paid Work: (Minutes per day; Mean Scores)*

	8 to 35 hrs per week	35.1 to 40 hrs per week	40.1 to 50 hrs per week	50.1+ hrs per week
Feeling of time pressure (1–21)	12.0	12.9	13.7	14.7
Perceived stress (1–5)	3.6	3.6	3.6	3.8
Index of leisure participation (1–100)	22.6	22.6	21.9	21.1
Satisfaction with work-family balance (1–4)	2.6	2.5	2.5	2.3
Satisfaction with time use (1–4)	3.1	3.1	3.0	3.0
Self-assessed health (1–5)	3.7	3.8	3.8	3.8

Correlation Between Hours of Paid Work, Feeling of Time Pressure, Perceived Stress, and Health (Pearson "r")*

	Time pressure	Perceived stress	Self-assessed health
Hours of paid work	0.08	0.60	0.50
Feeling of time pressure (1–21)	1.00	0.49	–0.13
Perceived stress (1–5)	0.49	1.00	–0.13

*Computed for employed population reporting 35 hours or more of paid work per week; all relationships are significant at .005 level.
Source: General Social Survey, Canada, 1998

crunched if they are not interested in what they are doing and have little control over their work. The presence or absence of the feelings of time crunch and stress is, therefore, associated not only with the length of working hours, but also with the type of the job and its occupational characteristics.

If different groups in modern societies are exposed to varying work pressures, can leisure help ease these pressures? A number of authors argued that it could. Iwasaki (76), suggested that leisure may be effective in dealing with stress, reducing stress and promoting satisfactory outcomes, regardless of stress levels. The research evidence in this regard is, however, not entirely conclusive. Peters and Raaijmakers (77) suggested that leisure time spent at home may ease the adverse effects of employed mothers' time crunch. Kay (78) showed, however, that for employed mothers paid work rather than leisure offsets the psychological drudgery of domestic work. Women reported that they feel that paid work givens them time "on my own". One interviewee said, "I go to work to be me. You could say that it is almost leisure (78).

Zuzanek and Mannell (79) concluded their analyses of the impact of leisure on mental and physical health by suggesting that the beneficial effects of leisure participation are unevenly distributed across different occupational and life cycle groups, and leisure may not be the first line of defense against severe work overload. Paradoxically, paid work rather than free time can counter domestic stress for employed women, whereas overworked professionals may gain relief from additional sleep or relaxed eating habits rather than from additional leisure. The stress-reducing and health-beneficial effects of leisure may thus manifest themselves not in situations when people are most pressed for time, but rather when they acquire some control over time, as for example in retirement.

WHAT CAN WE CONCLUDE ABOUT THE RELATIONSHIP BETWEEN WORK AND LEISURE?

The underlying assumption of most analyses of work-leisure relationships was that structural, organizational, and technological characteristics of work decisively affect or change the nature of leisure experiences. Born from an ideological reformist tradition, this approach seemed to promise radical improvement in human life as a result of technical restructuring of the work environment. Authors adhering to this position were looking for the sources of lifestyle changes in technological innovations, rather than in the social division of labor. In reality, work affects other aspects of human life primarily through social positioning of the workers in the labor market, including opportunities for upward mobility and social aspirations. From this perspective, analyses of work-leisure relationships could benefit from greater attention to the role of *occupational culture,* defined by technical, social, and cultural attributes associated with one's place in the occupational system.

The notion of a relatively stable *occupational culture* has been eroded, however, by the radical changes in the labor market in the 1980s and 1990s. According to Hutton (80), only 40% of the labor force today has secure full-time jobs. The rest of the jobs are part time, casual, insecure, and marginalized. Globalization of world economies and concerns with economic competitiveness resulted in the downsizing of many companies, which was often accompanied by an intensification of the job requirements for the reduced labor force (81). The "flexibilization" of working hours and the proliferation of part-time jobs resulted in shorter hours *per job,* but in the climate of social uncertainty people were often forced to carry more than one job, producing, paradoxically, longer working hours *per person* (82). Higher combined workloads of dual-career families also added to an acute sense of time pressure. As a result, the labor force of today has become more polarized along workload lines than it was in the past.

Factors other than the economy clearly have contributed to the growing time pressures in modern societies. Contrary to the predictions of the 1950s, the introduction of new household appliances and time-saving technologies, convenient or take-out foods, as well as the downsizing of families, did not result in the expected decline in domestic work. Maintenance and upkeep of time-saving devices takes time. The smaller size of families, in a social climate of growing concern with children's safety and well-being, was accompanied by *greater* care of *fewer* children. The growing number of smaller, nonfamily and single-parent households represents a loss of the scale in household production because, as Beckers indicated, there is an increasing number of people with household duties, but a decreasing number who benefit from them (83).

Responding to these developments, some authors raised the question about what will differentiate people with regard to leisure under the conditions of the declining importance of occupational status and work. According to Roberts and Veal, the lifestyle divide in postindustrial societies will be increasingly determined by people's value orientations rather than by a "bivariate" juxtaposition of work and leisure (38). It remains to be seen, however, whether lifestyle orientations will be able to counter the effects of repetitive and fragmented work that are still prevalent not only in industrially developing countries but in industrial societies as well. To put it differently, the concern about stifling effects of work on leisure and lifestyle will remain alive as long as there is room for de Tocqueville's question about expectations of people who spend twenty years making heads for pins (23). The question can be, of course, paraphrased and brought closer to our days: Can mindless computerized day trading of stocks induce a mindful lifestyle? (Day trading involves purchase of stocks when they begin to move up and their almost instantaneous sell-off for marginal profit. The job is done repeatedly, usually by low-paid employees working on commission. No thought or knowledge is required, just a swift reaction and some computer keyboard skills.)

Until de Tocqueville's or similar questions can be answered for large segments of the population, the effects of work on leisure will continue to attract the attention of researchers, reformers, and policy makers attempting—not unreasonably—to get *to the root* of the problem.

CHAPTER SUMMARY

Interest in the relationships between work and leisure dates back to the 19th century and the criticism at that time about industrialization and its adverse influences on worker's lives. Emerging concerns about this relationship spawned concepts about work/leisure relationships, such as the spillover, compensation, and compartmentalization hypotheses in which leisure is viewed as either something that relates to work (spillover), fills needs not met by work (compensation), or has no relationship with work at all (compartmentalization). The relationship with work may be negative or positive. Alternately, leisure and work may be independent domains. Empirical research has not been able to provide definitive answers to the various work/leisure hypotheses, and observers have recognized that the issues are complex and that more attention is needed to social and psychological factors that influence both work and leisure. Additionally, it is recognized that there are differences in the roles and lifestyles of various occupational categories and communities. Differences were highlighted in comparing leisure by *social class* based on underlying values to seek social equality, and by *sociooccupational status,* based on understanding the complexity of social and economic factors that have created different leisure patterns among different social groups. Moreover, the nature of work and leisure are changing rapidly and there is a trend toward polarization of the workforce, which influences time and resources available for leisure and creates perceived time pressures that can diminish workers' perceptions of their overall quality of life. There remains uncertainty, however, in how the relationship between leisure and work will change as globalization influences work practices, economics, and lifestyles in the current age.

STUDY GUIDE

Study Guide Author: Kristine Haertl

Summary of Main Points

Work and leisure are integral parts of our individual and collective existence. Patterns of work and leisure time use vary across cultures, socioeconomic classes, and eras. The author presents various theories that suggest relationships between paid work and leisure patterns, including the spillover (congruence), compensation (contrast), and compartmentalization (separate domains) theories. The contrast hypothesis suggests a significant variation or contrast of time use patterns between work and leisure activities. Conversely, the congruence hypothesis focuses on resemblances between work and leisure behaviors. As the nature of work and leisure evolve amid the emergence of technology and postindustrialized societies, continued research is needed to consider the relationships between work, leisure, time use, and their influence on personal health and well-being.

Application to Occupational Therapy

Occupational therapists often focus on enabling clients to experience lifestyle balance, time use, and quality of life. Therefore, an understanding of the relationships between leisure, work, and occupation is integral to facilitation of healthy lifestyle patterns. Overwork often includes increased stress, which may contribute to a number of overuse injuries or stress-related diseases. On the other hand, a lack of meaningful work or leisure may also contribute to ill health. A client-centered approach would consider individual, family, group, community, organization, or population daily lifestyle patterns, time use, and the overall relationship of work and leisure to health and well-being.

Traditional conceptualizations of occupational therapy were categorized to profile the occupational areas of paid work or productivity (including play and schooling for children and retirement occupations for seniors), self-care/self-maintenance (sometimes called activities of daily living or ADL), and play/leisure. The relationship between work and leisure differs, depending on the context and individual/societal factors. As the profession has reembraced occupation as its essence, studies of work, leisure, and occupation are integral to the advancement of evidenced-based practice on the prevention-intervention continuum. Integration of leisure in relation to or separate from work in the practice process would be done throughout from start to conclusion, and including assessment/evaluation, program planning, implementation, and evaluation.

Individual Learning Activities

1. Consider your own work/leisure history. What types of paid work have you had over the years? How did the type and amount of work you engaged in relate to your leisure patterns at the time? Create a time line graphing the following areas:

   a. Your historical history of paid and unpaid work
   b. Your favorite leisure activities (note leisure is related to, but not synonymous with, play—generally leisure is more structured as in a hobby or team sport)
   c. The relationship of your leisure participation to type and amount of work

   Following creation of your time line, write a two-page summary applying the concepts of the chapter to your time use patterns. Do you notice any work-leisure relationship? Do the contrast or congruence hypotheses apply? How did your work and leisure participation affect your overall health and well-being at the time?

2. Imagine yourself in the preindustrialized era. How would your work and leisure patterns have differed? Write a four-page creative story placing you in that period of time. Reflect on where and what type of work you choose to engage in and how your personal choices influence your choice of leisure occupations.

Group Learning Activity

Form groups of three to four individuals. Each group member should be assigned to a specific work sector (i.e., blue-collar/factory, professional business, social service). Locate potential interviewees from each category. Each group member should interview an individual from distinct work sectors. Construct interview questions related to their nature of work, leisure patterns, and daily time use. Upon completion of the interviews, group members should compare and contrast the relationships noted between work and leisure. Prepare a 20-minute presentation outlining the similarities and differences noted in each of the interviews. Apply chapter concepts, including theories, hypotheses, and concepts discussed.

Study Questions

1. The evidence of consistent relationships between work and leisure is conclusive.
   a. True
   b. False

2. An eight-hour day on the assembly line will likely lead a person to pursue monotonous leisure activities such as watching TV. The preceding statement is most in line with:
   a. Spillover hypothesis
   b. Contrast hypothesis
   c. Automation
   d. Segmentation

3. The W-O-L paradigm emphasizes
   a. The importance of daily ADLs on performance
   b. The importance of cognitive variables and personality traits on the work-leisure relationship
   c. The mediating effects of the organization on performance
   d. None of the above
4. "A set of technical, social, and cultural characteristics and attributes associated with one's place in the social division of labor and perception of one's self in the system."
   a. Organizational culture
   b. Contextual conceptualization
   c. Occupational culture
   d. Leisure culture
5. Personal control over one's use of time in the work environment affects health and well-being.
   a. True
   b. False

REFERENCES

1. Lundberg, G. A., Komarovsky, M., & McInerny, M. A. (1934). *Leisure: A suburban study.* New York: Columbia University Press.
2. Friedmann, G. (1961). *The anatomy of work, labour, leisure, and the implications of automation,* Glencoe, IL: Free Press.
3. De Grazia, S. (1962). *Of time, work, and leisure.* Garden City, NY: Doubleday.
4. Greenberg, C. (1958). Work and leisure under industrialism. In E. Larabee & R. Meyersohn (Eds.), *Mass leisure.* Glencoe, IL: Free Press.
5. Berger, B. M. (1963). The sociology of leisure: Some suggestions. In E. O. Smigel (Ed.), *Work and leisure: A contemporary social problem.* New Haven, CT: College and University Press
6. Dumazedier, J. (1967). *Toward a society of leisure.* Glencoe, IL: Free Press.
7. Riesman, D. (1950). *The lonely crowd.* New York: Doubleday Anchor Books.
8. Dubin, R. (1956). Industrial workers' worlds: A study in the central life interests of industrial workers. *Social Problems, 4,* 131–142.
9. Orzack, L. (1959). Work as a "central life interest" of professionals, *Social Problems,* Fall.
10. Goldthorpe, J. H., Lockwood, D., Bechefor, F., & Taylor, P. (1968). *The affluent worker: Industrial attitudes and behaviour.* London: Cambridge University Press
11. Galbraith, J. K. (1967). *The new industrial state.* New York: Signet Books.
12. Fourastié, J. (1965). *Les 40000 heures.* Paris: Robert Laffont.
13. Samuelson, P. A. (1967). *Economics.* New York: McGraw-Hill.
14. Kreps, J. M., & Spengler, J. J. (1966). *The leisure component of economic growth, the employment impact of technological change.* Prepared for the National Commission on Technology, Automation and Economic Progress. Washington, DC: U.S. Government Printing Office.
15. Owen, J. D. (1970). *The price of leisure. An economic analysis of the demand for leisure time.* Montreal: McGill-Queens University Press.
16. Linder, S. B. (1970). *The harried leisure class.* New York: Columbia University Press.
17. Schor, J. B. (1991). *The overworked American: The unexpected decline of leisure.* New York: Basic Books.

18. Hinrichs, K., Roche, W., & Sirianni, C. (Eds.). (1991). *Working time in transition.* Philadelphia: Temple University Press; Elchardus, M., & Glorieux, I. (1994). The search for the invisible 8 hours: The gendered use of time in a society with a high labour force participation of women. *Time & Society, 3*(1), 5–27; Breedveld, K. (1995). Measuring flexible working-time challenges from the Dutch case. *Statistics in Transition, 2*(4), 645–662; Garhammer, M. (1995). Changes in working hours in Germany: The resulting impact on everyday life. *Time & Society, 4*(2), 167–203; Gratton, C. (1996). Work, time and leisure in Europe: National differences and European convergence. In C. Gratton (Ed.), *Work, leisure and the quality of life: A global perspective.* Sheffield: Leisure Industries Research Centre.
19. Wilensky, H. (1960). Work, careers and social integration. *International Social Science Journal 12*(4), 543–560.
20. Wippler, R. (1970). Leisure behavior: A multivariate approach, *Sociologia Neerlandica 6*(1), 51–67.
21. Parker, S. (1983). *Leisure and work.* London: Allen and Unwin.
22. Marx, K. (1964). Economic and Philosophical Manuscripts (written in 1844). In K. Marx, *Selected Writings in Sociology and Social Philosophy* (T. B. Bottomore & M. Rubel, Eds.). New York: McGraw-Hill.
23. Tocqueville, A. de. (1954). *Democracy in America,* Vol. 2. New York: Vintage Books. (First Printing: 1838).
24. Howe, I. (1957). Notes on mass culture. In B. Rosenberg & D. M. White (Eds.), *Mass culture* (pp. 496–503). London: Collier-MacMillan.
25. Meissner, M. (1971). The long arm of the job: A study of work and leisure. *Journal of Economy and Society, 10*(3), 239–260.
26. Wilensky, H. L. (1964). The uneven distribution of leisure: The impact of economic growth on free time. In E. O. Smigel (Ed.), *Work and leisure* (pp. 107–145). New Haven, CT: College and University Press.
27. Friedmann, G. (1961). *The anatomy of work, labour, leisure, and the implications of automation.* Glencoe, IL: Free Press.
28. Theobald, R. (1961). *The challenge of abundance.* New York: C. N. Potter; McLuhan, M. (1964). *Understanding media.* London: Routledge and Kegan Paul Limited; Karasek, R., & Theorell, T. (1990). *Healthy work, stress, productivity, and the reconstruction of working life.* New York: Basic Books.
29. Taylor, F. W. (1947). *Principles of scientific management.* New York: Harper.
30. McLuhan, M. (1964). *Understanding media.* London: Routledge and Kegan Paul Limited.
31. Karasek, R., & Theorell, T. (1990). *Healthy work, stress, productivity, and the reconstruction of working life.* New York: Basic Books.
32. Kabanoff, B., & O'Brien, G. (1980). Work and leisure: A task attributes analysis. *Journal of Applied Psychology, 65,* 596–609.
33. Parker, S. (1971). *The future of work and leisure.* New York: Praeger.
34. Bacon, A. W. (1975). Leisure and the alienated worker: A critical reassessment of three radical theories of work and leisure. *Journal of Leisure Research,* 7(3), 186.
35. Roberts, K. (1999). *Leisure in contemporary society.* Wallingford Oxfordshire: CABI Publishing.
36. Kabanoff, B. (1980). Work and nonwork: A review of models, methods and findings. *Psychological Bulletin, 88,* 67.
37. Pennings, J. (1976). Leisure correlates of working conditions. Graduate School of Industrial Administration, Carnegie-Mellon University, Pittsburgh, PA: Unpublished manuscript (p. 2).

38. Veal, A. J. (2004). Looking back: Perspectives on the leisure-work relationship. In J. H. Haworth & A. J. Veal (Eds.), *Work and leisure, 107-120.* New York: Routledge.
39. Kabanoff, B. (1980). Work and nonwork: A review of models, methods and findings. *Psychological Bulletin, 88,* 60–77; Moorehouse, H. F. (1989). Models of work, models of leisure. In C. Rojek (Ed.), *Leisure for leisure.* London: Macmillan; Veal, A. J. (2004). Looking back: Perspectives on the leisure-work relationship. In J. H. Haworth & A. J. Veal (Eds.), *Work and leisure* (pp. 107–120). New York: Routledge.
40. Kando, T., & Summers, W. (1971). The impact of work on leisure: Toward a paradigm and research strategy. *Pacific Sociological Review* (Special Summer Issue), 312.
41. Kando, T., & Summers, W. (1971). The impact of work on leisure: Toward a paradigm and research strategy. *Pacific Sociological Review* (Special Summer Issue), 310–327; Pennings, J. (1976). Leisure correlates of working conditions. Graduate School of Industrial Administration, Carnegie-Mellon University, Pittsburgh, PA: Unpublished manuscript; Kabanoff, B., & O'Brien, G. (1980). Work and leisure: A task attributes analysis. *Journal of Applied Psychology, 65,* 596–609; Iso-Ahola, S. (1980). *Social psychology of leisure and recreation.* Dubuque, IA: Wm. C. Brown.
42. Wippler, R. (1970). Leisure behavior: a multivariate approach. *Sociologia Neerlandica 6*(1), 60.
43. Iso-Ahola, S. (1980). *Social psychology of leisure and recreation.* Dubuque, IA: Wm. C. Brown.
44. Mannell, R. C., & Iso-Ahola, S. (1985). Work constraints on leisure. In M. Wade (Ed.), *Constraints on leisure* (pp. 155–187). Springfield, IL: Charles C. Thomas Publishing.
45. Parker, S. (1971). *The future of work and leisure.* New York: Praeger.
46. Pennings, J. (1976). Leisure correlates of working conditions. Graduate School of Industrial Administration, Carnegie-Mellon University, Pittsburgh, PA: Unpublished manuscript.
47. Veal, A. J. (2004). Looking back. Perspectives on the leisure-work relationship. In J. H. Haworth & A. J. Veal (Eds.), *Work and leisure.* New York: Routledge.
48. Hoggart, R. (1957). *The uses of literacy: Aspects of working class life.* London: Chatto and Windus; Shostak, A., & Gromberg, W. (Eds.), (1965). *Blue-collar world.* Englewood Cliffs, NJ: Prentice Hall.
49. Lundberg, G. A., Komarovsky, M., & McInerny, M. A. (1934). *Leisure: A suburban study.* New York: Columbia University Press.
50. Szalai, A. (Ed.). (1972). *The use of time. Daily activities of urban and suburban populations in twelve countries.* The Hague: Mouton.
51. Quoted in Cheek, N. H., Jr., & Burch, W. R., Jr. (1976). *The social organization of leisure in human society.* New York: Harper & Row, Publishers.
52. Katz, E., & Gurevitch, M. (1976). *The secularization of leisure, culture and communication in Israel.* London: Faber & Faber.
53. Canadian 1992 General Social Survey. www.statcan.ca/english/Dli/Data/Ftp/gss/
54. Veal, A. J. (2004). Looking back: Perspectives on the leisure-work relationship. In J. H. Haworth & A. J. Veal (Eds.), *Work and leisure.* New York: Routledge.
55. Canadian 1998 General Social Survey. www.chass.utoronto.ca/datalib/major/gss/
56. Salaman, G. (1974). *Community and occupation. An exploration of work/leisure relationships.* London: Cambridge University Press.
57. Zuzanek, J., & Mannell, R. (1983). Work-leisure relationships from a sociological and social psychological perspective. *Leisure Studies 2,* 340.
58. Critcher, C., & Bramham, P. (2004). The devil still makes work. In J. H. Haworth & A. J. Veal (Eds.), *Work and leisure.* New York: Routledge.

59. Rojek, C. (2004). Postmodern work and leisure. In J. H. Haworth & A. J. Veal (Eds.), *Work and leisure.* New York: Routledge.
60. Hinrichs, K., Roche, W., & Sirianni, C. (Eds.), (1991). *Working time in transition.* Philadelphia: Temple University Press; Beck. U. (2000). *The brave new world of work.* Cambridge: Polity.
61. Wilensky, H. L. (1981). *Family life cycle, work and quality of life: Reflections on the roots of happiness, despair, and indifference in modern societies.* Report No. 442. Berkley, CA: Institute of Industrial Relations.
62. Schor, J. B. (1991). *The overworked American: The unexpected decline of leisure.* New York: Basic Books.
63. Bond, J. T., Galinsky, E., &. Swanberg, J. E. (1998). *The 1997 national study of the changing workforce.* New York: Families and Work Institute.
64. Zuzanek, J. (2000). *The effects of time use and time pressure on child-parent relationships.* Waterloo: Otium Publications.
65. Robinson, J. P., & Godbey, G. (1997). *Time for life: The surprising ways Americans use their time.* University Park: Pennsylvania State University Press.
66. Tremblay, D.-G., & Villeneuve, D. (1998). De la réduction a la polarisation des temps de travail; des enjeux de société. *Loisir & Societe/ Society and Leisure, 21*(2), 399–416.
67. Zuzanek, J., & Smale, B. J. A. (1997). More work-less leisure? Changing allocations of time in Canada, 1981–1992. *Loisir & Societe/Society and Leisure, 20*(1), 73–106.
68. Friedman, M., & Rosenman, R. H. (1974). *Type A behavior and your heart.* New York: Alfred A. Knopf.
69. Lehto, A.-M. (1998). Time pressure as a stress factor. *Loisir & Societe/ Society and Leisure, 21*(2), 491–512.
70. Nishiyama, K., & Johnson, J. V. (1997). Karoshi—Death from overwork: Occupational health consequences of Japanese production management. *International Journal of Health Services, 27*(4), 625–641.
71. Gleick, J. (1999). *Faster: The acceleration of just about everything.* New York: Pantheon Books.
72. Barnett, R. C. (1998). Toward a review and reconceptualization of the work/family literature. *Genetic, Social, and General Psychology Monographs, 124*(2), 125–182.
73. Canadian National Population Health Survey. w.statcan.ca/english/Dli/Data/Ftp/nphs/
74. Hill, M. S. (1988). Marital stability and spouses' shared time: A multidisciplinary hypothesis. *Journal of Family Issues, 9*(4), 427–451; Veenhoven, R. (1991). Questions on happiness: Classical topics, modern answers, and blind spots. In F. Strack, M. Argyle, & N. Schwartz (Eds.), *Subjective well-being: An interdisciplinary perspective,* 1–26. Elmsford, NY: Pergamon Press.
75. Karasek, R., & Theorell, T. (1990). *Healthy work, stress, productivity, and the reconstruction of working life.* New York: Basic Books; Zuzanek, J. (2004). Work, leisure, time pressure, and stress. In J. H. Haworth & A. J. Veal (Eds.), *Work and leisure,* 123–144. New York: Routledge.
76. Iwasaki, Y. (2002). *Examining rival models of leisure coping mechanisms.* Paper presented to the 2002 NRPA Leisure Research Symposium in Arlington, VA.
77. Peters, P., & Raaijmakers, S. (1998). Time crunch and the perception of control over time from a gendered perspective: The Dutch case. *Loisir & Societe/ Society and Leisure, 21*(2), 417–434.

78. Kay, T. (1998). Having it all or doing it all? The construction of women's lifestyles in time-crunched households. *Loisir & Societe/ Society and Leisure, 21*(2), 445.
79. Zuzanek, J., & Mannell, R. (1998). Life-cycle squeeze, time pressure, daily stress and leisure participation: A Canadian perspective. *Loisir & Societe/ Society and Leisure, 21*(2), 513–544.
80. Hutton, W. (1995). *The state we're in.* London: Jonathan Cape.
81. Handy, C. (1994). *The empty raincoat: Making sense of the future.* London: Hutchinson.
82. Gratton, C. (1996). Work, time and leisure in Europe: National differences and European convergence. In C. Gratton (Ed.), *Work, leisure and the quality of life: A global perspective.* Sheffield: Leisure Industries Research Centre.
83. Beckers, T. (1996). The hidden agenda. The expropriation of time in Europe. In C. Gratton (Ed.), *Work, leisure and the quality of life: A global perspective.* Sheffield: Leisure Industries Research Centre.
84. Veal, A. J. (2004). Looking back: Perspectives on the leisure-work relationship. In J. H. Haworth & A. J. Veal (Eds.), *Work and leisure,* 107–120. New York: Routledge.

Endnotes

[1]It is somewhat surprising that authors examining the nature of work-leisure relationship (Wilensky, 1960; Wippler, 1970; Parker, 1971) did not comment on the possibility of positive compensatory and spillover relationships.

CHAPTER 12

Occupational Deprivation: Understanding Limited Participation

Gail Whiteford

OBJECTIVES

1. Define occupational deprivation and distinguish it from occupational disruption.
2. Illustrate occupational deprivation through five globally recognizable examples: geographic isolation, extreme conditions of employment, incarceration, sex-role stereotyping, and refugeeism.
3. Identify environmental features that may contribute to occupational deprivation for people with special needs, impairments, and disabilities.
4. Consider how occupational deprivation may be addressed through the adoption of an occupational justice framework.

KEY WORDS

Cultural values and norms
Disability
Displacement
Environmental features
Geographic isolation
Incarceration
Occupational deprivation
Occupational disruption
Occupational justice framework
Overemployment
Refugeeism
Sex-role stereotyping
Unemployment
Underemployment

www.prenhall.com/christiansen
The Internet provides an exciting means for interacting with this textbook and for enhancing your understanding of humans' experiences with occupations and the organization of occupations in society. Use the address above to access the interactive Companion Website created specifically to accompany this book. Here you will find an array of self-study material designed to help you gain a richer understanding of the concepts presented in this chapter.

CHAPTER PROFILE

This chapter focuses on ways in which people are unable to participate in occupations due to structural as opposed to personal reasons. The concept of occupational deprivation is defined, contrasted with occupational disruption, and illustrated through examples relevant in the context of contemporary society. These examples include geographic isolation, employment conditions, incarceration, sex-role stereotyping, refugeeism, and disability. Implications of how occupational deprivation for individuals, communities, and societies can be addressed through adopting an occupational justice framework are explored.

INTRODUCTION

Previous chapters have shown how occupations provide structure, identity, and meaning in people's lives. As a way of understanding their experiences over time, people tell stories about themselves and their lives through accounts of what they have done, are doing, or are going to do in the future. A person's sense of self and his or her relationship with the world is very much influenced by participation in occupations chosen and performed during each stage of life. In turn, those occupations are shaped by the **cultural values and norms** of the societies in which people live as well as by prevailing economic and political factors.

What happens, then, when people are unable to do the things they want and need to do for extended periods of time? What consequences does this have for people individually, in families, in communities, and even in countries? In this chapter, we consider some of the factors and conditions that may prevent people from living out their occupational lives to the fullest extent. In so doing, we introduce the concept of occupational deprivation and provide some examples of deprived conditions and their causes.

The four major objectives for this chapter are as follows:

1. To define occupational deprivation and distinguish it from occupational disruption.
2. To illustrate occupational deprivation through five globally recognizable examples: geographic isolation, extreme conditions of employment, incarceration, sex-role stereotyping, and refugeeism.
3. To identify **environmental features** that may contribute to occupational deprivation for people with special needs, impairments, and disabilities.
4. To consider how occupational deprivation may be addressed through the adoption of an occupational justice framework.

The main sections of this chapter address the four objectives. The opening section offers a definition of occupational deprivation. The second section provides examples of occupational deprivation. Included in the second section is the example of extreme conditions of employment that have created a growing gap between people who experience considerable stress because they are doing too much and those who experience boredom, anxiety, or more severe consequences because they are doing too little. Discussed in the third section is the occupational deprivation created by disability and its consequent limitations to activity and social participation.

DEFINING OCCUPATIONAL DEPRIVATION

Occupational deprivation is a relatively new concept, but it has stimulated interest internationally. A pioneer in developing the theoretical concept of occupational deprivation, Ann Wilcock (1), suggested that not all people are afforded equal opportunities to participate in occupations of choice or in occupations having individual, familial, or cultural meaning. Using Wilcock's premise and through research conducted with prison inmates, occupational deprivation is defined here as "a state of prolonged preclusion from engagement in occupations of necessity and/or meaning due to factors which stand outside of the control of the individual" (2, p. 201).

The factors that produce occupational deprivation may be social, economic, environmental, geographic, historic, cultural, or political in nature, as discussed in the next section. It is important to emphasize that occupational deprivation occurs when someone or something *external* to the individual is creating conditions that lead to deprivation. It is important to note at this stage that an *internal* state, such as an illness, does not in itself cause occupational deprivation. This is an important distinction and one that will be covered later in the chapter in more detail.

A concept that is linked to occupational deprivation is **occupational disruption** (2). Occupational disruption may appear to be similar to occupational deprivation, but it refers to a different, common experience in most people's lives. The most important distinctions are, first, that occupational disruption is *temporary* or transient, such as having the flu. Second, disruption results from factors or situations over which the individual has some control, such as moving to a new town or changing jobs. In contrast, occupational deprivation is prolonged and due to external or environmental factors over which the individual has little or no control. Consider an example of occupational disruption that occurs frequently during ski season. A person falls on the slope during a ski trip and breaks a leg. With the leg in a plaster cast for eight weeks, the person's occupations are disrupted. During this time, going for a jog is impossible, as are many other pursuits, such as swimming or dancing. The person's normal pattern of occupational engagement is disrupted. However, when the leg has healed, the person returns to usual occupations (although the person may be less enthusiastic about skiing!).

Occupational disruption can also result from internal/individual circumstances. Examples might include grieving the loss of a loved one or electing to work a night shift. The most important things to remember about occupational disruption are that (a) it constitutes a temporary state and (b) given supportive conditions, this temporary state can be resolved (2, p. 201).

Interestingly, after a period of occupational disruption, people sometimes return to an enhanced level of occupational functioning. Their attitude toward certain occupations may change, or they may establish different priorities. This may result from their having spent time reflecting on the importance of certain occupations missing from their life during the disruption. Women, for example, after becoming a parent and getting through the occupational disruption associated with caring for a new infant, often report that they value and use their leisure time more highly than they did previously. Similarly, students who have experienced occupational disruption while preparing for and undertaking examinations may experience a renewed sense of pleasure in a range of restorative occupations when examinations are finished.

IDENTIFYING BARRIERS TO PARTICIPATION: FIVE ILLUSTRATIONS OF OCCUPATIONAL DEPRIVATION

In this section, examples of occupational deprivation are presented. Five illustrations of occupational deprivation were selected for their global relevance: geographic isolation, unsatisfactory conditions of employment (unemployment, underemployment, and overemployment), incarceration, sex-role stereotyping, and refugeeism. Each example reflects two essential features of occupational deprivation. First, that participation is limited by forces not within the immediate control of an individual, group, or community. Second, that occupational deprivation needs always to be interpreted within the historic, cultural, and social milieu and context within which it arises, in other words, occupational deprivation is a highly situated and complex phenomenon.

Geographic isolation results from the conditions of location that place some people at great physical distance from others or that separate them by terrain or climactic conditions. By way of contrast, people who live in large urban centers may have conditions of employment (or lack thereof) that make them vulnerable to occupational deprivation, the root cause of which is the prevailing economic climate in which they live. The remaining illustrations of occupational deprivation in this section (incarceration, gender stereotyping, and refugeeism) result from social, cultural, and/or political circumstances. As these concepts are presented, readers may think of other examples of occupational deprivation based on their own experiences and from the sociocultural contexts and environments in which they reside.

Geographic Isolation

Since earliest times, one of the most powerful constraints on people's opportunities to engage in occupations, particularly those of a social nature, has been **geographic isolation** (Figure 12-1 ■). It is hard to go to the cinema or meet friends at a café if you tend a lighthouse on a remote coastal peninsula and your nearest neighbor is a two-hour drive or boat trip away! Whereas some people actively choose to live in remote locations and accept the occupational deprivation that goes with it or enrich available occupations as a lifestyle choice, the impact of geographic isolation on other people may have very serious, long-term negative consequences.

What are the negative effects of geographic isolation, and why do they come about? One of the most important dimensions of occupations is that they locate us within the social world. Not being able to engage in occupations with other people

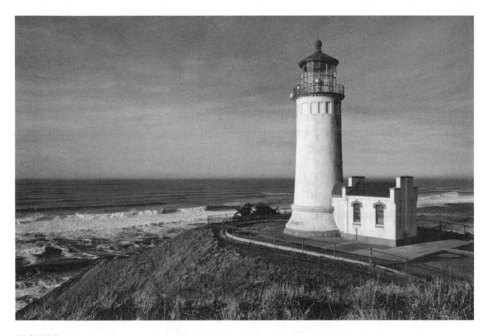

FIGURE 12-1 Occupational deprivation can be caused by restricted access to people, events, and places. Remote, isolated geographic locations can result in occupational deprivation. (Photodisc/Getty Images)

results in diminished opportunities for social interaction, a primary source of feedback about who we are and how others perceive us. Feedback from others is where we gain recognition for our efforts, and this feedback directly shapes our self-image and sense of self (3). Consider the following poignant account of geographical isolation as told by Australian aboriginal author Ruby Langford. Here she recounts her experiences of living in a camp in outback Queensland.

> The day came to pack up, we looked along the fence, the heat haze above the wires and said "well that's done, let's go to town" . . . this town was a Mecca of civilisation to me, look—here was a dress shop, I went right in. I needed a new dress. Halfway in the shop I saw myself in the shop mirror, close up. Here was a pregnant woman with blistered hands like a man's, her face peeling like flaky pastry and black . . . I stared at myself for a long time and then I bought a sleeveless cotton dress and went outside. I hadn't been to town for so long I was so lonely for another woman to talk to, so every woman who passed I said hello, hello, just to get them to talk to me. (4, p. 93)

Ruby's story is a poignant account of being desperate for interaction with other women whom she rarely encountered during her time in the outback. She is driven to seek feedback of any kind—even "Hello!" Although Ruby brings a touch of humor to this story, she does manage to highlight how being deprived of opportunities to do relatively normal, social things due to the tyranny of distance can lead to a sense of social isolation and the development of maladaptive coping strategies. Although not directly related to her story, problems such as alcohol abuse, petrol sniffing, domestic violence, and suicide tend to be more prevalent in rural and isolated communities (5). These problems are, without question, complex and multidimensional. Yet they do point to potentially adverse effects of the occupational deprivation brought about by prolonged geographic distance from others.

Another source of occupational deprivation related to geographic isolation is the lack of resources and occupational opportunities in some of the central desert communities in Australia. These remote communities, inhabited largely by aboriginal people who live west of Alice Springs, are, generally speaking, places in which there is little or nothing to do. Such geographic isolation is particularly problematic for the young people. In his inquiry into these communities, Paul Toohey described them as being places where

> life is sedentary and aimless . . . they are artificial hubs constructed from the imaginations of . . . people who hoped that people, who had only 30 years before lived in small wandering groups, could live happily next to a bore, church, generator and a store. It hasn't worked. The petrol sniffing is epidemic and proves that life in these desert communities holds little meaning for the teenage generation. In their traditional nomadic society, they had a great deal of autonomy. They have that same independence now that they live in big stationary groups with the result that they are bored stiff, so they sniff (petrol). (6, p. 3)

This is an extreme example, and one that has many layers of complexity, including the intersection of history, politics, race relations, and economics. The point about occupational deprivation is that there seems to be a link between being geographically isolated, being unable to participate in occupations that are meaningful and rewarding (particularly those that are socially oriented), and health. This is because, as Wilcock (1) pointed out, humans are inherently occupational by nature and being unable to "do" much for long periods of time is ultimately detrimental. It will be interesting to see how access to technologies such as the Internet will influence the sense of geographic isolation over time. The reality remains that, for many people currently living in remote communities, such technology is still inaccessible.

Problem Conditions of Employment

Another category of occupational deprivation relates to conditions of employment (**unemployment**, **underemployment**, and **overemployment**). The most common and visible type of employment problem is unemployment. Unemployment is one of the most challenging and complex problems of our time, and in many areas it is getting worse. In Western societies in particular, the occupation of paid employment has assumed a central position in how we think about and identify ourselves. One need only to think back to the last social gathering where inevitably someone asked the question, "What do you do?" and most often the response would be linked to paid employment (e.g., "I am a town planner" or "I'm a teacher"). Generally, people highlight their employment above other occupational pursuits, even when employment is not the occupation of most interest or importance to them. Accordingly, one rarely hears people respond with non-work-related roles, such as "I am a parent" or "I am a church volunteer." For most people in Western countries, paid employment is the occupation that most significantly influences social acceptance and social status. Declaring oneself to be a ski instructor will be met with a different response than one might receive from declaring oneself to be a graphic artist or a cardiologist. People's perceptions of us, at least initially, are strongly influenced by our primary occupations of paid employment. Such perceptions are shaped by social and cultural value systems and serve as a powerful reminder that occupations are a primary vehicle through which people interact in society and, in doing so, create or delimit opportunities for others to participate.

Given that one's vocation tends to influence social perceptions, what happens when people are deprived of the occupation of paid employment for long periods of time? What is the impact on sense of self or on general well-being? From research on long-term unemployed people, the effects are becoming understood. Most significant, unemployment seems to have a negative impact on both physical (1, 7–9) as well as mental (10–13) health. Platt (14) suggested that a link exists between unemployment and rates of self-harm and suicide. Psychologically and emotionally, unemployed people report that they are less confident, with lower self-esteem than employed people. At a skills level, it appears that the longer people remain unemployed, the more difficult it is to obtain employment due to diminishing skills and work-related behaviors. In short, unemployment imposes a huge price for people as individuals and for society at large (15). Thus, unemployment can be viewed as a primary contributor to occupational deprivation for multitudes of people worldwide.

Unemployment is viewed here as one form of occupational deprivation. To fully understand it, however, we need to consider the factors that influence employment participation rates and have an appreciation for the forces that preclude full employment for whole populations. To begin to understand these issues, we must recognize that declining workforce participation is a global phenomenon historically linked to rapid advances in technology, prevailing economic systems, and shifting demographics (16).

If we consider technology first, differing perspectives are needed for a rounded discussion. Considered simply, the rapid rise in technological advances may be seen as having released people from a whole range of backbreaking and monotonous, repetitive jobs. Paradoxically, although technological development may be viewed as representing progress for humankind, it can also be seen as the root cause of diminished employment opportunities for legions of semiskilled and unskilled workers. Jones (16) cited Drucker in describing the blue-collar working class as the fastest class to rise and fall that society has witnessed. Indeed, machinery, robotics, and computer-driven systems have replaced the blue-collar workforce in sectors as diverse as the manufacturing sector (especially the automotive industry), the agrarian sector, and the tertiary service sector. The impact of technology on the labor market has been unquestionably negative from an employment perspective, an outcome that economic forecasters were slow to predict and one for which there are few contemporary solutions (15). The financial viability of many industries has depended on their ability to embrace technology-reducing strategies to reduce the costs associated with large numbers of workers. Computerization, as well as the downsizing of workers and outsourcing of services, have inevitably resulted in fewer full-time employment opportunities for many people.

Let us consider a second influence on employment: global and national economic forces. Generally speaking, the financial viability of an industry depends to a large extent on the type of political and economic context in which it is located. Most First World, liberal democracies have capitalist economies based on the twin principles of competition and free-market trade. It has been argued that capitalist systems have commodified the labor force; that drives for increased productivity and a demand for the best (most profitable) bottom line have ultimately required substantive levels of unemployment. As Farnworth (17) suggested, "Unemployment is, in part, a consequence of the goals of capitalism" (p. 22). Governments in many countries appear to have recognized the social costs associated with unemployment. Typical government responses to this problem have been to introduce a variety of federally funded programs ranging from mutual obligation schemes (where you must work in exchange for receiving an unemployment benefit) to job creation programs, to mandatory retraining (18). However, these approaches have not been without unwanted consequences. The problem is that such employment assistance programs cannot help but have an impact on the labor force as a whole; such is the complexity of modern economies. In addition, care has to be taken to ensure that the individual and human rights of unemployed people are protected. Many people believe that well-intentioned, government unemployment programs can degenerate into a form of *slave labor*. Nevertheless, such programs exist, and full-time employment may never be available in future societies for all people, as Lobo (18) suggests pessimistically, but perhaps realistically.

> Many young people without jobs or underemployed live in deprivation, impermanence and temporary relationships in new ways. Emergent lifestyles include . . . welfare claimant careers, extended full-time education, and single parenthood. (19, p. 32)

A third factor that compounds occupational deprivation through unemployment is the pattern of shifting demographics of nations around the globe. Fundamentally, as a result of people living longer, healthier lives, the world has an increasing number of countries with burgeoning aging populations and shrinking younger generations. This means that there will be a huge gap in the future with increased populations having higher needs and smaller workforces capable of meeting them. This is a scenario that currently preoccupies policy makers and service providers, for example, in the area of health care. Accordingly, new, efficiency-driven models of service delivery are being developed alongside strategies directed at maximizing the exchange of skills and expertise between older, experienced workers and new entrants to the professional workforce. Across all sectors, the challenge will be to keep people working and being productive longer but in flexible ways that allow for planned and gradual transitioning between full-time work and retirement.

Neither futurists nor science fiction novelists are optimistic in their predictions of employment patterns in the coming decades. Consider this extract from Marge Piercy's account (20) of a future in which the world is no longer divided by national borders but by multinational zones. In Piercy's future world, people are either citizens/employees of a huge multinational corporation that controls all facets of their lives, or they live in the "Glop," a vast underworld of unemployed and unskilled people who have no access to education or reliable technology. Surviving, for those in the Glop, is the central occupation.

> Day workers and gang ninos and the unemployed lived in the Glop—the great majority of people on the continent. Most of the remainder were citizens of the enclaves . . . parts of the Glop were under domes, but the system had not been completed before governments stopped functioning . . . every quadrant was managed by the remains of the old UN, the eco-police, that had authority over earth, water, and air outside domes and wraps. Otherwise, the Multis ruled the enclaves, the free towns defended themselves as best they could and the Glop rotted under the poisonous sky, ruled by feuding gangs and overlords (20, pp. 45–46).

With this dramatic construction of a possible future, it is worth reflecting on some of the themes highlighted in Piercy's description of how the world could be. To what extent, for example, do we already have a global situation in which some people are being pressured to do more and more, while others are drifting further away from opportunities for paid employment, as well as other meaningful occupations? Indications are that this may already be happening in some countries. Due to the technological advances that many First World countries are experiencing, whole communities of people previously involved in industries, such as automobile manufacturing and mining, have been occupationally deprived by mass unemployment. Other industries, such as fishing and logging, have similarly left legions of people without work, without even the hope of work, in the wake of diminished natural resources and the absence of management for sustainability. In some communities it has become common for families to experience third-generation unemployment.

Simultaneously, the demands of employed people have changed dramatically in the last two decades, leading to overemployment for some. People are routinely being asked to work longer, unpaid hours, increase margins of productivity, and accept less annual leave than previously (21). The stress associated with greater work-related demands in increasingly competitive work environments is that people are constantly faced with the possibility of redundancy or downsizing. It is harder and harder for these people to live occupational lives that have a balance of work and leisure. Beder describes the situation, rather grimly.

> Millions of people are being encouraged and coerced to work long hours, devoting their lives to making or doing things that will not enrich their lives or make them happier . . . they are so busy doing this that they have little time to spend with their family and friends, to develop other aspects of themselves, or to participate in their communities as full citizens. And the best brains of a generation are engaged in persuading them to go on doing this without question (22, p. 3).

As Beder suggested, those caught up in the busy-ness of overemployment are materially rich but time poor. They do more and more (at work), though arguably, contribute less and less to their immediate communities. Overemployed people are chronically stressed because they are doing too much. The corollary is that increasing numbers of people are chronically stressed because they are doing too little. A strange inversion is occurring: Some people are materially rich but time poor, whereas others are materially poor but time rich.

It seems that a new two-class system of overemployed people versus unemployed or underemployed people is emerging. The economic conditions that surround this phenomenon are complex, but are easier to understand when the global distribution of wealth is examined. Huge differences in wealth exist between technologically developing and technologically advanced countries. In fact, it is estimated that U.S. $60 million is transferred every day from the world's poorest countries to repay the debts they owe to the richest (23).

What needs to be done to prevent the world from realizing Piercy's frightening depiction? This complex situation requires multifaceted approaches. Education, global economic reforms, and sustainable environmental practices are all part of the solution. Such a solution essentially involves changing the structural arrangements that keep people out of full levels of occupational participation and would therefore necessitate controversial major reforms in many countries to ensure greater equity and the redistribution of wealth. Accordingly, change on this scale would be neither swift nor painless.

In summary, employment patterns have changed dramatically during the last three decades, leaving large numbers of people at risk of occupational deprivation due to unemployment, underemployment, or overemployment. Overemployment is a new historically and economically situated phenomenon in which smaller numbers of people are working increasingly long hours and have little or no discretionary time. They experience occupational imbalance and a form of occupational deprivation that results when a single occupation dominates a life devoid of the rich tapestry of occupations available to us. A strange two-class inversion contrasts one group of people who are materially rich but time poor (overemployed) with another group of people who are materially poor but time rich (unemployed or underemployed). Occupational deprivation for both classes appears to be one of the most pressing global issues for the 21st century.

Incarceration

Prisons and detention centers in First World nations continue to grow at an alarming rate. **Incarceration** has long been viewed in Western countries as a deprivation of liberty (Figure 12-2 ■). The philosophic argument is that persons forfeit their right to freedom and are removed from society if they have committed acts defined as crimes. The rationale for such punishment is that through removal from society, convicts are unable to repeat the acts that constituted the original crime, and they are denied the freedom to engage in occupations at their discretion (24). From an occupational perspective, incarceration deliberately withdraws opportunities to participate in or choose occupational pursuits. Thus, through legal sanctions, societies determine that some people will be occupationally deprived through imprisonment. Such a sanction represents a powerful reminder that the right to *do* what one chooses, when, and where (within the confines of the law) is considered to be so central to our cultural understandings of what it is to be human, that to remove that freedom of choice and participation in occupations is considered the most severe punishment.

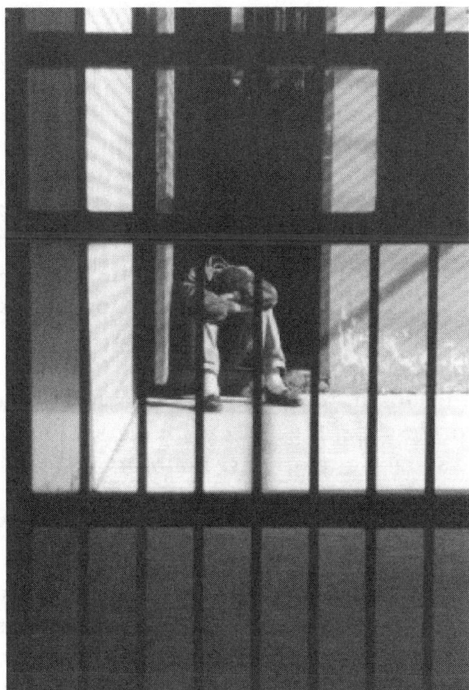

FIGURE 12-2 Social sanctions, such as imprisonment, create occupational deprivation as a type of punishment.
(Photograph courtesy of Francois Po Plessis)

Inside the institutional environment of prisons, inmates experience another level of occupational deprivation (to a greater or lesser extent, dependent on a number of factors). Prisons are institutions, and institutional life always imposes restrictions on occupational choice and patterns of engagement. One added feature to institutional life in prisons is security. Keeping inmates and prison staff safe restricts the types of occupations available and the timing of occupations. In many high-security units, tool use is restricted due to the risk of self-harm and the threat of injury to others. Total restriction of tool use, however, can compound problems associated with occupational deprivation (25). Another added feature of institutional life in many prisons is geographic isolation. Arguably community protection is increased when prisons are in geographically isolated places, but this isolation curtails any normative interaction with the "outside." Institutional policies, types of settings, and the severity of crimes all influence the extent to which inmates can interact through visits with the outside world and significant others.

What are the consequences of occupational deprivation during imprisonment? The term *stir crazy* is sometimes used to describe the negative effect of being deprived of opportunities for normal occupational engagement. One of the potential psychological consequences is disorientation and potential psychosis brought on by a combination of isolation, temporal dislocation, and inactivity (24, 26). Through everyday doing, we locate ourselves in time. The occupations of daily life form a temporal structure that provides predictable routines. For example, we prepare breakfast at the beginning of the day and may take the garbage out at night. Our occupations are also very much influenced by the social and cultural meanings associated with different days of the week. Generally speaking, we tend to do different things on Saturday and Sunday than we do on other days of the week. As for the weekdays, we experience Monday as being different from Friday. These important, yet subtle, distinctions of routine and meaning situate us in time and help to orient us to the external world, providing us with a rhythm and tempo to our daily lives. In prison, there is little differentiation between hours, days, weeks, and months. One day is much the same as the next, punctuated by normal variations (sleeping in on a holiday, for instance). Incarceration also deprives inmates of the opportunity to participate in special occasions and the occupations that accompany them, such as shopping for family birthdays. Such deprivation of occupational engagement, experienced as living in an apparently endless, featureless sea of time, can be detrimental to mental health. Psychosis and increased suicide attempts are major mental health risks of imprisonment (27), as are depression and increased aggression (28). Rioting in prisons has even been interpreted as a response to diminished occupational opportunities (29).

Changes in correctional policy over the years in some countries reflect the sentiment that dehumanized prison environments and unnecessary incarceration are ultimately counterproductive to the long-term interests of societies. Studies supporting this point of view have been equivocal. This has made it easier for critics of correctional reform to assert that the purpose of incarceration is punishment, not rehabilitation. Winston Churchill observed, "The mood and temper of the public in regard to the treatment of crime and criminals is one of the most unfailing tests of the civilization of any country" (30). Yet, educational programs and other humane efforts that may be conducive to preventing recidivism are not universally adopted.

Harsh conditions during incarceration can lead to prison unrest and violence and have not clearly demonstrated their value as a compelling deterrent to crime (31). An occupational perspective on prison life appears necessary both to understand the consequences of incarceration and to reduce the recidivism of repeat offenders who are unprepared to contribute to society outside prison. An understanding of occupational deprivation and the contrasting concept of occupational enrichment are critical in planning for the community and occupational reintegration of those who have been incarcerated.

In summary, incarceration leads to a condition of occupational deprivation that varies across inmates. When occupational restrictions are too severe, the effects are highly detrimental, ranging from boredom to psychosis, suicide, and rioting. Severe forms of occupational deprivation actually mitigate against inmates' future abilities to reintegrate successfully into communities. With rates of incarceration growing internationally, this form of occupational deprivation requires ongoing monitoring, research, and continued debate and dialogue.

Sex-Role Stereotyping: Gendered Constructions of Occupational Deprivation for Women

Geographic isolation and incarceration are fairly obvious contributors to scenarios of occupational deprivation, but being of a particular gender is not. **Sex-role stereotyping** refers to the social judgments made about what men and women typically should and should not do. A historical examination of sex-role stereotyping in different cultural contexts shows that women have been deprived from engagement in a vast array of occupations otherwise available to men. Wilcock began to explore the impact of sex-role stereotyping on women when she wrote that "women, too, have generally suffered occupational deprivation for hundreds of years" (1, p. 147).

One of the most obvious reasons that women experience occupational deprivation is due to religious and cultural sanctions (32). Historically, many religions have prescribed which occupations are acceptable for women to engage in and which are not (Figure 12-3 ■). Prohibited occupations for women have been as diverse as manual labor of certain types, creative pursuits (such as playing music or painting), building, hunting, or socializing. Whereas some occupations have been forbidden because of religious law, other occupations have been historically viewed as unacceptable for women because of prevailing social and cultural belief systems. The right to vote, play certain sports, socialize in a public bar, fly an airplane, or work in a mine are all occupations that have been denied to women in some national/cultural contexts until recent times, in which some countries (but not all) have moved to ensure equity of access and participation (32).

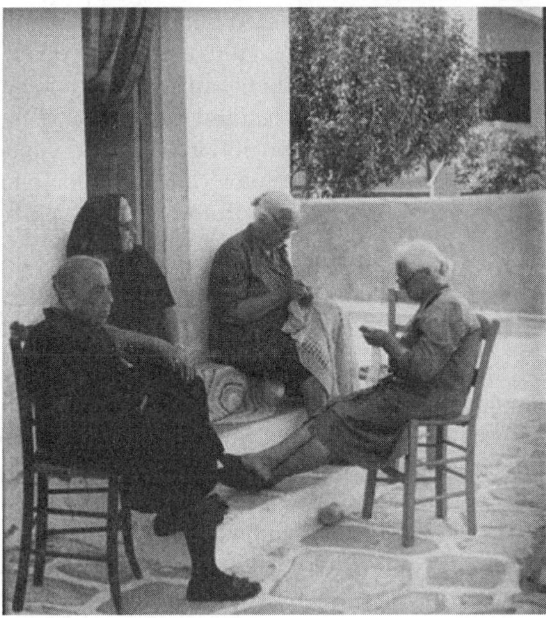

FIGURE 12-3 Some cultures have defined expectations for the occupations of women. These sex-role stereotypes are sometimes slow to change. (Copyright by Hava Gurevich, July 1987, Antiparos, Greece, Summer of 1987)

The biological argument for depriving women of the opportunity to engage in some occupations has been and, in some situations, continues to be reproduction and fertility cycles. Health risks associated with reproduction may also contribute to diminished levels of occupational engagement and performance (33). Following childbirth, the raising of an infant is most likely to be the occupational responsibility of the mother. Despite the postmodern context in which we live, child rearing is still regarded by most societies as the occupational domain of women. Primeau (34) pointed to research undertaken in the United States indicating that even in households where both partners are employed in paid work, women still assume the majority of responsibility for child-care-related tasks. A "second shift" of household and child-rearing-related tasks appears to deprive employed women of opportunities (in the form of free time) to participate in leisure occupations (35).

Economically, the work of women is of central importance in most countries. In their historically important examination of the workloads of women in sub-Saharan Africa, Barrett and Brown (33) pointed out that women are the major contributors to agricultural production. They cite several studies that point to differences in time spent in agricultural occupations between men and women. For example, among the Beti people of Cameroon, men spend 7.3 hours per day in agricultural occupations, whereas women spend 10.6 hours. When such workloads are coupled with child rearing and other domestic duties, it is evident that women may be occupationally deprived because they have very little discretionary time for more than work occupations.

Three main ideas have been presented to highlight the occupational deprivation experienced by women because of inherent, historical sex stereotyping. First, women, as a subgroup of society, are vulnerable to sustained states of occupational deprivation through both the overt exclusions of some religions and the influence of cultural and social values that deny certain occupational behaviors. Second, biological imperatives, particularly women's reproductive cycles and responsibilities, influence women's occupational participation rates, most notably in leisure occupations. Third, discrepancies in divisions of labor in both technologically developing and technologically advanced countries deprive women of opportunities to participate in leisure and discretionary occupations.

Refugeeism: Displacement and Dislocation of Refugees

It is difficult for someone who has not been a refugee to imagine what it is like to be deprived of participation in lifelong valued occupations. Many refugees are escaping from situations in which they have been victims of violence or persecution, such that they have often undergone a level of trauma from which they never fully recover (Box 12-1). Often added to the trauma is a period of sustained deprivation from opportunities to participate in a whole range of familiar occupations that would ordinarily provide structure, meaning, and coherence on a daily basis. Refugeeism is a large and complex problem internationally. Here, we will briefly consider some factors that contribute to the occupational deprivation of refugees.

When refugees escape the situation from which they have fled or been ejected, the first experience of **displacement** is one of transitory living in which most occupations differ, whether in form or location, from those that were habitual. Refugees may live in numerous temporary facilities, including camps, for periods sometimes extending to years. Their fate is often uncertain, as numerous bureaucratic processes unfold to determine their ultimate destination and fate. In these temporary and transitional facilities, it is very difficult for refugees to engage in the occupations of meaning that characterized their lives in their home country. Lack of facilities, space, artifacts, and tools and dislocation from a normative sociocultural context create great difficulties for doing the things that previously imbued life with purpose and meaning. Even the basic occupations associated with self-care and maintenance may assume a radically different form in the environment of a refugee camp. Food preparation, for example, may afford little opportunity for family involvement, given the large numbers of people in a camp. Too much time, too little to do, a lack of objects and tools, and the effects of trauma all contribute to a state of occupational deprivation in the short term for refugees. Though we may tend to think of refugee camps as safe havens (albeit temporarily) for people fleeing often violent upheavals, the experience of living in one can be very different. A snapshot of what life is like in a refugee camp follows (36).

> There was a lot of things happening every minute in the camp—people getting depressed, people were getting . . . crazy. Some of the people just got crazy and they couldn't control themselves, so there was a lot of people, but it was good that we had a lot of people which we could help . . . needed to help them settle, to keep calmed down and to help them with food and whatever they needed . . . we had had too much trauma. When we got there we came from some warm place which was our place which was our life but in which you could be killed. But when we came here we felt we survived that, but we couldn't survive now. The conditions of the life in the camp and when you see someone else starving and going crazy, when you see other things you just forget about yourself and try to help them . . . when the bread came there was so many people trying to grab the bread (p. 82).

Upon resettlement in a host country, some conditions change for refugees. They may, however, continue to face occupational deprivation due to cultural, social, and economic isolation. Language, for instance, is a huge barrier for many newly arrived refugees in their new home country. Insufficient language skills limit educational opportunities and diminish refugees' opportunities to engage in occupations of paid employment. Sharing a language creates opportunities for interaction and the development of understanding of the occupations of a sociocultural milieu. Not sharing a language with local residents isolates and deprives people of interaction and the development of occupational opportunities.

Differences in cultural and religious orientations can compound occupational deprivation when a host country isolates refugees, expresses indifference toward them, or responds with outward hostility to the beliefs and specific practices of refugee groups. Understandably, national and ethnic communities then form where values and belief systems can be shared rather than challenged, compounding refugees' isolation from mainstream society.

BOX 12-1 What is Refugeeism?

According to the 1951 Convention Relating to the Status of Refugees, a refugee is a person who "owing to a well-founded fear of being persecuted for reasons of race, religion, nationality, membership in a particular social group, or political opinion, is outside the country of his nationality, and is unable to or, owing to such fear, is unwilling to avail himself of the protection of that country." Refugeeism pertains to attitudes that restrict appropriate aid to refugees for various social, political, and cultural reasons. For example, restrictive immigration policies may be implemented within a climate of hostility and fear toward refugees, asylum seekers, and migrants (Figure 12-4 ■). Refugees and migrants may be unfairly blamed for the social and economic ills of society, including rising crime and unemployment. Such reactions contribute to an increase in racism, violence, and unwarranted fear and prejudice against refugees, asylum seekers, and migrants.

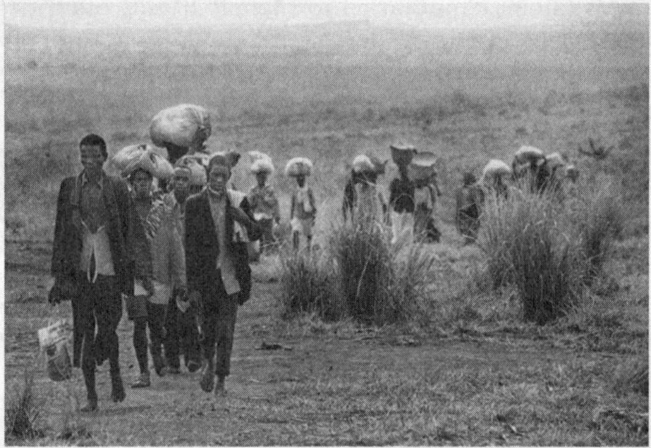

FIGURE 12-4 War and internal political strife within nations can deprive people of the safety and support of community. A column of Hutu refugees escape from Burundi into Tanzania with cooking pots, food, and a few chickens.

Social isolation, coupled with economic pressures, means that many refugees face limitations to their full participation in occupations of meaning and necessity in the context of a new, dominant culture. Not all refugees experience such isolation, but common issues do exist that need to be understood and addressed, particularly because national and ethnic tensions will likely continue if not increase the dislocation of people from their communities of origin. Refugees typically experience occupational deprivation because they are dislocated physically and socially from familiar environments. Their linguistic, economic, and cultural isolation in host countries is understandable, but compounds the occupational deprivation that characterizes refugee life. Importantly, people who have lived through the experience really aspire to the re-creation of a peaceful and occupationally normative life. Certainly, as is suggested here, they want to transcend the label refugee, and assume a rightful place in society again (36).

> I mean when I hear the word refugees, I don't take it as only refugees, its "remember me—I have a long story" I've had many time when people turn on the TV and look at the news which I don't look at any more, I just watch the sport, something which is normal. When it comes to war and that stuff I just put it somewhere else, I change the channel, I don't watch it. Personally, I don't like to be called refugee (p. 85).

DISABILITY AND OCCUPATIONAL DEPRIVATION

Occupational deprivation refers to situations and conditions that exist external to an individual or group, depriving them of important occupational opportunities beyond their immediate control. Geographic isolation suggests how the physical environment can lead to occupational deprivation. Refugeeism offers a prime example of how political situations can lead to occupational deprivation. Cultural forces that create sex-role stereotyping and the social and economic factors that bring about wide-scale unemployment, underemployment, or overemployment have also been considered with reference to occupational deprivation.

Occupational deprivation may also arise from social and cultural practices related to individual characteristics. Some conditions that exist within individuals constitute barriers to occupation because "someone or something external to the individual is doing the depriving" (2, p. 201). Of concern here are conditions that have a physical causation and those that are psychological, emotional, or cognitive in nature. Occupational deprivation is *not inherent in limited physical, psychological, emotional, or cognitive abilities.* The point needs to be emphasized that deprivation from occupations of meaning or cultural significance is made worse by *someone or something external* to the individual (i.e., the human and nonhuman environment). Having schizophrenia, for example, in and of itself does not create occupational deprivation; the social exclusions faced by people with schizophrenia because of the stigma of mental illness may also contribute to their experience of occupational deprivation.

Being born with or acquiring a chronic illness or a **disability** is a reality that confronts many people. Being blind, having cerebral palsy, contracting multiple sclerosis, becoming depressed, sustaining a brain injury or having schizophrenia (as suggested earlier) are only some of the examples of situations that represent a challenge to people trying to live full and rewarding occupational lives. In the past, disabling conditions, whether these were physical, psychological, emotional, or cognitive, were often synonymous with social isolation and severely restricted occupational opportunities. Even aging has historically precluded engagement in certain occupations. The central question is whether various types of disabilities in themselves are barriers to participation in occupations or whether human and physical environments are the real impediments. We need to ask how social attitudes have precluded participation in occupations by people with disabilities. How have social attitudes constrained people with various types of disabilities from self-expression through action?

Narrative accounts of life with a physical disability point to the attitudes of other people as one of the biggest barriers to participation in the world around them. Stereotyped perceptions, limited expectations, and subtle marginalization all serve to constrain people who have chronic physical illness or physical disability from accessing and fully engaging in occupations of meaning and choice. Attitudes of the physical able-bodied population may have changed in recent times due to better education and increased opportunities for interaction (e.g., through mainstream schooling). Yet, it still seems that many able-bodied people have definite views on what people with disabilities should and should not do. People with disabilities have reflected on the difficulties they have had in *breaking out* of society's stereotyped perceptions. Some prevailing attitudes may have changed, but they tell people with able bodies that there is still a long way to go before people with disabilities can participate fully in leisure and work occupations as diverse as flying a plane, dating, dancing, or being a competitive athlete.

The physical or built environment can either enable or inhibit occupational engagement for people with some form of physical limitation. People with physical disabilities have chronicled their frustrations with physical environments that, on a daily basis, prevent them from doing what they want and need to do. They may not use the language of occupation, but they are referring to their everyday experiences of occupational deprivation. A perspective often taken by people with so-called disabilities is that it is not shortcomings in their personal characteristics and abilities that create the disability; rather, it is the shortcomings of the physical environment that disable them. As Gerhart suggested, "Often, a change in the environment can foster independence far more readily than a change in the individual" (37, p. 139).

How, then, can environments enable or constrain opportunities for occupational engagement? For a start, the conceptualization of a physical environment determines who can participate. Free-flowing space with unrestricted access should be the ultimate aim of public places so that everyone can participate, regardless of whether they are elderly persons with walkers, toddlers, or persons using electric wheelchairs. Ensuring that things like signage, switches, doors, parking, seating, and ramps are user friendly to a range of people (not just the able-bodied), facilitates engagement in the occupations we enjoy in public places. Occupations such as shopping, having a picnic, listening to an outdoor concert, or browsing in the botanical gardens should be possible for all people if the physical environment has been conceptualized and accordingly designed to be barrier free. This is the premise for universal design.

Assistive technology is another facet of the physical environment that can be introduced to enable occupation. A wide range of technology is available to assist people with the instrumental aspects of occupational performance such as opening a door, switching on a computer, or holding a fork. The use and availability of such technology within the environment can facilitate opportunities for all people to engage in occupations that are meaningful. Technology can actually transform occupational opportunities. An example of technology creating opportunities for social occupations is the Internet. Because of instant messaging, social networking websites, blogsites, and interactive games, the Internet has created a new range of social occupations that enable persons with and without physical disabilities to participate in social networks and to greatly reduce the social isolation that disability previously often created.

What occupational deprivation is experienced by persons with disabilities that arise from a psychological disorder, a cognitive difficulty, or a mental illness? Such biological conditions may impair occupational performance, but they need not be, in themselves, barriers to occupational engagement and satisfaction, if the human environment is supportive. The conceptualization and construction of the physical, nonhuman environment is important, but the social environment is what really enables or constrains occupational opportunities for people with nonphysical impairments and disabilities. In the not-so-distant past, people with mental illnesses and intellectual disabilities were often subjected to alienating and marginalizing treatments including heavy medication and surgery. In addition, opportunities to be involved in the everyday occupational world of so-called normal people were denied them through the process of physical isolation brought about by institutionalization.

The extent to which society has changed its understanding and tolerance of nonphysical impairments is still a matter of some debate. From the excellent book *I Always Wanted to Be a Tap Dancer* (a collection of stories by women with disabilities about their lives), one narrator's comments on her experiences with disability are compelling. In the following excerpt, Meg reflects on her experiences of having manic depression, and on the attitudes of others toward her disorder and their perceptions of the "doing" dimension of her life.

> Having once had a mental illness, everything you do in the future becomes suspect. I sat through a committee meeting where the issue of mature-age people returning to study was being debated. One committee member spoke scathingly about "fruitcakes" who come to study as therapy . . . I never really decided to make the choice to be open about my experiences, they are part of me and my qualifications just as much as my university qualifications and my employment experience. When I applied for my position . . . I was asked why did I start the Manic Depressive self help group . . . so I told them. I am grateful for the tolerance and understanding that has been extended to me in my job. But why should I be grateful? . . . I do my job well, yet I am always conscious of needing to prove that I am as good as anyone else or that I have to make up for the years I lost to illness, and most importantly, never appearing to be mad or high or nervous in any way (38, p. 112).

From this account, it is clear that the attitudes and beliefs of others still exert a strong influence on the daily occupations of the lives of people with mental illness. From Meg's story it is evident that because of her history of mental illness, all her actions became "suspect." Accordingly, going about everyday activities for people having been so affected is complicated by needing to appear "OK," including how happy or sad she can be in her interactions with others.

From accounts such as the one just presented, it is clear that facilitating greater occupational opportunity for people dealing with such conditions is a shared responsibility. Through increased community education and by enacting pragmatic strategies in the workplace, it should be possible to create a future wherein the occupational potential of people with mental illness or cognitive or emotional disorders can be more fully realized. The challenge is to heighten awareness in communities; that it is the attitudinal barriers that most often restrict people with non-physical disabilities from participation in occupations, particularly outside the home. Principles such as *reasonable accommodation* can go a long way toward enabling people to be involved in numerous everyday occupations, particularly in paid employment. *Reasonable accommodation* refers to the modification of a physical, social, or emotional environment to enable the occupational performance of individuals or groups. For example, reasonable accommodations are made when work environments allocate specific tasks, rather than whole occupations, to persons with diminished concentration due to a cognitive impairment or the effects of antidepressant medication.

In this section, the occupational deprivation produced by conditions in the physical, social, and emotional environments has been explored. Special attention was given to the deprivation experienced by persons with disability, highlighting the observation that constraints to occupational engagement in disability are imposed by the human and nonhuman environment. They are not inherent in the disability itself. Recent advances in technology, education, and attitudinal shifts have all helped to reduce the occupational deprivation of people with disabilities. We are now exposed to images of people in wheelchairs hang gliding, people with leg amputations climbing mountains and snow skiing, and people in nursing homes lifting weights. Such images have the power to improve awareness that all people, regardless of age and status, have a fundamental human need to live meaningful occupational lives—to create and recreate themselves through what they do.

USING AN OCCUPATIONAL JUSTICE FRAMEWORK TO ADDRESS OCCUPATIONAL DEPRIVATION

In 2004, Townsend and Wilcock published a groundbreaking work that synthesized and further developed many years of thinking about inequities in levels of occupational participation around the globe. Their exploratory theory of occupational justice (39) represents an important contribution to how we might better understand and begin to address occupational deprivation. In this volume, Chapter 13 by Stadnyk, Townsend, and Wilcock suggests that the occupational determinants of a given country, which include its economic, policy, and cultural environment, influence the accepted forms of, and opportunities for, occupational engagement. This in turn, they assert, can create scenarios of injustice leading to occupational imbalance, occupational alienation or (of most interest to us in this chapter) occupational deprivation.

We can test their model with some real-life examples. Vietnam is a liberal, communist country. It is still resource poor but developing rapidly. Its policy environment is strongly influenced by communist ideals and values, which put collective needs above those of the individuals and prioritize community development. The government recently started building massive Internet access facilities, free for every citizen to use for several hours per week. This is based on a belief that all Vietnamese citizens need to be technologically literate so that they are not at a disadvantage now or in the future. Creating mass Internet access (tens of millions of people) has developed skills and opportunities for people to participate in technologically based occupations. Imagine what this has cost! In essence, changes in the political and policy environment have enabled people who may have been disadvantaged to access technology and the occupations associated with it. Vietnamese people will not experience occupational deprivation as a result of not having adequate access to low-cost technology.

Also in Vietnam, with its complex mix of culture, history, and politics, persons with disabilities are not automatically given rights of citizenship. With a focus on the collective rather than the individual, and with a concern for the multitudes of able-bodied people in Vietnam, the policy environment does not allow for the mobilization of (comparatively) high levels of resources to be made available to individuals with disabilities. Accordingly, they have minimal access to education and experience occupational deprivation in terms of diminished opportunities to develop their skills and knowledge, including diminished Internet access compared to able-bodied Vietnamese citizens. Without an education, it is difficult to work, socialize, or even communicate effectively, as highlighted by Whiteford and McAllister (40).

Occupational justice as an explanatory framework may be a work in progress, but, as we have seen in the examples from Vietnam, it may have real application in understanding occupational deprivation. Indeed, occupational deprivation is a very emotionally laden phenomenon and can benefit from scrutiny using an **occupational justice framework** to interpret research, using different methodologies and involving those who actually experience forms of occupational deprivation.

CHAPTER SUMMARY

In this chapter, the concept of occupational deprivation was described as a condition in the environment in which individuals, for reasons beyond their control, are unable to participate or engage in occupations necessary for their spiritual, mental, physical, or economic well-being for extended periods.

Examples of conditions that illustrate occupational deprivation were provided, including geographic isolation, unsatisfactory conditions of employment (unemployment, underemployment, and overemployment), incarceration, sex-role stereotyping, and refugeeism. Occupational deprivation was contrasted with occupational disruption, which is described as a temporary condition that can be resolved through supportive efforts that may be initiated by the individual affected.

The special case of occupational deprivation that occurs for people with special needs, who have permanent, acquired, or congenital disabilities, was also described. In this instance, deprivation is often a consequence of social conditions, such as attitudes and policies that lead to environmental designs that fail to make occupations accessible for people with the diversity of physical, mental, and cognitive abilities that exist within a population. Improved awareness of the importance of occupations in daily lives will lead to a more widespread appreciation of the effects of occupational disruption and deprivation when these occur. Understanding deprivation from the standpoint of occupational justice may enable this to be done more consistently and effectively.

STUDY GUIDE

Study Guide Author: Julie Bass Haugen

Summary of Main Points

Developing a full understanding of humans as occupational beings living in social structures that influence occupational participation requires us to examine both positive and negative dimensions of occupational experiences. Earlier chapters have introduced rich descriptions of human occupations across the life span and in different contexts. We have learned how occupational engagement can provide meaning and purpose in life and can contribute to identity. In this chapter, occupational deprivation was explored as an example of diminished participation due to factors that are external to persons. Appreciation of the influencing factors and effects of deprivation in specific examples helps to develop an awareness of unjust situations in communities and globally.

Application to Occupational Therapy

When occupational therapy practitioners work with individuals and populations to address occupational issues, they carefully examine all the personal and environmental factors that influence performance and engagement. This discussion of occupational deprivation provides an occupational perspective for interpreting many social issues in the newspapers as well as in occupational therapy practice. As well, the concept of occupational deprivation provides language to define occupational issues, goals and outcomes in occupation-based practice. In medical settings, the primary focus is often on the person or internal factors that contribute to occupational problems. Many health conditions are temporary states and may be viewed as disruptions in a typical occupational profile.

When occupational therapy is used to address larger world issues (like the ones discussed in this chapter), the emphasis must significantly shift from a cursory review of the immediate environment to the social, economic, environmental, geographic, historic, cultural, and political factors that influence the situation. Many of these external factors are complex and have not been made explicit in occupational therapists' client documents, texts or public descriptions of the profession. To eliminate occupational deprivation and serve as an effective change agent, the occupational therapist would talk about occupations and their impact on individuals, populations and societies whenever possible. Occupational therapists would adopt an occupational lens for viewing the situations of individuals and families, and raise questions and consider solutions to change local conditions, such as occupational opportunities for new immigrants, or reasonable accommodations in workplaces. As well, occupational therapists can speak out collectively in the media or public situations through professional associations about social, political and economic conditions that result in the occupational deprivation of particular groups in their communities.

This discussion of occupational deprivation raised awareness of environmental factors that are not typically addressed in an occupational therapy text. It challenged readers to look beyond the physical barriers that are associated with inaccessible environments to include complex societal factors that were prevalent in these case studies. Consideration of the impact of geographic isolation, unsatisfactory conditions of employment, incarceration, sex-role stereotyping, and refugeeism on occupations emphasized avenues for occupational therapy practice beyond the typically funded areas covered by health insurance. The implication is for occupational therapists to make prospective new funders more aware of the potential value of occupation-related intervention, from immigration programs that are attempting to assist refugees to settle to probation services and women's programs. Occupational therapists may enable re-integration into society by those who have been imprisoned and energize women to recover from abusive, isolating, or other deprived situations.

This expanded view on the influence of environment on occupational engagement is also important when working with people having disabilities. Occupational therapy may realize its full potential if interventions target the societal barriers (whether policy based or attitudinal) that result in occupational deprivation.

Individual Learning Activities

1. Conduct an environmental scan of health and socio-cultural issues and current events in the news.
   a. Describe three examples of occupational disruption and three examples of occupational deprivation. For each example, identify the characteristics that provide evidence of disruption versus deprivation.
   b. Select one example of disruption and one example of deprivation to explore further. Propose an occupational therapy intervention for each example. Compare and contrast your interventions for these two examples.
2. Identify an issue for which there may be controversy, whether it is an example of occupational disruption or occupational deprivation. Write a five-paragraph essay that summarizes the issue and presents alternative views. Document your references.

Group Learning Activity

Select a historical event that provides an example of occupational deprivation. Conduct a review of the literature on this event. Write a group paper and make a presentation that includes

a. A summary of the historical event that includes a brief description, the population, the time period, the geographic area, and areas of occupational deprivation.
b. The characteristics of this event (i.e., social, economic, environmental, geographic, historic, cultural, or political) that provide evidence of occupational deprivation.
c. The effect of occupational deprivation on the health, quality of life and opportunities to participate equitably of individuals who experienced the historical event.
d. Develop a question worthy of study related to this event that is consistent with an occupational science and occupational justice framework.
e. Propose an occupational therapy evaluation or intervention that may have helped in this situation.
f. Document your references for the paper.

Study Questions

1. All of the following are characteristic of occupational disruption EXCEPT
   a. The contributing factors are typically beyond one's control
   b. Can result from internal/individual circumstances
   c. Is temporary or transient
   d. Resuming normal activities is expected
2. In Stadnyk, Townsend, and Wilcock's exploratory theory of occupational justice they suggested that the determinants of occupational engagement in a country include all of the following environments EXCEPT
   a. Economic
   b. Policy
   c. Cultural
   d. Geographic
3. An essential feature of occupational deprivation is that
   a. Participation is not within the immediate control of an individual, group, or community.
   b. It needs to be interpreted within the historic, cultural, and social milieu and context within which it arises
   c. None of the above
   d. Both a and b above
4. All of the following were described as influencing factors on unemployment EXCEPT
   a. Changes in technology
   b. Motivation for work
   c. Global and national economic forces
   d. Shifting demographics of nations around the globe
5. All of the following were identified as **increased** risks for prisoners associated with occupational deprivation EXCEPT
   a. Suicide attempts
   b. Aggression
   c. Recidivism
   d. Rioting

REFERENCES

1. Wilcock, A. A. (1998). *An occupational perspective of health.* Thorofare, NJ: Slack, Inc.
2. Whiteford, G. (2000). Occupational deprivation: Global challenge in the new millennium. *British Journal of Occupational Therapy, 63*(5), 200–204.
3. Mead, G. H. (1934). *Mind, self and society.* Chicago: University of Chicago Press.
4. Langford, R. (1988). *Don't take your love to town.* Ringwood, VIC: Penguin.
5. AIHW (Australian Institute of Health and Welfare). (1992). Health in rural and remote Australia (Report No. AIHW Cat. No. PHE 6). Canberra: Australian Institute of Health and Welfare.

6. Toohey, P. (2000, August 5–6). Another generation stolen by the fumes. *The Australian,* 3.
7. Cook, D. G., Cummins, R. O., Bartley, M. J., & Shaper, A. G. (1982). Health of unemployed middle aged men in Great Britain. *Lancet,* 1290–1294.
8. Beale, N., & Nethercott, S. (1985). Job loss and family morbidity. A study of factory closure. *Journal of the Royal College of General Practitioners, 280,* 510–514.
9. Government of Australia. (1992). *Enough to make you sick: How income and environment affect health* (Australian National Health Strategy Research Report No. 1). Canberra: Ministry of Health.
10. Colledge, M., & Bartholemew, R. (1980). *A study of the long term unemployed.* London: Manpower Services Commission.
11. Jackson, P. R., & Warr, P. B. (1984). Unemployment and psychological ill health: The moderating role of duration and age. *Psychological Medicine, 14*(1), 605–614.
12. Warr, P. (1987). *Work, unemployment and mental health.* Oxford: Oxford University Press.
13. Smith, R. (1987). *Unemployment and health: A disaster and a challenge.* Oxford: Oxford University Press.
14. Platt, S. (1984). Unemployment and suicidal behaviour: A review of the literature. *Social Science & Medicine, 19,* 93–115.
15. Toulmin, S. (1995). Occupation, employment and human welfare. *Journal of Occupational Science: Australia, 2*(2), 48–58.
16. Jones, B. (1998). Redefining work: Setting directions for the future. *Journal of Occupational Science, 5*(3), 127–132.
17. Farnworth, L. (1995). An exploration of skill as an issue in unemployment and employment. *Journal of Occupational Science, 2*(1), 22–29.
18. Botsman, P., & Latham, M. (2000). *The enabling state.* Sydney, Australia: Pluto Press.
19. Lobo, F. (1998). Social transformation and the changing work–leisure relationship in the late 1990s. *Journal of Occupational Science, 5*(3), 147–154.
20. Piercy, M. (1991). *Body of glass.* London: Penguin.
21. Bittman, M., & Rice, J. (1999). Are working hours becoming more unsociable? *Australian Social Policy Research Centre Newsletter, 74*(1–4).
22. Beder, S. (2000). *Selling the work ethic.* Carlton, Australia: Scribe.
23. Roodman, D. M. (2001). *Still waiting for the jubilee: Pragmatic solutions for the Third World debt crisis* (Worldwatch Paper 155). Washington, DC: Worldwatch Institute.
24. Molineux, M., & Whiteford, G. (1999). Prisons: From occupational deprivation to occupational enrichment. *Journal of Occupational Science, 6*(3), 124–130.
25. Whiteford, G. (1995). A concrete void: Occupational deprivation and the special needs inmate. *Journal of Occupational Science, 2*(2), 80–81.
26. Whiteford, G. (1997). Occupational deprivation and incarceration. *Journal of Occupational Science: Australia, 4*(3), 126–130.
27. Liebling, A. (1993). Suicides in young prisoners: A summary. *Death Studies, 17*(5), 381–409.
28. Zamble, E. (1992). Behaviour and adaptation in long term prison inmates: Descriptive longitudinal results. *Criminal Justice and Behaviour, 19*(4), 409–425.
29. Useem, B. (1985). Disorganization and the New Mexico Prison riot of 1980. *American Sociological Review, 50*(5), 677–688.
30. Churchill, W. S. (1910). Statement of the Rt. Hon Winston. S. Churchill, Secretary of state for the Home Department. In *Hansard Column. London: The Stationery Office,* British Government.
31. Andrews, D. A., Zinger, I., Hoge, R. D., Bonta, J., Gendreau, P., & Cullen, F. T. (1990). Does correctional treatment work? A clinically relevant and psychologically informed meta-analysis. *Criminology, 28,* 369–404.

32. Rowbotham, S. (1996). *Hidden from history: 300 years of women's oppression and the fight against it.* Sydney, Australia: Pluto Press.
33. Barrett, H., & Brown, A. (1993). Workloads of rural African women: The impact of economic adjustment in sub-Saharan Africa. *Journal of Occupational Science, 1*(2), 3–12.
34. Primeau, L. (1996). Work vs nonwork: The case of household work. In R. Zempke & F. Clark (Eds.), *Occupational science: The evolving discipline* (pp. 57–79). Philadelphia: F. A. Davis.
35. Zuzanek, J., & Mannell, R. (1993). Gender variations in the weekly rhythms of daily behaviour and experiences. *Journal of Occupational Science, 1*(1), 25–37.
36. Whiteford, G. (2005). Understanding the occupational deprivation of refugees: Case Study from Kosovo. *Canadian Journal of Occupational Therapy, 72*(2), 78–88.
37. Gerhart, K. (1998). Consequences for personal independence. In M. A. McColl & J. E. Bickenbach (Eds.), *Introduction to disability.* London: W. B. Saunders.
38. Smith, R. (1989). Meg's story. In A. Lawrence (Ed.), *I always wanted to be a tap dancer.* Parramatta, NSW: New South Wales Womens' Advisory Council.
39. Townsend, E., & Wilcock, A. (2004). An exploratory theory of occupational justice. In C. Christiansen & E. Townsend (Eds.), *Introduction to occupation: The art and science of living* (pp. 243–273). Upper Saddle River, NJ: Prentice Hall.
40. Whiteford, G., & McAllister, L. (2007). Politics and complexity in intercultural fieldwork: The Vietnam experience. *Australian Occupational Therapy Journal,* 54, S*1*, S74–S83.

CHAPTER 13

Occupational Justice

Robin L. Stadnyk, Elizabeth A. Townsend, and Ann A. Wilcock

OBJECTIVES

1. Understand the evolving concept of occupational justice.
2. Relate the concept of occupational justice to concepts such as social justice and equal opportunity.
3. Identify examples of situations where people are deprived of meaningful occupation.
4. Describe conditions in an "occupationally just" world.
5. Identify societal changes that would be necessary in moving toward a world that would be more occupationally just.

KEY WORDS

Capabilities
Enablement
Justice of difference
Occupational alienation
Occupational apartheid
Occupational deprivation
Occupational imbalance
Occupational marginalization
Occupational rights
Occupationally just world
Meaningful occupations
Theory of occupational justice

CHAPTER PROFILE

This chapter unites the concept of justice with the broad view of occupation presented throughout this book. Starting from the premise that humans are occupational beings and that just societies are guided by ethical, moral, and civic principles,

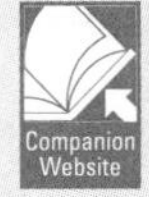

www.prenhall.com/christiansen
The Internet provides an exciting means for interacting with this textbook and for enhancing your understanding of humans' experiences with occupations and the organization of occupations in society. Use the address above to access the interactive Companion Website created specifically to accompany this book. Here you will find an array of self-study material designed to help you gain a richer understanding of the concepts presented in this chapter.

Our appreciation is extended to research assistants Tammy Cole and Chloé Buckley. Appreciation is also extended to participants in occupational justice workshops and presentations, whose challenging discussions helped to refine the ideas presented in this chapter.

principles of occupational justice that focus on peoples' occupational rights, needs, strengths, and potential are introduced. New insights on the evolving theory of occupational justice which was published in the first edition of this book are presented to link ideas, reasoning, beliefs and principles related to this concept. Explored are situations in which occupational injustices such as occupational imbalance, deprivation, marginalization, alienation, and apartheid occur. Relationships between occupational justice and social justice are explored.

INTRODUCTION

Occupational justice arose as an intriguing topic for consideration in the 1990s (1–8). Contemplation of occupational justice grew from research on the occupational foundations of human existence (2–5) and on the principles of empowerment and justice that implicitly inform practices that strive to be person centered (1, 6, 7). Townsend and Wilcock (8–10) sought a language and concept to raise concerns about the unfairness of some people flourishing in what they do, whereas other people are leading unhealthy, empty, marginalized, or dangerous lives.[1]

Occupational justice was first described as complementary to social justice, "Whilst social justice addresses the social relations and social conditions of life, occupational justice addresses what people *do* in their relationships and conditions for living" (8, p. 84). Motivating this exploration is a utopian vision of an **occupationally just world.**

An occupationally just world is envisioned as one that would be governed in a way that enables individuals to flourish by doing what they decide is most meaningful and useful to themselves and to their families, communities, and nations (8). Many questions are prompted by such a vision. One could ask: what if people do not want to do something meaningful or useful? How can individuals decide what is meaningful, just, or unjust when they do not fully appreciate how families, communities, or nations work? Is justice about society, individuals, or power relationships? Likely the chapter will raise as many questions as it answers.

Whereas earlier publications about occupational justice introduced the terminology and concepts related to occupational justice (8–12), this chapter provides a reexamination of issues and literature for an investigation of occupational justice as a concept of importance to occupational science, philosophy, political science, sociology and other fields, including occupational therapy. First, ideas from literature about justice that inform the concept of occupational justice are presented. Then, the evolving theory of occupational justice is described. Stories of occupational injustice and questions for continuing a dialogue on this topic complete the chapter.

DEFINING OCCUPATIONAL JUSTICE

What is occupational justice? The concept of occupation is grounded in a belief that humans are occupational beings. Humans participate as interdependent, active agents in culturally defined occupations that determine their health and quality of life. From this perspective, humans' occupations are more than what the marketplace defines as work. The concept of occupational justice juxtaposes moral, ethical, and political ideas of justice on occupation. A focus on occupational justice means that we look at diverse occupational needs, strengths, and potential of individuals and groups, while at the same time considering issues of rights, fairness, empowerment, and enablement of occupational opportunities.

Occupational justice offers a new lens for looking at and acting on local and world struggles from an *occupational* perspective. That is, considering these struggles from the standpoint of what meaningful and purposeful occupations (tasks and activities) people want to do, need to do, and can do considering their personal and situational circumstances.

Occupational therapists have long been interested in issues of social justice (1), which has as its focus the social relations and social conditions of life, particularly in relationship to the equitable distribution of resources and power. Occupational justice diverges from social justice through an interest in individual as well as group differences; a concern for the enablement of diverse participation in society as well as the distribution of rights and goods; and, a focus on the relationships between occupation, health, and quality of life.

IDEAS ABOUT JUSTICE

Justice is generally accepted to be an ideal vision of society expressed through ethical, moral, and civic principles (13–20). Justice has been debated since the earliest humans recognized the need for principles to adjudicate disputes over food, land, women, men, children, and their possessions (13–15). Definitions of justice have developed over time to adjudicate the sharing of resources and land.

Other definitions have outlined expectations for acceptable and unacceptable behavior among families, communities, nations, and more recently, global communities. In his 1971 classic book *A Theory of Justice,* the American philosopher John Rawls highlighted individual rights, responsibilities, and liberties as moral principles of justice (16). Jürgen Habermas, a German philosopher, focused on ideas of liberty and free expression. He proposed an ideal speech situation in which everyone can express opinions without restriction, and disputes would be settled through argumentation rather than violence (17, 18), an ideal that Armstrong contends has not yet been achieved in reality (19). Tara Smith has explored justice as a personal virtue of respect and fair treatment of others (20).

Social justice in modern society has a variety of meanings (16). Procedural justice is concerned with dispute resolution to hear the views of all parties. Restorative justice is concerned with the restoration of perpetrators of wrongdoing and with restitution to victims. Distributive justice is primarily concerned with the morally proper distribution and redistribution of resources in society. Distributive justice is prominent in laws and policies that address fair distribution of income, pensions, housing, resources such as health care, and social services. The *social safety net* is an example of a distributive form of social justice that indicates that resources such as social assistance income, public housing, and other subsidies will be reserved for those "in need," which generally means those without sufficient income to purchase these necessities. Funding for a social safety net is usually procured through taxation. Therefore, many poorer countries face a double jeopardy because they neither raise taxes nor fund social programs to help redistribute resources to vulnerable groups, such as those who are elderly, have disabilities, or live in poverty.

Laws and policies encouraging the redistribution of resources are not the only influences on justice as experienced by individuals in societies. Governance is regulated by many types of texts, extending to the texts of films, media advertising, Web sites, and cultural materials that convey a message about social expectations (21–23). When people experience justice or injustice, they are not fully aware of the invisible decisions about policy, professions, health, economics, social welfare, education, transportation, and industry that determine possibilities for participating or not in various occupations or the function of the state in regulating or otherwise influencing what they do.

Governments, agencies, businesses, or organizations regulate what a population can and cannot do beyond the interpersonal decisions one makes in private life. Adult international sports provide an example to show how political dimensions of social justice have public as well as private ramifications. Adult international sports funding and regulations are powerful determinants over which athletes will be supported for competition. Public policy and laws play a large part in determining athletes' empowerment not only to participate in sports but also to travel, accept certain kinds of financial sponsorship, make choices about the use of performance-enhancing drugs, and visit countries on scholarships and visas. The public regulation of justice in sports sets the stage for the interpersonal experience of justice (or injustice) during competition, although this ruling apparatus is invisible and unconscious in everyday experience. It is true that individual motivation and energy make a difference, but the organization of society is a powerful force in determining whether or not there will be unfair advantage, mistreatment, exclusion from opportunity, and domination by some adults while others are disempowered to act (24). A socially just society would be enacted through everyday life if and when people insist on respect, fairness, equitable opportunity, and shared responsibility in what they do as well as in their social relationships (25).

Many critiques demonstrate how visions of justice could be more enlightened by looking beyond the distribution of resources. Three authors who discuss power, enablement, rights, capacities, and meaningful work in relation to social justice are particularly noteworthy in contemplating occupational justice.

Iris Marion Young was a philosopher with an interest in contemporary political theory, feminist social theory, and public policy analysis. She argued that power is a central feature in defining justice. To illustrate her point, she contrasted distributive justice with a politics of difference that suggests consideration of a **justice of difference** (26). Her distinction was between a focus on *possession* in distributive justice and a focus on justice based on *opportunity* regardless of difference. She defined opportunity as a concept of *enablement,* and justice to *enable* individuals to play, work, and live without exploitation or violence in the everyday world. Public interests in *possession* are congruent with public support for equal distribution of rights, responsibilities, liberties, and goods. For instance, distributive justice supports equal access for everyone to the same health services (27–34). Young's concept of a politics of difference as a basis for justice is congruent with writers in the 1980s, such as Labonte and McKnight, who argued that empowerment, not just access to services, is closely linked with health and quality of life (35, 36).

Distributive justice, in Young's view, addresses principles of allocation in which biological or social differences cannot be taken into account. In particular, she raised concerns of justice and injustice that are rooted in unequal power relations wherein some are empowered to direct their lives, whereas others remain exploited, marginalized, disempowered, culturally subordinated, or abused. To illustrate these features of injustice, she pointed to the everyday experiences of persons with disabilities, persons of color, women, and others. She highlighted the alienating experiences of members of small groups struggling for a voice in a dominant cultural context, even if some individuals from these groups gain power.

Martha Nussbaum (37, 38) is an American philosopher with an interest in political philosophy and ethics. Her theory of capabilities, developed with Amartya Sen, addresses the topic of occupational rights. Looking at the United Nations Declaration of Human Rights (39), one can see how many of the rights described refer to occupations. For example, most readers will be familiar with articles (rights) such as freedom of speech, presumption of innocence, and freedom from slavery or torture. But the articles in this document also include the right to start a family, choose employment, work, have rest and leisure, pursue education, and participate in the cultural life of a community. However, the Universal Declaration of Human Rights is a vision document, with many articles yet to be enacted in most countries.

Nussbaum (37, 38) encourages others to move beyond thinking about rights to thinking about capabilities, or what people are actually able to do or be. Her list of capabilities includes items such as life and bodily integrity. It also includes complex capabilities such as the ability to use the senses, imagine, think, and reason, as well as the ability to use imagination and thought in connection with experiencing and producing works and events of one's own choice. Other capabilities include having control over one's environment, including political participation, being able to seek employment on an equal basis, and being able to hold property. All the capabilities described speak to the process of being occupied in one's environment. A capabilities approach to justice necessarily focuses on how one acts in the world, an important component of occupational justice.

Vicki Schultz is a professor of law with an interest in gender and work. Writing in the *Columbia Law Review* (40), she developed a feminist critique of paid and unpaid work that is applicable to other marginalized groups. She is interested in the potential of work to be reshaped in positive ways to empower, rather than constrain, people's lives. Her writing recognized the importance of integrating work and family life for women and men and emphasized the importance of work not just as a means of earning income, but also as a way for people to experience identity, community, and citizenship. She envisioned a "social order in which work is consistent with egalitarian conceptions of citizenship and care" (p. 1886). Schultz's writing stimulates thinking about how occupational opportunities shape, and have the potential to be shaped by, individuals in an occupationally just society.

AN EVOLVING THEORY OF OCCUPATIONAL JUSTICE

A discussion of an evolving theory of occupational justice, is now presented, along with the ideas, reasoning, and set of beliefs and principles that have guided its development. Also discussed are distinctions between occupational and social justice.

Historical Evolution of Occupational Justice Theory

There is never a clear starting point for the development of complex concepts, although in the case of occupational justice there is some historical sequence. In formulating a concept of occupational justice, ideas about humans as occupational beings led Wilcock to propose an occupational perspective of justice (2–5). Concurrently, ideas about the democratic, collaborative underpinnings of client-centered practice, focused on enabling meaningful occupation, led Townsend to propose that the everyday practice of justice involves enabling empowerment through occupation (1–6, 7, 11, 12). The relationship between occupation and justice was a mutual interest when Townsend and Wilcock met in 1997 (8–10).

Critique and reflection on intersecting ideas led to the development of reasoning summarized in a framework of occupational determinants, occupational forms, and outcomes of occupational injustices. As ideas and reasoning advanced, it became clear to Townsend and Wilcock that interests in occupational justice were based on certain beliefs and principles. With an evolving outline of beliefs and principles came a growing awareness of features that seem to distinguish occupational justice as complementary to, but different from, social justice.

From 1999 to 2006, Townsend and Wilcock conducted a series of workshops and presentations on occupational justice to generate open discussion, development, and critique of ideas, beliefs, and principles related to occupational justice. Presentations were held in Australia, Britain, Canada, Portugal, Sweden, and the United States, with contributors primarily from the fields of occupational science and occupational therapy, but also from sociology, planning, social work, and nursing (41).[2]

The theory of occupational justice presented in this chapter is considered to be evolving because the need for questioning, testing, refinement, and critique of the ideas, reasoning, beliefs, and principles related to occupational justice is recognized. Building on the original work of Townsend and Wilcock (8–10), this chapter presents a synthesis of ideas about occupational justice emerging from the occupational justice workshop discussions (41), and ongoing work by Townsend (11, 12), Townsend and Whiteford (42), Kronenberg and Pollard (43), Stadnyk (44), Stadnyk, Townsend, and Jurczak (45), Wilcock (46), and others.

Intersecting Ideas About Occupational Justice

Intersecting ideas that gave rise to an evolving theory of occupational justice are illustrated in Figure 13-1 ■. The concept of occupational justice rests on the idea that individuals are different and have different needs. Different needs are

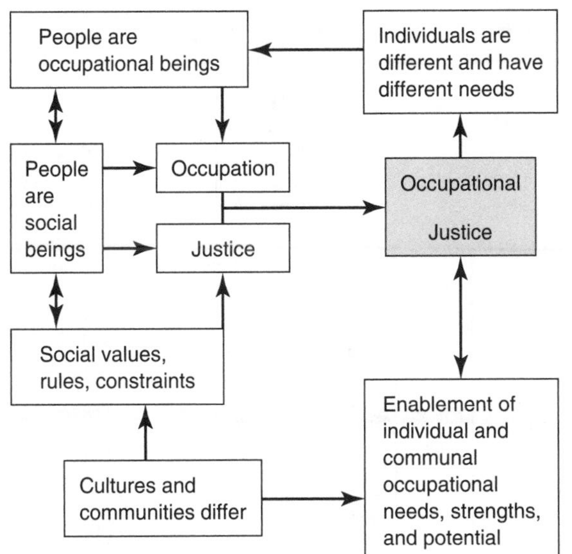

FIGURE 13-1 A Framework Exploring the Creation and Outcomes of Occupational Justices and Injustices

expressed through the occupations that comprise daily life because humans are autonomous, occupational beings. Humans need and want to be occupied for purposes of health, quality of life, and the sustenance of families and communities. Humans' drive to participate in occupations derives from many needs. Although occupational classifications vary greatly, there is a common recognition that the range of purposes for occupation may encompass looking after the self or others, enjoying life, or doing something that feels or is acknowledged by others to be productive.

Humans are also social beings whose lives are embedded in social values, rules, constraints, cultures, and communities. In real life, humans are interdependent with each other in diverse contexts. A major challenge in the survival of the human race is to reconcile differences in social values, rules, constraints, cultures, and communities. A social perspective on enabling empowerment with oppressed groups would recognize difference and diversity (6, 26). To reconcile ideas that humans are simultaneously occupational and social beings and that individual differences require a justice based on enablement, Wilcock and Townsend proposed the juxtaposition of occupation and justice to form the concept of occupational justice.

A process of reasoning has been used to expand ideas about occupational justice and their relationships. A fundamental component of this reasoning process is to explain how occupational injustices occur, and what the outcomes of occupational injustices might be. Figure 13-2 ■ shows how occupational determinants and forms interact with the contexts of individuals, groups, or communities to produce occupational outcomes related to occupational justice or injustices.

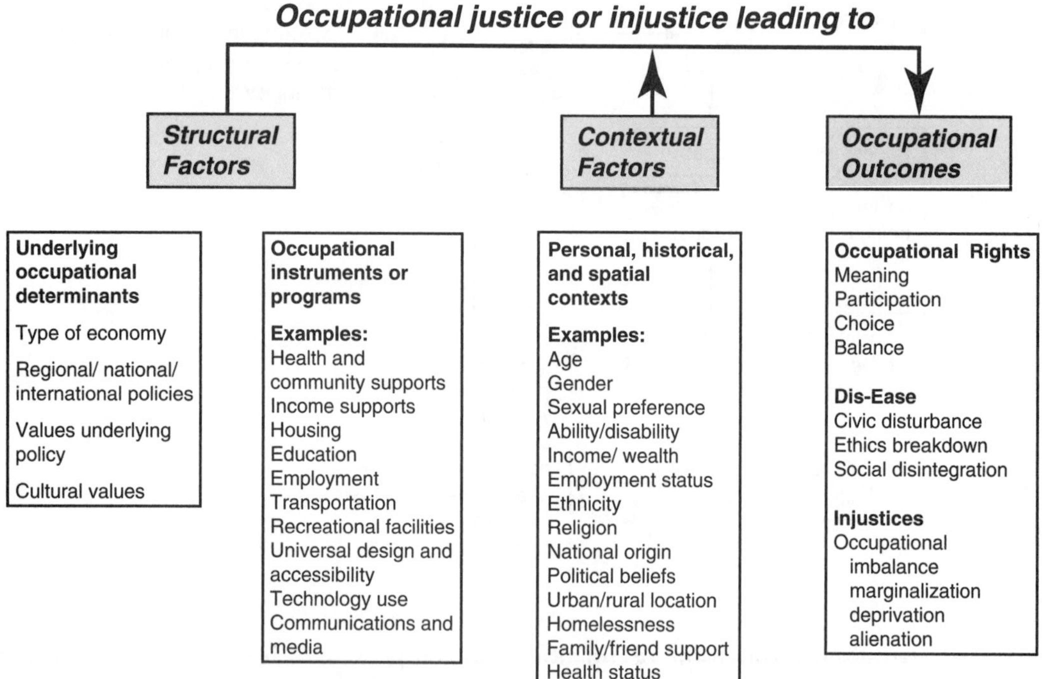

FIGURE 13-2 A Framework of Occupational Justice
Source: R. L. Stadnyk. A Framework of Occupational Justice: Occupational Determinants, Instruments, Contexts and Outcomes.

Structural Factors

Two levels of structural factors contribute to conditions of occupational justice or injustice. Underlying **occupational determinants** are factors such as the type of economy, national and international policies, policy values, and cultural values. The economic structure determines which occupations are economically rewarded and which occupations are private or of social rather than economic value. Policies (and their underlying values) such as employment conditions, pensions, health and social care systems, and environmental protection determine the ways in which certain occupations are conducted. Farming and fishing, for instance, are highly regulated in some countries to bring consistency to the economic market and/or to protect the environment. Cultural and policy values may determine what work will be given the highest and lowest prestige or wages. Moreover, cultural values are translated into decisions about what rituals and routines will be followed in a particular community or nation. Such values also define who will be included in occupations based on gender, race, age, or other distinctions. In essence, occupational determinants regulate through economics, law, policy, or culture what people do and how they are rewarded. Hence, the particular structure of these determinants sets out the possibilities and limits of occupational justice or occupational injustice.

An example of underlying occupational determinants with devastating occupational outcomes can be found in Kronenberg and Pollard's description of *occupational apartheid.* Occupational apartheid is an enduring characteristic of societies in which "some people are of different economic and social value than others" (43, p. 65). They emphasize the "unresponsive, collusive, or exploitative policy measures maintaining privilege over poverty" (p. 66) in the deliberate and systemic creation of conditions of occupational apartheid. They note that systemic constraints can extend to legal, economic, social, and religious organization.

Occupational determinants are operationalized in **occupational forms**. Occupational determinants are often experienced as funding priorities that inhibit or enhance occupational forms, which in turn will affect how work, parenting; play, recreation, sports; and supportive care are organized and fostered. For example, an occupational determinant such as a commitment to health promotion (both as a value and as a funding priority) may be operationalized in terms of a good primary health-care system, opportunities for physical activity in communities, community development initiatives, or employment initiatives. Occupational forms in the market may determine types of technology used in daily life, the division of labor, and employment practices, including social services and job creation schemes. Depending on how they are organized, occupational forms may create conditions of occupational justice or injustice.

Contextual Factors

Contextual factors are individual, group, or community characteristics that mediate the effect of occupational determinants and forms on outcomes (47). These characteristics are given meaning by the individual's societal and cultural context. Research in diverse areas such as policy analysis (44, 47), determinants of health, social justice (26, 37, 38), and occupational apartheid (43) remind us that particular contextual factors can create conditions in which people do not have equal access to resources, programs, and services. The inclusion of contextual factors in this occupational justice framework reminds us that occupational determinants and forms are experienced differently by different people, a state of affairs that may be intentional or unintentional. For example, some income support programs are targeted explicitly to older adults or persons who are unable to work. Kronenberg and Pollard (43) provide compelling stories to remind us how people in chronic poverty experience structural factors in a way that excludes their participation in meaningful occupations. The list of contextual factors presented here is not exhaustive, but rather suggestive of factors to consider looking at the relationship between structural factors and occupational outcomes.

Occupational Outcomes

The outcomes of occupational justices or injustices can be discussed by examining the achievement of occupational rights, the potential for creation of dis-ease, or the outcomes of injustice.

Townsend and Wilcock (9, 10) proposed four occupational rights: the right to experience occupation as **meaningful** and enriching; the right to develop through **participation** in occupations for health and social inclusion; the right to exert individual or population autonomy through **choice** in occupations; and the right to benefit from fair privileges for diverse participation in occupations **(balance).** A positive set of occupational outcomes is important to articulate if society is to move toward a vision of an occupationally just world.

What if structural and contextual factors do not create conditions for occupational outcomes that meet the occupational rights of individuals, groups, and communities? Occupational injustices are experienced through the occupations of daily life as ongoing, unresolved stress. Occupational injustices are thus socially structured, socially formed conditions that give rise to stressful occupational experiences. The need is to consider injustices that may result from or lead to **dis-ease.** Dis-ease is experienced individually, in families, in communities, nationally, or internationally. People develop symptoms of dis-ease that can range from individual fatigue and immune system disorders, to international civic disturbance and social disintegration of health, education, and other systems.

Understanding of occupational injustices continues to evolve as more occupational scientists and occupational therapists undertake scholarly work and practice in areas related to occupational justice. Four outcomes of occupational injustice highlighted in this discussion are **occupational imbalance, occupational deprivation, occupational marginalization,** and **occupational alienation.**

Occupational imbalance is a temporal concept because it refers to allocation of time use for particular purposes and is based on the reasoning that human health and well-being require a variation in productive, self-sustaining, and leisure occupations (48–50). For individuals, an occupational imbalance may occur when an individual has no time for occupations other than paid work, or conversely, when survival, family, and parenting responsibilities present such a burden that a person lives in poverty, unable to develop skills or time for work or leisure (51, 52). Within societies, an occupational imbalance is seen when some people are overoccupied and others are underoccupied. Within the marketplace, this is called overemployment versus underemployment or unemployment. Although individual motivation, ability, and other personal factors may explain occupational imbalance in part, the hierarchical classification of occupations drives a labor market in which those with particular skills and knowledge are paid well and have lots of work, whereas others are unable to find paid work at all.

In the preceding chapter by Whiteford the concept of **occupational deprivation** was introduced, whereby the engagement of individuals, families, groups, communities or populations in occupations of necessity and/or meaning are limited due to external factors that are generally outside their control. Examples of occupational deprivation occur when children are deprived of opportunities and resources to play because of poverty, childhood disability, or economic and social forces that lure them into child labor. Such children fail to fully develop their physical and mental talents, and they fail to learn about themselves and others in the world (53, 54). When adults are isolated in prison, refugee camps, or institutions with a limited range of occupations that are unconnected to the real world, they become mentally depressed and physically frail, and they are unable to participate in the cultural occupations that bind families and communities. Injustice results when societies tolerate occupational deprivation for some while others have full rein to play, go to school, remain active while in institutions, or participate fully in family and community.

Occupational marginalization occurs when people are not afforded the opportunity to participate in occupations and to exert choices and decision making related to occupational participation. Occupational marginalization often operates invisibly, through expectations of how, when, where, and which persons should participate in occupations. Occupational marginalization serves to exclude individuals or groups from the opportunity to participate in society's valued occupations, relegating them to invisible or less-valued occupations in which they have very little choice or control. Marginalization often occurs because individuals or groups are discriminated against, explicitly or implicitly, because of one or more of the contextual factors described earlier, such as gender, age, or ability. Occupational marginalization at its worst is a form of occupational apartheid, in which "occupations are paid, valued, and enhance life for some, while in the same places and times occupations are taken for granted, exploited and trivialized for others" (11, p. 10).

People experiencing occupational marginalization may be occupationally imbalanced, but often their occupations are not visible in the dominant political and economic systems. The societal focus on paid productive occupations means that important occupations across the life span are underrecognized, such as children's play, adolescents' need to experience adventure, or adults' unpaid caregiving to persons with disabling conditions. Other occupations important to survival of some persons, such as prostitution or scavenging for food or items that can be sold, are so negatively valued by society as to not be recognized as legitimate and life sustaining.

Occupational alienation is the outcome when people experience daily life as meaningless or purposeless. Take the example of those with chronic illness (55). There is increasing interest worldwide in using health resources to repair, heal, and replace body parts (kidneys, knees, hearts, joints, stem cells). There is an injustice in such practices when societies expend so many financial and social resources on fixing the body and mind of a select few people that there are insufficient resources to enable these same and other people to do something in life that is important to them (27, 28). We may value life enough to expend resources on its preservation through medical and surgical interventions, but if people are alienated from themselves and others because of limited occupational opportunities, why is life being preserved? Occupational alienation can also be a concern for those involved in paid work occupations. Beyond their economic value, some occupations may enrich people mentally and spiritually, whereas other occupations are experienced by some or all people as boring or lacking in meaning (56). Participation in occupations is a major force in shaping identity, so lack of positive experiences in occupation can distort identity formation (57). Repetitive, mind-numbing occupations may suit some people, whereas for others they generate a sense of occupational alienation. These are usually occupations that are highly standardized, rigidly repetitive, and without opportunities for individual choice, control, decision making, or creativity. To be regimented, confined, and possibly exploited in daily occupations at work or elsewhere becomes a matter of justice when some people are privileged while others are alienated (58).

Kronenberg and Pollard (43) described a form of occupational alienation that they term *occupational absurdity*. In situations of occupational absurdity, the work has lost its connection with meaning not only for the individual, but also in the broader social context. An example of occupational absurdity was observed in a sheltered workshop setting in which the work of people in one room was to put nuts on bolts, while people in another room removed the nuts from the bolts. Conditions of occupational absurdity can reinforce occupational marginalization.

Beliefs and Principles about Occupational Justice

A third component of an exploratory theory of occupational justice is beliefs and principles. Four beliefs and four principles are introduced next (Table 13-1 ■). The beliefs in this theory of occupational justice are based on ideas, values, and assumptions about humans as autonomous, yet interdependent, occupational beings who participate in occupations in social conditions that determine health and quality of life.

Beliefs

Humans are Occupational Beings Occupational justice is conceptually grounded in the belief that humans are occupational beings (2–4). Humans need and want to be occupied in various ways and for various purposes. In an early description of occupational science, Johnson and Yerxa (59) stated that individuals are most true to their humanity when engaged in occupation. They supported their belief that occupation is central to virtually everything human by citing research on human curiosity (60), the behavior of East African primates (61), and adaptation in daily living (62).

TABLE 13-1 *An Exploratory Theory of Occupational Justice: Beliefs and Principles*

Beliefs
• Humans are occupational beings
• Humans participate in occupations as autonomous agents
• Occupational participation is interdependent and contextual
• Occupational participation is a determinant of health and quality of life
Principles
• Empowerment through occupation
• Inclusive classification of occupations
• Enablement of occupational potential
• Diversity, inclusion, and shared advantage in occupational participation

Quoting from Karl Marx (63), Wilcock (2) referred to occupation as "man's species nature" (p. 19). In her initial publication of a theory of the human need for occupation, historical and contemporary research sources are used to illustrate occupation's three major functions in species survival. These are to (1) provide for immediate bodily needs for sustenance, self-care, shelter, and safety; (2) develop skills, social structures, and technology aimed at gaining superiority over predators and the environment; and (3) exercise and develop personal capacities enabling the organism to be maintained and to flourish (2, p. 20). Furthermore, she asserted that the human development of an "occupational brain encompasses, integrates and tries to balance the social, selfish, physical, emotional, intellectual and spiritual nature of people" (3, p. 71). Drawing from her study of a history of ideas about occupation, Wilcock (4) concluded that "occupation is so central to the study of the origins and *development* of humans in society that much of the evolution of the human species, from pre–*Homo sapiens,* is traced by studying occupations, such as tool usage, food production, creativity, and domestic and communal activities" (p. 72).

A rapidly expanding literature on occupational science is illuminating what occupation and lack of occupation mean to humans, although many other disciplines are also interested in participation, activity, involvement, and community action. What occupational science contributes is the broad understanding that these interests can be united through the concept of occupation. Also new is the assertion of occupational scientists that, at our core, humans are occupational beings and that the organization of societies shapes the meanings, values, opportunities and resources for participation in occupations.

One area of study has shown that community, identity, and occupation are closely related. In a study of urban community action planning, Ross and Coleman (64) involved teenagers in occupations for the purpose of developing their communities and their identities. It seems that individual humans have a need for occupation in part for growth of mind, body, and spirit for development of the self as well as for engagement with other individuals in groups and communities. Occupations are "enfolded," blurring distinctions between what is considered to be work, leisure, parenting, and more (65). Jackson found that humans, in old age, use occupation as a means of connecting with others to avoid loneliness and loss of meaning (66). In her ethnography of 20 elderly individuals with disabilities, Jackson identified a human need for occupation in the adaptive strategies used to deal with loss. Elderly healthcare advocates took up new occupations or let others go in their need for risk and challenge, and they ordered their time and routines by considering what they wanted and needed to do each day.

Humans Participate in Occupations as Autonomous Agents In the need for occupation, humans are individual, autonomous, active agents (persons) with differing capacities to choose and participate in occupations (67). This belief rests on the concept of personhood and rational will. Kant and other western philosophers proposed that human agency, the will and drive to act, lies in individuals. From this perspective, individuals are active agents who hold the power to allocate resources as a means toward a visionary or *ideal* goal such as justice (16, 68). The idea of personhood has given rise to the belief in the equal worth of individuals regardless of difference, a point debated in public services such as health care (28). Individual persons experience that "occupational participation is important because it undergirds much of our temporal sphere of existence" (69, p. 144).

Individuals' will and drive to participate in occupations has a biological and an environmental basis. Individuals possess the biological power to act and to reflect on, assess, and make decisions about participation in occupations. The spirit informs choices to seek meaning and purpose in the range of occupations that constitute daily life. Human needs and power to participate in occupation differ greatly because human bodies and minds are individually unique (70).

The active, autonomous power of humans to act is an important point. If all active agents are worthy, one is prompted to ask whether participation in all occupations is also worthy, regardless of the results people accomplish through their occupations. The question Wilcock posed is: Do those who lack particular physical, intellectual, or emotional capacities deserve less material wealth, or fewer opportunities to work, enjoy life, and live in families or communities than others? (5).

Occupational Participation Is Interdependent and Contextual Although humans are autonomous occupational beings, participation in occupations is interdependent and contextual. Occupations do not occur in a vacuum; rather, interdependent participation occurs. Because occupations are more than an abstraction of the mind, occupations occur in real-life contexts grounded in real time and real places, using real equipment, materials, and supplies, with real people. Furthermore, occupations occur in a context of invisible occupational determinants and forms that determine possibilities and limits for occupational participation.

Beyond biological traits that determine autonomous interest, ability, and will, occupational participation involves interaction with other humans in a physical, social, cultural, and institutional context. As Davis and Polatajko asserted in presenting occupational development earlier in this book, an interplay is seen between individual autonomy and interdependence in doing things with others. Humans are both biological entities and products of society. Whereas Kant explored the autonomous self, Giddens (21) and Habermas (17, 18) are examples of modern philosophers who presented the self and society as interwoven and interdependent—the self being shaped by society, and society being shaped by the concerted will of the many selves who comprise a society. Conceptions of social and occupational justice hinge on debates that have been documented by the World Health Organization on the responsibility of the state to mediate on matters, such as structural determinants of health, that are beyond individual control (71, 72).

Socially defined occupational determinants and occupational forms, such as health services, have been put in place to respond to particular ideas about health and the use of economic resources for health. Occupational determinants and forms shape what humans decide about the real places, methods, and tools that humans recognize as the technology of daily life. The interdependence and contextual nature of occupations may not be visible and immediate, but humans are nonetheless dependent on what others have done before or are doing around us. Even when humans engage in solitary occupations, such as reading a book, there is an interdependence with the author who wrote it and the publisher and workers who produced it. The chair or bed used to read is most likely built by someone other than the reader. Although some people do make their own furniture, it is highly likely that others have fashioned the tools used to exert the self-sufficiency required of reading. Humans have designed communities and societies, and humans have created the opportunities or constraints for people to play sports, attend school, or build cars. Conversely, the presence of sports facilities encourages sports, and the presence of an automotive factory in a community determines that many people will look for paid occupations in the automotive industry.

Occupational Participation Is a Determinant of Health and Quality of Life A belief that humans are occupational beings who participate as autonomous yet interdependent agents in a context prompts one to ask why humans participate in occupations? Wilcock's *An Occupational Perspective of Health* (1st and 2nd editions) (4, 46) presents a history of ideas and evidence that participation in a broad range of occupations is a determinant of health. This is apparent when health is defined as the ability and opportunity to live, work, and play in safe, supportive communities as outlined in the Ottawa Charter for Health Promotion, a Canadian and World Health Organization definitive statement about health (71).

The terms *leisure-rich* and *leisure-poor* convey the belief that wellness is about more than the absence of disease (52). Time influences health in important ways because humans have biologically determined temporal rhythms that are necessary for mental health and the regulation of sleep (73–75). Gendered differences in time use point to gendered differences in occupations and health status and quality of life (76). "Activity" is so widely known to enhance health that communities are being urged to use urban planning and public transportation as tools to encourage more physical activity within the built environment as a strategy for health promotion (77). Moreover, we know that humans need to feel useful, and that we fail to flourish and remain healthy when we feel that there is nothing useful to do (78).

Health can be promoted through occupation. However, occupation does not always promote health. Participation in some occupations may be degrading or debilitating, a point argued in Braverman's classic analysis of 20th-century work (79). The concept of occupational risk provides a framework for exploring the chronicity of illness, such as the persistent mental illness experienced by people who use community mental health services and who are often unemployed (55). The impacts of occupational participation on families, communities, and the world are just beginning to be understood, but it is clear that communities struggle to survive when industries leave or the natural environment is destroyed.

Principles

The principles in this theory outline rights, responsibilities, and freedoms of enablement. They derive from a recognition that individuals have occupational needs, strengths, and potentials that affect health and quality of life.

Empowerment Through Occupation The concept of occupational justice is based on a principle described here as *empowerment through occupation.* This principle takes a stand in favor of equality in power sharing. Power sharing refers to power exerted and accepted through horizontal collaboration and partnership (80). The contrast with collaborative power sharing is hierarchical, authoritative control of power, whether this is done with benevolence or cruelty. Hierarchical, authoritative behavior both reflects and perpetuates hierarchical structures. A more equitable distribution of power would reduce the hierarchical dominance of some while generating the empowerment of everyone (81-83).

Empowerment has many meanings that refer to taking on power (7). One use of this term describes the growth of individual or group feelings of power. To feel empowered is to generate feelings of personal drive, motivation, purpose, confidence, identity, and even joy. A second use of the term empowerment describes everyday behavior. To act in an empowered way is to behave assertively, to be decisive, or to be reflective and confident about the actions of oneself or a group, family, or community. A third use of the term empowerment refers to social structures and organization. To organize empowering structures, one brings an empowerment lens to policies, procedures, laws, media images, language, or funding priorities.

To employ an empowerment lens requires asking questions about power. One might ask, for instance, Who has power and whose interests are served or not served? Who has control and privilege, who is expected to comply, and what are the consequences for not complying? The principle of empowerment through occupation emphasizes that the structure and organization of society determine possibilities for feeling or acting empowered in everyday occupations.

The reasoning that links empowerment with injustice (see Figure 13-2) is that occupational determinants, such as economic practices, policies and laws, and cultural forces are also determinants of empowerment. In turn, occupational determinants shape occupational forms, such as the division of labor, the managerial regulation of services, professions, or wars that shape possibilities for empowerment to choose and participate in various occupations. Disempowerment leaves people alienated and with diminished power to shape what they do with their lives.

People experience empowerment or disempowerment in everyday actions and feelings. Empowerment through occupation might be experienced, therefore, as occupational participation, choice, meaningfulness, balance, and enrichment. Disempowerment through occupation would be experienced as occupational deprivation, alienation, marginalization, or imbalance.

The principle of empowerment through occupation to enable feelings, behaviours and social structures and organization of empowerment through action is congruent with Iris Morton Young's analysis of power (26). Her critique of distributive social justice is that the concept does not address the domination and oppression that is experienced in everyday life by women, immigrants, persons with disabilities, the poor, and other groups. Her concerns with power are in "five faces of oppression": exploitation, marginalization, powerlessness, cultural imperialism, and violence. Restated as occupational injustice, some women, older adults, immigrants, racialized minorities, persons with disabilities, and persons in poverty are oppressed by requiring them to participate in occupations that exploit their talents for someone else's gain, keep them on the economic margins because of low pay, or are associated with violence if they do not comply with expectations, policies, or laws.

Inclusive Classification of Occupations If one accepts that an occupationally just world would empower everyone to participate as they need and want to do in society, one accepts the need for a more inclusive classification of occupations. From the perspective of occupational justice, the principle of an inclusive classification of occupations is supported by Young who recognized that justice "concerns the definition of the occupations themselves" (26, p. 23). Occupational injustices appear to arise in the separation of work from other occupations and in the hierarchical definitions of occupations. Therefore, one needs to reflect on how some occupations historically became paid work while other occupations were considered private and unpaid. When occupations are classified hierarchically, inequalities in status and wages perpetuate a social class structure between the haves and the have-nots. From an occupational perspective, one would question the definitions of occupations that are included or left out of the hierarchical classifications of work. What part do hierarchical occupational classifications play in creating a world where some people have too much to do while others are underemployed or unemployed?

Some people may seek greater occupational participation, choice, meaningfulness, balance, and enrichment beyond, as well as through, their paid work. Yet occupations outside paid work may be dismissed as unproductive, frivolous, or a backdrop to what is really important—paid work. Those who succeed at paid work generate greater income and greater influence in the organization of society. Conversely, those who are occupationally deprived become disempowered, particularly where they are deprived of paid work. Additionally, there is a long-standing problem with the (under)valuing of unpaid work that is often the domain of women: child care, care to other family members, and household maintenance. There is a fundamental injustice in the discrepancies of pay, privilege, and status allocated to these occupations. Those who are interested in social justice have already raised concerns about gender, racial, and other segregation in the division of labor (79). Occupational justice adds a critique of the actual definitions of occupations. The concern is with the hierarchical advantages in status and wages accorded to intellectual and managerial occupations over occupations for creativity, environmental sustainability, family support, or community building.

Enablement of Occupational Potential The principle of enablement of occupational potential builds on the previous principles and, particularly on the idea of individual difference. A positive definition of enablement refers to approaches and conditions that can be developed to support all people individually and collectively in developing their occupational potential (84). Enablement of occupational potential is interconnected with the principles of empowerment through occupation and an inclusive classification of occupations. Enablement processes would focus on those who are currently disempowered or occupationally deprived and would aim to engage all people regardless of differences as participants in the decision making about their occupational performance and occupational engagement in society.

Enablement approaches emphasize collaborative interpersonal forms of helping, combined with the development of enabling policies, laws, and economic practices (84, 85). An example of enablement through occupation would be to advocate with and for children with various talents, and to coach and coordinate them to participate in a school play. Without enablement, assertive and vocal children do well, but those who lack occupational development or opportunities to learn dramatic and artistic skills because of poverty, disability, cultural attitudes, or other reasons would likely be left out.

The development of enabling conditions would involve writing policies that attend to the empowerment of all participants or stakeholders in a particular issue. An example would be involving professionals, managers, and the public in policy making and budget decisions concerning playgrounds. The aim would not necessarily be to develop the most efficient playground measured in terms of successful sports teams or resource management. Rather, the aim would be to develop the most participatory and inclusive playground operated within a defined budget. Enabling policy would be written with broad stakeholder input to ensure reasonable accommodations. That is to say that playground and community buildings would be physically and attitudinally accessible for parents with children, for persons of diverse cultural backgrounds, for older people, and for people who use mobility aids.

Similarly, legislation to enable healthy participation in occupations could require health services to focus on population health promotion equally with individualized, acute health services. Enabling economic practices would reorganize accounting systems to calculate social production as well as economic production. Evaluation of the effectiveness of enablement would focus on whether or not there were equitable opportunities and resources for all to participate. An advocate for occupational justice might envision all citizens participating to empower themselves and others to draw out their full potential as humans.

An important point to include in a discussion of enablement is the matter of choice. Basic to the idea of occupational justice is an assumption that humans ought to have some choice about what to do with their lives. Choice is also the means by which humans decide what occupations are priority, and more to the point, what occupations they consider to be most useful and meaningful to them. In enabling occupational justice, one would foster a culture of choice while acknowledging social constraints on choice. In the most restrictive or exploitive situations, people make choices to deliberately work slowly or to make mistakes that delay the production of goods. As expressions of limited but real choice, humans risk tremendous pain, injury, and losses to escape violence to live a safer life in exile. The language of choice fits with the language of occupational justice and enablement because it reminds humans that the withdrawal of participation in occupations is the ultimate choice, even in the most restrictive of conditions such as prisons and refugee camps. The principle of enablement of occupational potential would emphasize the development of opportunities and resources with and for individuals, groups, communities and populations to expand their choices. This would be particularly true where unequal choices are available to different individuals or groups because they have different abilities or different circumstances.

Diversity, Inclusion, and Shared Advantage in Occupational Participation Diversity follows on the principle of enablement. In an occupationally just world, there would be clear recognition that individuals are also members of social groups. In introducing the terminology of occupational justice, Wilcock and Townsend stated that "occupational justice implies that societies value different occupational capacities and different occupational meanings. Rather than sameness, occupational equity and fairness demand respect for differences that arise in different, individual capacities, and different meanings derived from both personal and cultural meanings" (8, p. 84).

The implication of this statement is that inclusion and shared advantage are linked principles within the concept of occupational justice. An occupationally just community or nation would be socially inclusive—that is, in an occupationally just society all persons would be entitled to participate in occupations that they need or want to do to contribute to individual or community life. The corollary to social inclusion is shared advantage. Everyone in an occupationally just community or nation would share the social and economic advantages of that community or nation. Privilege would be equalized, not only as a social principle, but through the use of an inclusive classification of occupations that would flatten the hierarchical system of privileges that go with some work and leisure occupations but not with others.

The combined principles of diversity, inclusion, and shared advantage pose challenges to ideas about entitlement. One is left wondering if more equal recognition of the worth of all occupations means that everyone would have a similar income or even a guaranteed income. The clearest implication is that these combined principles oppose social exclusion and differential privileges that create different classes of people. A recognizable example is the social exclusion of people of lower socioeconomic status from the occupations associated with healthy eating. This principle leads to questions about the occupational differences of those with and without financial resources. Whereas families with financial resources have many occupational choices for purchasing a variety of foods or eating at restaurants, hungry children and hungry mothers are economically deprived of the occupation of shopping at will and of cooking the proteins, vegetables, fruits, and other foods that are required for good physical and mental health (54).

The combined principles of diversity, social inclusion, and shared advantage would guide an occupationally just society to watch out for individuals or groups who are excluded from choosing and participating in the typical and valued occupations of that society. For example, an occupationally just community might work to minimize the exclusion of diverse immigrants from certain kinds of employment, or the exclusion of persons with mental illness from the occupations of political office.

DISTINCTIONS BETWEEN OCCUPATIONAL AND SOCIAL JUSTICE

Complementary features as well as distinctions between occupational and social justice are becoming clearer as ideas, reasoning, beliefs, and principles are articulated. As summarized in Table 13-2 ■, occupational justice seems to be more than a subcategory of social justice. *Social* justice is a concept that recognizes humans as social beings who engage in social relations (16). The advocacy in this concept favors equitable access to opportunities and resources to reduce group differences related to characteristics such as age, ability, culture, gender, social class,

TABLE 13-2 *An Exploratory Theory of Occupational Justice: Distinctions Between Occupational and Social Justice*

Occupational Justice
• Humans are occupational beings
• Interests in health and quality of life
• Different opportunities and resources
• Enablement
• Individual differences
Social Justice
• Humans are social beings
• Interests in social relations
• Same opportunities and resources
• Possession
• Group differences

and sexual orientation. *Occupational* justice, in contrast, is a concept to guide humans as occupational beings who need and want to participate in occupations to develop and thrive. The advocacy in this concept favors the enablement of *different* access to opportunities and resources to acknowledge individual differences resulting from human biology and human interaction with the natural and human environment.

USING STORIES TO CONSIDER AN EVOLVING THEORY OF OCCUPATIONAL JUSTICE

This section presents three stories illustrating ideas, reasoning, beliefs, and principles related to occupational justice.

Story 1: Cared For, but Occupationally Marginalized (86)

Amy is a young woman who lived in her own home, with the assistance of attendants. Amy had a job as a teaching assistant in a school. Living expenses started to overwhelm her. She consulted a credit counselor who told her that work-related expenses exceeded her income, so she should give up her job. "It crushed me to give up my job, it really did, because it meant everything to me." Soon, Amy was told that it was too expensive to provide her with attendant care in her home. She would have to move to a long-term care center. "It was like they put the brakes on my life." Amy strives to be a full participant in her community, but funding priorities create barriers to her participation. Although there is money to pay for attendants to travel with her to medical appointments, there is no money to pay for assistance to go to meetings or events outside the facility she lives in. "It almost seems like you've got your food and roof and you still have a roof over your head and you should be grateful you have that." Occupational determinants ensure food and shelter for someone like Amy, but not a living situation of her choice. When policy values emphasize custodial care of persons with disabilities, opportunities to engage in meaningful, chosen occupations are seen as a luxury instead of a right.

Story 2: Unemployment and Employment: The Interplay of Occupational Imbalance, Deprivation, Marginalization, and Alienation

Omar was recently laid off from the local steel mill where he had worked for 30 years. When the steel mill closed, many of the men in the town found themselves unemployed. Employment opportunities in other industries were not available in the local area. The steel mill and local employment agencies offered retraining, but Omar, like many of his former workmates, refused it. He had no interest in computer-based work at a desk after working with his hands for so many years. He spent most of his days at the coffee shop with his former buddies from work, returning home each evening to spend time with his wife, Amira.

Although Omar and Amira's two children were grown and out of the home, the youngest, at 22, needed help financially to attend university. The oldest daughter, age 24, needed to work full time and could not afford day care for her two children, so Amira was babysitting them.

Amira and Omar quickly depleted their savings during his first year of unemployment. Amira went back to work as a nurse, a career she had put on hold to take care of her grandchildren. By working night shifts, she was able to continue to babysit for her daughter. Amira was overoccupied and exhausted. She valued babysitting far more than nursing but felt compelled to work as a nurse because her husband was "doing nothing." Amira resented that Omar did not take over the care of his grandchildren. Omar remained immobilized, unable to see child care as a meaningful alternative to working at the plant. He halfheartedly helped with cooking, cleaning, and laundry in the evenings, as his wife rested or prepared to go to work.

In this scenario, Amira made occupational sacrifices so that two families could manage financially. In many ways her occupational contributions were marginalized. Societal values assume that family members will step in to deal with financial and child-care issues, and the family-sustaining work of women is often invisible. Occupational forms to address this family's need for child care and employment choices did not fit with their needs and preferences. Omar had opportunities to be occupied but remained unoccupied, alienated by the limited choices available to him.

Story 3: Alienated from a Cultural Community of Occupations

This story was provided, with permission, by an occupational therapist reflecting on a professional experience during a workshop in Brisbane, Australia during 2001.[2]

I know a woman who experienced a brain injury related to anoxia following routine surgery. She was a valued elder in her rural, aboriginal community. Now she is unable to remember and communicate well and has great difficulty walking the 4 kilometers from her cabin to the nearest town where she has sold her crafts to support herself. The result is that she is now alienated from her cultural community as their elder, and alienated as an impoverished, disabled woman who was formerly a proud, financially self-sufficient leader. A local interpreter has volunteered to help me work with her.

Her situation is made worse by the normative expectations and standards of my own profession of occupational therapy and my culture. My standard assessment tools are culturally bound, and thus invalid, so my assessment of her lacks the formal data expected by health services before home support services can be approved. As well, she needs her caregiver to collect firewood, hunt for food, and take her to town, but these are not culturally expected duties in the standard list of approved caregiving services. Her rural life creates nonstandard needs. This is a woman who could continue to be financially self-sufficient and a proud community leader if support services were available to address her culturally-specific and rural needs. Instead, our current system provides home support only to help her with bathing and cooking occupations. The impact on this woman is that she is both occupationally and financially deprived.

Reflections on Stories

The three stories all implicitly recognize that humans are occupational beings, that social structures and organization shape occupational possibilities and constraints, and that justice is related to health and quality of life. The stories focus on different needs for opportunities and resources and on the importance of enabling the diverse occupational potential of individuals. Each story points to occupational injustice issues that go beyond having basic needs met. All three stories indicate availability of services and supports, but resources were not attuned to the occupational rights of the individuals concerned. Amy lacked the support she needed to participate in community occupations that had meaning for her. Services were instead focused on provision of shelter and care. Omar had opportunities for retraining, but they did not fit with his preferences and skills. Amira and her daughter had access to child care, but it was too expensive for them to afford. The aboriginal woman lacked opportunities to earn money through culturally based crafts. Neither the aboriginal community nor state services were in a position to offer transportation or a helper for her to resume her income-generating occupations.

The three stories point out the importance of enablement approaches to achieve occupational justice. Social justice might define access to services, but social justice cannot speak to the specialized resources needed to enable some people to accomplish what they need or want to do.

Furthermore, the stories illuminate the overvaluing of some occupations and undervaluing of others. Calls for social justice have produced changes in occupational classifications to reduce gender, race, and other discrimination in the workplace. Occupational justice can extend the analysis of justice issues to address differences in ability, differences in the division of labor, and differences in the value of occupations in the private as well as the public, paid work-oriented realms of society.

Those who are interested in occupational justice are encouraged to continue this exploration through a dialogue for raising awareness. An exploratory theory of occupational justice presents the authors' analysis of ideas, reasoning, beliefs, and principles. Through a dialogue around questions, such as those suggested in Table 13-3 ■, others will consider whether occupational justice is a viable concept on its own, or whether the concerns for justice raised here are actually within the realm of social justice. If occupational justice is a viable concept, the next steps will be to consider appropriate education, research, and activism to bring occupational justice to greater public attention.

TABLE 13-3 *Occupational Justice: A Dialogue for Raising Awareness*

Are all occupations worthwhile? Are occupations an economic or social issue? Should all occupations be paid in order to achieve occupational justice? Are income averaging and guaranteed minimum income occupational justice policies? Should people be paid to enjoy themselves? Should manual occupations (such as cleaning) and nonmanual occupations (such as research) be accorded equal prestige and pay? Do any criteria or conditions justify occupational privilege of prestige or pay?
What rights, responsibilities, and freedoms should govern the enablement of occupational potential? Should society be responsible for enabling individuals to achieve their occupational potential? What if the enablement of some to do what they want, such as driving a car, disables others who cannot do what they want, such as exercise outside because of car exhaust fumes and smog? What priorities should be given to using economic resources for enablement? How should enablement of community and family occupations be balanced with enablement of economic occupations?
How can a society deal with the concepts of diversity, social inclusion, and shared advantage? Why are there different economic rewards for being a chef in a restaurant and cooking meals for a large family? Both engage in similar occupations of food purchasing, preparation, and presentation, but one is paid and the other is not. Why is this? What if the person cooking for a large family is living in poverty associated with lack of education rather than lack of hard work? Would occupational justice be done if the family was paid to cook nutritious, economical meals to ensure healthy occupational development of the children and any grandparents who live there? What if social inclusion undermines the occupational potential of some people; for instance, should children with a disability be included or segregated in schools if the aim is enablement of their occupational potential?
Is occupational justice really different from social justice? Are physically inaccessible buildings a matter of occupational injustice or social injustice? Does occupational injustice or social injustice occur when employers cannot or will not offer flexible hours and locations for people with disabilities?

CHAPTER SUMMARY

The discussion in this chapter has presented occupational justice as a concept that is complementary to but different from social justice. Based on early workshop discussions on occupational justice, the literature, and critical analysis of historical and ethnographic data, the authors proposed an evolving theory of occupational justice. The foundations of this theory are ideas, reasoning, beliefs, and principles that lead to distinctions between occupational and social justice. The concept of occupational justice diverges from social justice through an interest in individual as well as group differences, through a concern for enablement of diversity contrasted with the equal distribution of rights and goods, and through a focus on the relationships between health, quality of life, and meaningful occupation. Readers are left to contemplate occupational justice as a new formulation of justice that would define the rights, responsibilities, and civic principles of an occupationally just world.

STUDY GUIDE

Study Guide Author: Kate Barrett

Summary of Main Points

This chapter provides an introduction to the evolving concept of occupational justice. Ideas about how principles of justice might apply to opportunities for individuals and communities to participate in occupation are explored. An appreciation for how societal and contextual structures can foster as well as prevent or discourage occupational justice promotes understanding of the constraints and opportunities for occupational participation. Occupational behavior is often shaped by social policies, laws, and expectations; policies may determine who can and who cannot participate, or when an occupation may be performed, or where it may be performed. From an occupational perspective, these polices may be either just or unjust.

Application to Occupational Therapy

Understanding the concept of occupational justice gives occupational therapists a wider lens from which to view the people with whom we work. As occupational therapists work with individuals, it is important that they understand how their social, cultural, and economic situations shape the occupations in which they participate and why. As occupational therapists work with families, groups, communities and populations, it is important to keep the concept of occupational injustice and justice as a way of presenting health and social equities from an occupational perspective. In occupation-based practice, one would want to raise occupational issues, goals and outcomes that address population-based injustices, from lack of appropriate transportation, inaccessible workplaces, and so on.

What would the practice of occupational therapy look like if occupational therapy personnel started with the basic premise that everyone has the occupational rights to experience meaning, have choice, participate in occupations that foster health and inclusion, and participate in diverse occupations? The concept of occupational justice calls the occupational therapist to work not only with the abilities and challenges of an individual, but also to become an advocate for just policies that foster participation for everyone.

The concept of occupational justice and the profession of occupational therapy are closely linked. Both maintain that participation in occupation is a desirable outcome. Thinking about occupational justice as a right of humanity forces us, as occupational therapists, to go beyond the idea of physical and mental disabilities and consider other reasons for restricted participation in occupation. Occupational therapists possess unique knowledge about how people and communities experience meaning. They understand the importance of participation and how to build contexts to facilitate opportunities for doing.

Individual Learning Activities

1. Think of an occupation that is meaningful to you. Identify societal conditions that permit you to participate in that occupation. Are there people restricted or discouraged from participating in this occupation? Explore possible societal factors that influence this occupation.
2. Identify a local or national policy related to education, health care, or social policy that you believe needs to be changed or improved to work toward an occupationally just society. Find out who is an influential person in the area of the policy. Write a letter to that person describing the issue and how the policy could be improved.

Group Learning Activity

Occupational determinants consist of factors such as economy, national and international policies, policy values, and cultural values. In your group, reflect on the society in which you live. Identify rules, attitudes, and policies that promote an occupationally just society. Identify rules, attitudes, and policies that contribute to occupational marginalization, deprivation, and alienation. What steps would you take to foster a more occupationally just society?

Study Questions

1. Described as "the opportunity and resources (personal, environmental, societal) for individuals and communities to select and engage in a range of purposeful occupations that are culturally and personally meaningful" is the following term:
   a. Social justice
   b. Occupational enrichment
   c. Occupational justice
   d. None of the above
2. The authors advocate which of the following as the means to occupational justice?
   a. Policy changes
   b. Activism
   c. Enablement approaches
   d. All of the above

3. All of the following are outcomes of occupational injustice highlighted by the authors EXCEPT
   a. Occupational preference
   b. Occupational alienation
   c. Occupational imbalance
   d. Occupational marginalization

4. Distributive justice refers to the fair distribution of all of the following EXCEPT
   a. Income
   b. Housing
   c. Physical abilities
   d. Social services

5. The two theorists credited with developing the concept of occupational justice are
   a. Christiansen and Townsend
   b. Townsend and Wilcock
   c. Wilcock and Christiansen
   d. Rawls and Townsend

REFERENCES

1. Townsend, E. A. (1993). Muriel Driver Memorial Lecture: Occupational therapy's social vision. *Canadian Journal of Occupational Therapy, 60,* 174–184.
2. Wilcock, A. A. (1993). A theory of the human need for occupation. *Journal of Occupational Science: Australia, 1*(1), 17–24.
3. Wilcock, A. A.(1995). The occupational brain: A theory of human nature. *Journal of Occupational Science: Australia, 2*(1), 68–73.
4. Wilcock, A. A. (1998). *An occupational perspective of health,* Thorofare, NJ: Slack, Inc.
5. Wilcock, A. A. (1998). Reflections on doing, being and becoming. *Canadian Journal of Occupational Therapy, 65*(5), 248–256.
6. Townsend, E. A.(1996). Enabling empowerment: Using simulations versus real occupations. *Canadian Journal of Occupational Therapy, 63,* 113–128.
7. Townsend, E. A.(1998). *Good intentions overruled: A critique of empowerment in the routine organization of mental health services.* Toronto, ON: University of Toronto Press.
8. Wilcock, A. A., & Townsend, E. A. (2000). Occupational justice: Occupational terminology interactive dialogue. *Journal of Occupational Science, 7*(2), 84–86.
9. Townsend, E. A., & Wilcock, A. A. (2004). Occupational justice. In C. Christiansen & E. Townsend (Eds.), *Introduction to occupation: The art and science of living* (pp. 243–273). Upper Saddle River, NJ: Prentice Hall.
10. Townsend, E. A., & Wilcock, A. A. (2004b). Occupational justice and client-centered practice: A dialogue in progress. *Canadian Journal of Occupational Therapy, 71*(2), 75–87.
11. Townsend, E. A. (2003, October 31). *Occupational justice: ethical, moral and civic principles for an inclusive world.* Paper presented at Annual meeting of European Network of Occupational Therapy Educators, Prague, Czech Republic. www.enothe.hva.nl/meet/aco3/acc03-text03.doc.

12. Townsend, E. A.(2003). Reflections on power and justice in enabling occupation. *Canadian Journal of Occupational Therapy, 70*(2), 74–87.
13. Adelson, H. L. (1995). The origins of a concept of social justice. In K. D. Irani & M. Silver (Eds.), *Social justice in the ancient world* (pp. 25–38). Westport, CT: Greenwood Press.
14. Irani, K. D. (1995). The idea of social justice in the ancient world. In K. D. Irani & M. Silver (Eds.), *Social justice in the ancient world* (pp. 3–8). Westport, CT: Greenwood Press.
15. Pitkin, H. F. (1981). Justice: On relating public and private. *Political Theory, 9,* 327–352.
16. Rawls, J. (1971). *A theory of justice.* Cambridge, MA: Belknap Press of Harvard University Press.
17. Habermas, J. (1995). *The philosophical discourse of modernity: Twelve lectures* (F. Lawrence, Trans.). Cambridge, MA: MIT Press.
18. Habermas, J. (1990). *Moral consciousness and communicative action* (Christian Lenhardt & Sherry Weber Nicholsen, Trans.). Cambridge, MA: MIT Press.
19. Armstrong, H. (2000). Reflections on the difficulty of creating and sustaining equitable communicative forums. *Canadian Journal for Studies in Adult Education, 14,* 67–85.
20. Smith, T. (1999). Justice as a personal virtue. *Social Theory and Practice, 25,* 361–384.
21. Giddens, A. (1991). *Modernity and self-identity: Self and society in the late modern age.* Stanford, CA: Stanford University Press.
22. Smith, D. E. (2005). Institutional ethnography: A sociology for people. Walnut Creek, CA. Altima Press.
23. Gough, I. (1979). *Political economy of the welfare state.* London: Macmillan Press.
24. Callan, E. (2000). Liberal legitimacy, justice, and civic education. *Ethics, 111,* 141–155.
25. Marshall, G., Swift, A., & Roberts, S. (1997). Social justice. In *Against the odds? Social class and social justice in industrial societies* (pp. 7–20). Oxford: Clarendon Press.
26. Young, I. M. (1990). *Justice and the politics of difference.* Princeton, NJ: Princeton University Press.
27. Cookson, R., & Dolan, P. (2000). Principles of justice in health care rationing. *Journal of Medical Ethics, 26*(5), 323–329.
28. Daniels, N., Kennedy, B. P., & Kawachi, I. (1999). Why justice is good for our health: The social determinants of health inequalities. *Daedalus, 128*(4), 215–251.
29. Emanuel, E. J. (2000). Justice and managed care: Four principles for the just allocation of health care resources. *Hastings Center Report, 30*(3), 8–16.
30. Jennings, B. (1990). Democracy and justice in health policy. *Hastings Center Report, 8*(1), 22–23.
31. Maynard, A. (1999). Inequalities in health: An introductory editorial. *Health Economics, 8,* 281–282.
32. McGary, H. (1999). Distrust, social justice, and health care. *Mount Sinai Journal of Medicine, 66*(4), 236–240.
33. Moskop, J. C. (1983). Rawlsian justice and a human right to health care. *Journal of Medicine and Philosophy, 8,* 329–338.
34. Veatch, R. M. (1990). Justice in health care: The contribution of Edmund Pellegrino. *Journal of Medicine and Philosophy, 15,* 269–287.
35. Labonte, R. (1989). Community empowerment: The need for political analysis. *Canadian Journal of Public Health, 80,* 87–88.
36. McKnight, J. L. (1989). Health and empowerment. *Canadian Journal of Public Health, 76*(suppl 1), 37–38.
37. Nussbaum, M. C. (2003). Capabilities as fundamental entitlements: Sen and social justice. *Feminist Economics 9*(2, 3), 33–59.

38. Nussbaum, M. C. (2004). Beyond the social contract: Capabilities and global justice. *Oxford Development Studies 32*(1), 3–18.
39. General Assembly of the United Nations. (1948). *Universal Declaration of Human Rights.* Retrieved April 27, 2006, from http://www.un.org/Overview/rights.html
40. Schultz, V. (2000). Life's work, *Columbia Law Review, 100*(7), 1881–1964.
41. Howard, L., Gamble, J., Bye, R., Arblaster, K., Dean, P., & Casley, L. (1999). Unpublished. Occupational Justice Workshop. Notes from Australian Association of Occupational Therapists Conference; Canberra, Australia.
42. Townsend, E., & Whiteford, G. (2005). A participatory occupational justice framework: population-based processes of practice. In F. Kronenberg, S. S. Algado, & N. Pollard (Eds.), *Occupational therapy without borders: Learning from the spirit of survivors* (pp. 110–127). Toronto: Elsevier Churchill Livingstone.
43. Kronenberg, F., & Pollard, N. (2005). Overcoming occupational apartheid: A preliminary exploration of the political nature of occupational therapy. In F. Kronenberg, S. S. Algado, & N. Pollard (Eds.), *Occupational therapy without borders: Learning from the spirit of survivors* (pp. 58–86). Toronto: Elsevier Churchill Livingstone.
44. Stadnyk, R. (2005). *Personal contributions to the cost of nursing home care: Policy differences and their impact on community-dwelling spouses.* Unpublished doctoral thesis, University of Toronto, Toronto, Ontario, Canada.
45. Stadnyk, R., Townsend, E., & Jurczak, S. (2005). Public policy analysis considering occupational justice issues: A framework for therapists. *Canadian Association of Occupational Therapists Annual Conference, Vancouver, BC.* (National)
46. Wilcock, A. A. (2006). *An occupational perspective of health, 2nd ed,* Thorofare, NJ: Slack, Inc.
47. Fast, J., Eales. J., & Keating, N. (2001). *Economic impact of health, income security and labour policies on informal caregivers of frail seniors.* Edmonton, Alberta: Department of Human Ecology, University of Alberta.
48. Willis, P. (1977). *Learning to labor: How working class kids get working class jobs.* New York: Columbia University Press.
49. Primeau, L. A. (1995). Work versus non-work: The case of household work. In R. Zemke & F. Clark (Eds.), *Occupational science: The evolving discipline* (pp. 57–70). Philadelphia: F. A. Davis.
50. Christiansen, C. (1996). Three perspectives on balance in occupation. In R. Zemke & F. Clark (Eds.), *Occupational science: The evolving discipline* (pp. 431–451). Philadelphia: F. A. Davis.
51. Gramm, W. S. (1987). Labor, work and leisure: Human well-being and the optimal allocation of time. *Journal of Economic Issues, 21,* 167–188.
52. Bernard, M. (1988). *Leisure-rich and leisure-poor: Leisure lifestyles among young adults.* In *Leisure studies* (pp. 131–149). New York: Taylor & Francis.
53. Doyal, L., & Gough, I. (1991). *A theory of human need.* London: Macmillan.
54. McIntyre, L., Connor, S. K., & Warren, J. (2000). Child hunger in Canada: Results of the 1994 National Longitudinal Survey of Children and Youth. *Canadian Medical Association Journal, 163*(8), 961–965.
55. Fieldhouse, J. (2000). Occupational science and community mental health: Using occupational risk factors as a framework for exploring chronicity. *British Journal of Occupational Therapy, 63*(5), 211–217.
56. Farnsworth, L. (1998). Doing, being, and boredom. *Journal of Occupational Science: Australia, 5*(3), 140–146.

57. Christiansen, C. H. (1999). Defining lives: Occupation as identity: An essay on competence, coherence and the creation of meaning. *American Journal of OccupationalTherapy, 53*(6), 547–558.
58. Westwood, S. (1985). *All day, every day: Factory and family in the making of women's lives.* Chicago: University of Illinois Press.
59. Johnson, J. A., & Yerxa, E. J. (1989). *Occupational science: The foundation for new models of practice.* New York: Haworth.
60. Berlyne, D. E. (1966). Curiosity and exploration. *Science, 153,* 25–33.
61. Goodall, J. (1996). Occupations of chimpanzee infants and mothers. In R. Zemke & F. Clark (Eds.), *Occupational science: The evolving discipline* (pp. 31–42). Philadelphia: F. A. Davis.
62. Montgomery, M. A. (1984). Resources of adaptation for daily living: A classification with therapeutic implications for occupational therapy. *Occupational Therapy in Health Care, 1,* 9–23.
63. Marx, K. (1843). Economic and philosophical manuscripts. In E. Fisher (Ed.), *Marx in his own words* (p. 31). London: Allen Lane, The Penguin Press.
64. Ross, L., & Coleman, M. (2000). Urban community action planning inspires teenagers to transform their community and their identity. *Journal of Community Practice,* 7(2), 29–45.
65. Bateson, M. C. (1996). Enfolded activity and the concept of occupation. In R. Zemke & F. Clark (Eds.), *Occupational science: The evolving discipline.* Philadelphia: F. A. Davis.
66. Jackson, J. (1996). Living a meaningful existence in old age. In R. Zemke & F. Clark (Eds.), *Occupational science: The evolving discipline* (pp. 339–361). Philadelphia: F. A. Davis.
67. Sheldon, K. M., Ryan, R. M., & Reis, H. (1996). What makes for a good day? Competence and autonomy in the day and in the person. *Personality and Social Psychology Bulletin, 22,* 1270–1279.
68. Metz, T. (2000). Arbitrariness, justice, and respect. *Social Theory and Practice, 26,* 24–45.
69. Carlson, M. (1995). The self perpetuation of occupations. In *Occupational science: The emerging discipline* (pp. 143–158). Philadelphia: F. A. Davis.
70. Derber, C. (1979). *The pursuit of attention: Power and individualism in everyday life.* Boston: G. K. Hall.
71. Messick, D. M. (1991). Social dilemmas, shared resources, and social justice. In H. Steensma & R. Vermunt (Eds.), *Social justice in human relations, Vol. 2: Societal and psychological consequences of justice and injustice* (pp. 49–69). New York: Plenum Press.
72. World Health Organization, Health and Welfare Canada, Canadian Public Health Association. (1986). *Ottawa Charter for Health Promotion.* Ottawa, Canada.
73. Clark, F. (1997). Reflections on the human as an occupational being: Biological need, tempo and temporality. *Journal of Occupational Science: Australia, 4*(3), 86–92.
74. Aronoff, M. S. (1991). *Sleep and its secrets: The river of crystal light.* Los Angeles: Insight Books.
75. Moore, A. (1995). The band community: Synchronizing human activity cycles for group cooperation. In R. Zemke & F. Clark (Eds.), *Occupational science: The emerging discipline* (pp. 95–106). Philadelphia: F. A. Davis.
76. Bird, C. E., & Fremont, A. M. (1991, June). Gender, time use, and health. *Journal of Health and Social Behavior, 32,* 114–129.
77. Frank, L. D., & Engelke, P. O. (2001). The built environment and human activity patterns: Exploring the impacts of urban form on public health. *Journal of Planning Literature, 16*(2), 202–218.

78. do Rozario, L. (1994). Ritual, meaning and transcendence. The role of occupation in modern life. *Journal of Occupational Science: Australia, 1*(3), 46–53.
79. Braverman, H. (1975). *Labor and monology capital: The degradation of work in the 20th century.* New York: Monthly Review Press.
80. McQuarie, D., & Spaulding, M. (1989). The concept of power in Marxist theory: A critique and reformulation. *Critical Sociology, 16*(1), 3–26.
81. Byrne, C. (1999). Facilitating empowerment groups: Dismantling professional boundaries. *20*(1), 55–71.
82. Illich, I., Zola, I. K., McNight, J., Caplan, J., & Shaiken, H. (1977). *Disabling professions.* London: Marion Boyers.
83. Zacharakis-Jutz, J. (1988). Post-Freirean adult education: A question of empowerment and power. *Adult Education Quarterly 39,* 41–47.
84. Townsend, E. A., Beagan, B., Kumas-Tan, Z., Versnel, J., Iwama, M., Landry, J., Stewart, D., & Brown, J. (2007). Enabling: Occupational therapy's core competency. In E. A. Townsend & H. P. Polatajko. Enabling occupation II: Advancing an occupational therapy vision of health, well-being and justice through occupation (pp. 87–171). Ottawa, ON: CAOT Publications ACE.
85. Townsend, E., & Landry, J. (2004). Interventions in a societal context: Enabling participation. In C. Christiansen & C. Baum & J. Bass Haugen (Eds.), *Occupational Therapy: Performance, Participation and Well-being* (pp. 494–521). Thorofare, NJ: Slack.
86. Hidden Costs/ Invisible Contributions Research Program. (2004). *Stakeholders perceptions of the role contributions make to aging well: Persons with disabilities focus group.* Unpublished raw data.

Endnotes

[1]Certainly declarations of *social* justice tend to generate controversies when societies set out principles for adjudicating rights, responsibilities, and liberties (17, 72). The introduction of *occupational* justice has also generated strong reactions. Some reactions may be to rejoice in the prospect of revisiting justice from an occupational perspective. Other reactions may be negative viewing the topic as *political ideology.* Be assured that the discussion is in fact small "p" political because it raises questions about power, but it does not take a stand with a large "P" Political Party. It is true that the discussion is about ideology, but we are considering small "i" ideology—a set of ideas, not large "I" Political Ideology.

[2]Townsend and Wilcock have led workshops and given presentations on occupational justice in Canberra, Australia (1999), London, England (2000), Brisbane, Australia (2001), Calgary and Prince Edward Island, Canada (2001), and Los Angeles, California (2002), and Stockholm, Sweden (2002). To date, more than 300 people have been directly involved in our exploration of this concept. Not surprisingly, interest in occupational justice was particularly strong in two groups who are already exploring occupation. Leading this exploration are occupational scientists, who explore occupation as a field of academic interest, and occupational therapists, who use occupation as a medium of therapy with individuals, groups, agencies, or organizations, and who focus on outcomes of therapy related to a broad range of occupations that are contextually defined, including occupations to look after the self and others, occupations to enjoy life, and occupations to enhance social or economic productivity.

CHAPTER 14

Occupational Science and Occupational Therapy: Occupation at Center Stage

Matthew Molineux

OBJECTIVES

1. Define, compare, and contrast the fields of occupational science and occupational therapy.
2. Examine the relationship between occupational science and occupational therapy.
3. Discuss the concept of occupation as central to both occupational science and occupational therapy.
4. Provide a brief historical review of the evolution of occupational science and occupational therapy, and how the fields have evolved.
5. Present an overview of research on the value of occupation and its use in therapy.

KEY WORDS

Occupation
Occupational science
Occupational therapy

CHAPTER PROFILE

Occupation and the relationship between occupation and health are of interest to both occupational science and occupational therapy. Although the two fields share a concern with occupation and health, the relationship between the science and the therapy is still being negotiated. Some suggest that the two fields should be different; some suggest that there is no need for occupational science; others argue that

Companion Website

www.prenhall.com/christiansen

The Internet provides an exciting means for interacting with this textbook and for enhancing your understanding of humans' experiences with occupations and the organization of occupations in society. Use the address above to access the interactive Companion Website created specifically to accompany this book. Here you will find an array of self-study material designed to help you gain a richer understanding of the concepts presented in this chapter.

they are both important and should coexist. This chapter will provide an overview of occupational therapy and demonstrate how occupation has been a central concern for the profession, although the prominence of occupation has waxed and waned over the years. The field of occupational science will also be described, including its development from within occupational therapy. Although the alternative arguments will be discussed, this chapter will present both occupational science and occupational therapy as valuable, and discuss how both place occupation at center stage.

INTRODUCTION

As readers of this book will realize, occupation can be a broad construct that is readily understood by most people, once it is explained. Those who recognize that all humans are occupational beings can easily recognize the importance of occupation and the dynamic that exists between what people do and their health, at least from the standpoint of their own lives. Readers with particular disciplinary or professional backgrounds will also see links between the idea of occupation and their own fields. For example, geographers already understand much about how humans exist within and how we use space and time. By considering the occupations that take place within particular contexts, geographers are likely to appreciate human experiences in a different way. Although occupation may be a peripheral construct in many fields, it takes center stage in two fields: occupational science and occupational therapy. The relationship between those two fields is still being negotiated, but it is well accepted worldwide that occupation is the core construct of both. This chapter will explore the place of occupation in both fields. It will begin with occupational therapy, move on to occupational science, and end with a brief overview of the relationship between them, while acknowledging the debates that continue about this relationship.

OCCUPATIONAL THERAPY

A Brief Historical Overview

The history of the occupational therapy profession in two of the founding countries, Britain and the United States, is well documented elsewhere (see, for example, 1–7). Although it is beyond the scope of this chapter to trace the profession's history, a brief history of occupational therapy will provide some useful background. Although Wilcock (2, 3) has shown that the roots of occupational therapy reach back before the 20th century, it is generally accepted that the modern profession was formally founded in the United States in 1917, when the National Society for the Promotion of Occupational Therapy was established (8). That organization was founded by a group of people (including architects, doctors, nurses, and social workers) who agreed that what is now labelled "occupation" was important for humans and health. The founders' views were informed either by their own personal experiences of the restorative nature of occupation or by their experiences of seeing occupation have a positive impact on the patients with whom they were working. The work of Americans who became known as occupational therapists was underpinned by several core assumptions: the essential role of occupation in human life, the link between mind and body, the belief that lack of occupation could lead to poor health and dysfunction, and conversely that participation in occupation could maintain or restore health and function (8). Early occupational therapy practice was, therefore, focused on providing opportunities for people to engage in occupations. This may have been providing opportunities for people to participate in arts and crafts while restricted to a hospital bed, or encouraging long-term residents in psychiatric institutions to participate in the daily tasks of washing, cooking, and gardening.

Since that early period, the profession has undergone various changes and developments in response to internal and external factors, and this evolution in the United States has been well documented by Kielhofner (8). One of the major influences in the history of occupational therapy has been the medical profession. Physicians and psychiatrists in particular have played central roles, including: being founders of the National Society for the Promotion of Occupational Therapy; articulating an early philosophy for the field; and, holding leadership positions in early professional organizations. Although the profession retained a focus on occupation for a number of decades after it was founded, the powerful influence of medicine meant that toward the middle of the 20th century, occupational therapists began to reduce the focus of practice to the minutia of body structures and functions. This reductionist approach fit well with the medical model's concern for diseases of the body and within physical rehabilitation and psychiatric settings in which many occupational therapists were working. Occupational therapists soon came to realize, however, that a narrow focus on physical and psychological components often did not enable them to address the occupational needs of their patients and clients, particularly those with long-term difficulties (8). For example, a woman may be able to move around with a walking stick (cane) following a stroke and so should be able to join her friends at a coffee shop. But she may not do so because she is still unable to accept the new image of herself as a woman with a walking stick.

The inadequacies of a reductionist view of humans and health have been long recognized, and many American occupational therapists (9–13) have called for the profession to reengage with its foundational concepts and return occupation to the center of occupational therapy practice. Kielhofner (8, 14, 15) proposed that since about the 1970s the occupational therapy profession has been attempting to renegotiate its professional paradigm. He has suggested that the profession has reengaged with an occupational perspective and reinterpreted it for the current time, and so defined the contemporary paradigm. The core assumptions of the contemporary paradigm are that humans have an occupational nature, humans may experience occupational dysfunction, and occupation can be used as a therapeutic agent (8). Although it is true that there has been a renaissance of interest in occupation (16), there remains a tension between the philosophy and current practice of occupational therapy. For example, not so long ago I was visiting an

and rank issues that are either more pressing or are prerequisites for other occupations on a client's list.

At this point in the assessment, the occupational performance or other issues have been identified, but the exact nature and cause of the strengths and difficulties are likely to be unknown. The next stage is to determine why those occupations present challenges for the person. With a continuing focus on occupation as the domain of concern, the next phase of assessment would address one or more of the following:

1. The person's capacities, abilities (e.g., muscle strength, attention span, sensory perception, impulse control), as well as the person's interests, motivation, sense of self, sense of meaning and purpose in life, attitudes to making choices and exerting control in their lives, and more;
2. The environment (e.g., physical barriers such as steps, social barriers such as stigma, political barriers such as persecution due to religious beliefs, and legislative barriers such as limited employment opportunities due to refugee status);
3. The occupation (e.g., the occupation may be particularly complex, time consuming, occur in particular settings with others or alone, or be dependent on access to specific tools, materials, or environments.

The outcome of the full-assessment process will be a list of prioritized occupational performance and other issues with a detailed understanding of what strengths are present and what factors are causing the difficulties. For example, Susan may be unable to play with her young daughter since having a stroke that left her with a weak right upper limb and reduced endurance. In addition, the usual play location for Susan and her daughter is on the floor, and Susan finds it difficult to sit down, and move around on the floor, and stand up again, partly due to her reduced right lower limb strength and postural instability. Moreover, Susan is struggling with a new identity and social situation as someone who has a visible, physical restriction and an invisible drive to prove to herself and others that she can be a good mother, worker, and citizen.

Therapeutic Planning

Once the occupational performance and other issues and their underlying causes are known with individual clients, it is possible to plan an individualized or group therapeutic program. One of the first factors to consider at this stage is the desired outcome, that is, what is the likelihood that the underlying cause will improve and what vision of new occupational opportunities will energize the person to action? These are important considerations, as they determine the focus of therapy.

Broadly speaking, the two possible foci of occupational therapy are to improve (or maintain) the person's capacities (attitudes, purpose, etc.) or to adapt the occupation and/or the environments. Figure 14-1 ■ provides an illustration of the possible relationship between these two approaches. If the person is likely to make changes in their occupations, then it is appropriate to spend time in therapy focused on enabling the person to make the changes and to reconstruct their occupational life. This approach would be suitable if a person is living with depression and is unable

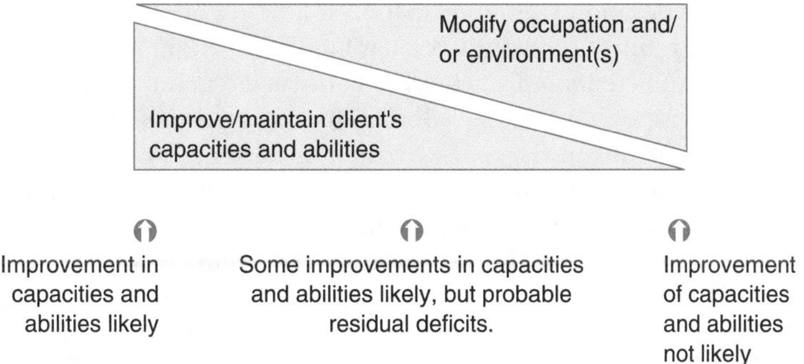

FIGURE 14-1 Two Approaches to Occupational Therapy

to manage their work and leisure occupations with any sense of hope. Alternately, when the environment restricts, marginalizes, or actually deprives the person of desired or necessary occupations, therapy would focus on modifying the occupation and/or environments with communities, organizations or populations as well as with individuals. Broad community action with an advocacy group for persons with spinal cord injuries would be one example of an appropriate approach for enabling participation in society by a person who was a wheelchair user following a spinal cord injury and who was in need of a more accessible community, workplace, and home setting. Of course, few clients will fall neatly into one of those two options: enabling a person to increase capacity and enabling change in their occupations and the environment. Thus much occupational therapy involves a combination of both approaches. Whatever the approach adopted with a particular client, the ultimate aim of occupational therapy is to enable the person to engage in the occupations he/she wants and needs so that the person can participate fully in everyday life as a respected member of society.

Whatever the approach, best practice in occupational therapy is to produce goals and objectives for each client following assessment, because these make the aims of intervention explicit. As suggested earlier, goals and objectives will relate to the occupational performance and other issues of the person, based on the earlier example of working with individuals. For occupation-based practice, the goals would focus on occupations, such as cooking, work, child care and others, rather than on increasing range of motion, developing problem-solving skills, or extending concentration span, all of which are components of performance, but which need to be considered in the context of participation in occupations. That is not to say that addressing these issues is not of concern; it is just that they are the subtext and not the primary goal when using occupations as therapy. Once the person and occupational therapist have identified occupation-based goals and objectives, it is necessary to plan the actual occupations of therapy. Working in an occupation-based way would mean that therapy sessions will consist of engaging the client in a range of occupations. Factors that must be considered when identifying the occupations for therapy include the interests of the client, the resources of the occupational therapist, the environment, and the occupations that are available for use to achieve the person's goals and objectives.

Another consideration is *how* occupation will be used as therapy. For example, a client may want to return to cooking a Sunday lunch for his family, and that is the agreed priority goal. The intervention plan could be constructed in two ways. First, each session could focus on an aspect of cooking a Sunday lunch for the family: planning the meal, going shopping, cooking the first course, roasting a chicken, and making a cake. An alternative approach would be to undertake a range of occupations, which would enable the client to develop the underlying abilities and to make environmental adaptations in order to enable preparation of the Sunday lunch. For example, one session might draw on an interest in woodworking to develop upper limb strength, another might use washing and dressing to improve sequencing difficulties, another might have the client cook a moderately complex lunch—all in a therapeutic, simulated home/kitchen/workshop environment (such as is often established within an Occupational Therapy Department in a health-care setting). Various "transfer learning" strategies would then be used to enable the person to practice the skills at home or to integrate them into the sequenced occupation of actually preparing a trial Sunday meal if the client is still in the health setting. A third option would be to design a group program for persons with disabilities to cook for each other, or to cook for their families or friends. The approach might link people with a self-help community group or a consumer organization that advocates with and for people with a disability. None of these approaches is better than the other; they each engage the client in occupations and so are legitimate occupational therapy interventions. The decision of which one to follow will depend on the client, the therapist, resources, policies, and the therapeutic environment.

A final aspect of planning is probably the most difficult and also the most important. Although any of us can engage another person, or indeed a group of people, in an occupation (e.g., we go out for dinner, attend parties, and undertake sport/leisure pursuits with other people), not all such experiences are therapeutic. The initial planning stages outlined earlier will help to maximize the chance that an occupational therapy encounter will be beneficial for the person, for example, the initial plans highlighted the need for being client centered and responding to the person's needs and priorities. The occupational therapy session needs to maximize the benefit for the person(s) involved. Planning involves the occupational therapist and person (where possible) in considering how to structure the environment and the session, how they will interact, and what information they will both share. These enabling approaches that engage the client in all aspects of occupational therapy are a distinguishing feature of this profession.

Reed and Sanderson (26) have provided one way of understanding some ways in which an occupational therapy session may be shaped (see Table 14-1 ■). An example of this aspect of planning is presented in Table 14-2 ■, drawing on the suggestions of Reed and Sanderson.

Implementation and Evaluation of Occupational Therapy

An occupational therapy plan is implemented as it evolves and evolves as it is implemented. Clearly the aim, initially at least, is to provide sessions as planned, but occupational therapy practice is not a linear process, and so the therapist must remain aware of the person's mood, changes in priorities, changes in occupational performance and

TABLE 14-1 ***Intervention Strategies (Adapted From Reed and Sanderson [1992] 26)***

Methods	Teaching/Learning Methods
"Normal"	Demonstration and performance
Adapted individual	Exploration and discovery
Adapted environmental	Explanation and discussion
	Role playing/simulation
Occupational Media	Problem solving and decision making
Inanimate: Products and Materials	Audiovisual aids
Creative arts and crafts occupations	Practice and repetition
Manual arts and crafts occupations	Behavioral management
Leisure, games and sports occupations	Education
Everyday living occupations—home, community	
Everyday living occupations—work-based	**Therapeutic Approaches**
Education and learning tasks	Normal developmental sequencing
Toys or other play occupations	Normal activity sequencing
Computer or other technology-based occupations	Task analysis
Animate: Persons Interacting with Clients	Graded occupations
Self	Adapted occupations
Dyad, Group, Family, Community, etc.	Occupational groups
Group	Normal environment
Animals	Adapted environment
Plants and nature	One on one
	Consulting
Modalities	Adapted therapy equipment
• Functional activities	
• Self-care activities	
• Work-related activities	
• Leisure/avocational activities	
• Homemaking activities	

underlying issues, and changes in the person's environment and in the service and societal contexts. Thus there is rarely a neat demarcation between assessment, planning, implementation, and evaluation. An ongoing process of reassessment, individual evaluation of outcomes, and overall program evaluation occurs so that occupational therapy can be modified if and when necessary. Occupational therapy is complex, and to maximize effectiveness, efficiency, and cost-benefit, the therapist will need to draw on various types of reasoning (27, 28, 29). Mattingly (27) and Mattingly and Fleming (28) provide very useful discussions that demonstrate the complexity of occupational therapy, to which readers are directed for further consideration of these issues.

In summary, this section has presented a brief introduction to client-centered, occupation-based occupational therapy. It began by providing an overview of the profession's history and the way in which the profession has held occupation centrally, except during the reductionist period. The historical part ended with an acknowledgment that, although there is a desire to take an occupational approach in modern

TABLE 14-2 *Extract From a Sample Intervention Plan*

Session 4	0930 – 1100 Friday
Goal	Mrs. Jones will bake a cake for her granddaughter's birthday in five weeks.
Objective	After a further session, Mrs. Jones will prepare and cook a fish pie with minimal verbal and physical prompting.

Methods

Will use "normal" technique unless it is clearly too difficult and will then introduce adaptations to method and/or environment as appropriate (e.g., nonslip mats); hold bowl while she stirs, food processor

Occupational Media/modalities

Occupation that Mrs, Jones is familiar with—cooking.
Dyad—Mrs. Jones and therapist so she can concentrate and be given full attention.

Teaching Methods/Therapeutic Approaches

Lay out all the necessary tools and equipment before the session begins.
Begin by making sure Mrs. Jones is familiar with kitchen.
As she is making the pie, make suggestions about how Mrs Jones might do it differently so that she can complete it independently.
Educate her about the recovery of motor function post stroke as necessary and appropriate.
Acknowledge all her achievements and give her positive feedback wherever appropriate, recognizing that she is anxious about this session.
Discuss further as appropriate the sort of cake she wants to bake for her granddaughter.
Be vigilant for instances where Mrs. Jones neglects her left hand.
Ensure that therapist's nonverbal communication is positive and supportive.

practice, it does not always happen. Key stages of the occupational therapy process with individual clients were then outlined, and in doing so, the central place occupation can have in practice was demonstrated, with awareness that the principles and processes of engagement in occupations and client priorities are key points in working with family, group, community, organizational, or population clients as well. Occupation can be a powerful focus from the occupational therapist's first contact with a person/group/community and throughout assessment, planning, implementation, and evaluation. Although this section acknowledged the ongoing tension between current practice and the philosophy of the profession, it illustrated one example of working with an individual in a manner that uses occupation at center stage in practice.

OCCUPATIONAL SCIENCE

What is Occupational Science?

In the late 1980s occupational therapy academics at the University of Southern California were developing a new doctor of philosophy program and so debated the nature and focus of that program. Those involved in planning the program believed that the profession would be usefully served by educating scholars in the science of occupation. The commencement of that doctoral program and the publication of the first paper that proposed occupational science marked the formal recognition of a new discipline (30). A closer examination of the history of occupational therapy reveals that the naming of occupational science was merely the culmination of a slow but steady movement within the profession (31, 32, 33, 34). Almost 20 years later, the field of occupational science has developed significantly, and the most recent milestone was the first International Occupational Science Think Tank held July 19–21, 2006, at the Australasian Occupational Science Centre in Nowra, New South Wales, Australia.

Occupational science was defined by Yerxa and colleagues (30, p. 6) in the first paper on the topic as "the study of the human as an occupational being including the need for and capacity to engage in and orchestrate daily occupations in the environment over the lifespan." Although that original definition is clear, it is worth highlighting several aspects to further clarify the nature of the discipline. First, occupational science is a *field of study* that draws on a range of research methodologies and approaches due to the complexity of humans and the multifaceted nature of occupation (30, 35). Second, the perspective adopted by those working in the field is that *humans are occupational beings.* This statement asserts not only that humans engage in occupations, but also that humans have an innate occupational nature. Yerxa (36) coined the term "*Homo occupatio*" in contrast to *Homo sapiens,* to capture the intrinsically occupational nature of humans. The third aspect of the definition worth highlighting is the suggestion that humans have *a need to engage in occupations* as well as the necessary capacities to do so. Finally, humans not only engage in occupations over the life span but also manage or *orchestrate their occupational engagement in their environment.*

As the initial definition suggests, occupational science was originally seen as a field of study, not an occupational therapy theory and not a form of practice. Furthermore, although occupational science grew out of, and had strong links with, occupational therapy, the profession and study of the science of occupation are separate entities. The distinction made is that occupational science is a basic science dealing with the nature and structure of occupation and the relationship between occupation and health, broadly defined (30). In contrast, occupational therapy is an applied science that focuses on the therapeutic application of knowledge about occupation and health, also broadly defined (37). Despite this distinction, early proponents of occupational science saw clear benefits of occupational science for occupational therapy. For example, Yerxa and colleagues (30) argued that occupational science would provide support for what occupational therapists did in practice and so would enable them to provide better services to clients, help occupational therapists differentiate themselves from other health and social care professionals, and enable occupational therapists to contribute to the eradication of societal problems. In fact, the early proponents suggested that the knowledge generated by occupational science would "underline the profound importance of the occupational therapy profession to society as a whole in the twenty-first century" (30, p. 14). Wilcock (38, pp. 299–300) was similarly convinced of the link between the two fields, and she suggested that "the potential for growth and development of occupational therapy, if based on occupational science, is almost overwhelming." Even those who have questioned the value of occupational science and the utility of the knowledge generated by the field have seen its potential value (15, 39–43).

Explaining occupational science as a field is relatively easy, as the preceding paragraphs demonstrate. It is an interdisciplinary field of study concerned with understanding human occupation in context and the relationship between occupation and health viewed broadly to include optimal well-being and equitable participation in the everyday life of a society by all citizens. Given the growth in occupational science, since it was first named, it is now possible to read numerous theoretical discussions and research papers that explicate the growing knowledge about occupation and health. These include papers in the *Journal of Occupational Science*, books that focus on occupation, such as this text offering an *Introduction to Occupation*, or occupation and health and/or occupational therapy practice, which is grounded in occupation (1, 44–50). Increasingly, reviews and critiques of the literature on occupation and occupational science are also now available (51–53).

Occupational Science Research

Occupational science has now been developing, formally at least, for nearly 20 years, with a growing body of theoretical and empirical research to explore topics of interest to the field. To provide a taste of occupational science research and to demonstrate its value, some examples of research are presented here. It is worth noting that some of the research may not be labeled by its authors as occupational science, although it is included because it adds to the growing knowledge base about the nature and structure of occupation and the relationship between occupation and health. Inclusion of such research demonstrates the multidisciplinary nature of occupational science and highlights the value of looking beyond the boundaries of occupational therapy. It does not, however, negate the need for research that explicitly focuses on occupation from the outset, as discussed later.

The complexity of occupation means that several examples of research seek to understand the essential experiential elements of occupation, and from this research, it is clear that there are different experiences of engagement in occupation. For example, Iwarsson, Samuelsson, and Hagberg (54) showed that, at a conceptual level at least, there is support for the idea of occupation. Using soft modeling techniques, the researchers examined a preexisting data set for evidence to support a proposed model of occupation and its relationship to factors such as gender, personality, social network, and physical health. Although the analysis did not produce support for occupation as a broad construct, it did support a more limited variable, that of "household and work occupations." In addition to theoretical research, one significant body of evidence comes from a relatively large number of quantitative studies that have compared performance of three different types of human "doing" (55–62). The terminology used to describe the three different types of human "doing" has varied between investigators, but can be broadly described as occupation, imagery-based occupation, and rote exercise. This research is based on the premise that humans, as occupational beings, will perform quantitatively differently in an occupation compared to a nonoccupation.

These studies, and others, have demonstrated that when humans engage in an occupation compared to a rote exercise,[2] they complete a greater number of repetitions, report experiencing greater enjoyment, have greater tolerance for pain, rate their experience higher in semantic differential scales, make fewer errors, remember more of the steps involved in the occupation, and display better overall quality of performance (55–62). In addition, it is interesting to note that when given the choice, people choose to engage in an exercise that resembles an occupation rather than a rote exercise (63). It seems that being able to exert choice and control over the occupations in which one engages may influence whether or not they have a positive impact on health (64–66).

Rudman et al. (64) demonstrated that when people discuss their participation in occupation, they describe different activities in different ways. In their qualitative research, elderly men and women living in the community were interviewed about their occupational performance and well-being. Although the participants talked of occupation as being defined in terms of physical, mental, or social doing, or some combination of these, it was clear that not all instances of doing were considered an occupation. The extent of engagement associated with the doing determined how it was perceived. In a smaller, in-depth study, Rebeiro and Allen (67) described the benefits of engaging in voluntary work for the second author, a man living with schizophrenia. The benefits of his voluntary work in a library will be discussed below. What is interesting in relation to the current discussion is that John Allen was very clear that he would not have benefited from just any type of voluntary work. He had chosen library work deliberately because it best met his needs and had maximal positive impact on his mental and overall health. Law et al. (68) also found that characteristics of an activity or occupation, such as choice, control, and intrinsic motivation affect how it is perceived by the person.

The way in which occupation enables individuals to create, re-create and express their self-identity is also well documented (64, 66, 67, 69–77). For example, in a qualitative study of 12 community living seniors in Canada, one of the findings was that, when seniors spoke about engaging in occupation, it was clear that they used the word *occupation* to demonstrate aspects of their identity, to describe themselves, and to achieve social recognition (64). Occupation can also provide a means by which individuals, perhaps particularly those who have some form of disability, are able to challenge themselves and achieve competence and mastery, thereby enhancing their self-image, self-esteem, and sense of accomplishment (66, 67, 69, 75, 78–81).

The way in which humans experience and orchestrate time is influenced greatly by engagement in occupation (64). Habitual and routinized ways of managing occupational engagement can, in fact, be "adaptive strategies that contribute to well-being" (82, p. 216). This can occur on an hour-to-hour or day-to-day basis, but can also span an entire life by enabling the preservation or recollection of treasured memories (64, 78). Occupation can even permit individuals to last beyond their own physical existence and exist in a future time by leaving behind a legacy (64). Occupation has aesthetic benefits in that it can provide pleasure through opportunities to create and/or enjoy beautiful objects or experiences (78, 83). Furthermore, occupation can serve as a coping mechanism, or a means of adjustment, when faced with distressing or difficult times. For example, women with breast cancer have identified how they used gardening as a way of coping because it gave them a release, acted as a means of escape, gave them back some control, and was relaxing (78).

Perhaps due to the cumulative effect of the benefits just outlined, engagement in occupation has been shown to have a positive impact on health and well-being. When talking about engagement in occupation, people identify that participation is ". . . essential to one's continued existence and to the quality of that existence" (64, p. 642). Vrkljan and Miller-Polgar (80) found that the three women living with breast cancer who participated in their study reported that the ability to engage in occupations "served to reinforce the notion that they were alive" (80, p. 240). From their experience of working with people with dementia, health-care staff have recognized the benefits of engagement in occupation to themselves and their clients (84).

It has also been demonstrated that engagement in occupation positively affects survival. A study by Iwarsson, Isacsson, Persson, and Scherston (85) used longitudinal data from a 25-year study of 192 elderly people living in rural Sweden. The data collection began in 1969–1970 when the subjects were 67 years old. A large amount of data were collected on this group of people from medical, psychological, and socioeconomic assessments. There was no occupational therapy input into the design of the study or type of data gathered. For the study reported by Iwarsson et al. (85), the research team devised an "index of active participation in daily occupations," which drew on 33 of the 134 items in the socioeconomic assessment. Although the study was retrospective and the items measured were specific to cultural differences between participation in household work of men and women in rural Sweden, the team found that those women who were more active survived longer than those who were less active. No differences in survival rates were found for active or inactive men.

In contrast, a large-scale, longitudinal study by Glass, De Leon, Marottoli, and Berkman (86) involved over 2,800 elderly men and women living in New Haven, Connecticut. The data collection began in 1982, and subjects were followed annually for 13 years. The researchers were interested in the impact that three different types of activity had on survival: social (e.g., attending church, visits to the cinema and restaurants), productive (e.g., gardening and shopping), and fitness (e.g., walking and physical exercise). Information on participation in these activities during the previous month was gathered via a baseline interview. The results were reported in 1999 and described the subjects' participation in activities gathered during the baseline interviews and the outcome measure of death. Glass and colleagues found that those people who were more active survived longer. Of greater interest is the analysis of the three different types of activities in relation to survival. "Social and productive activities were observed to confer equivalent survival advantages compared with fitness activities. This observation is important because it suggests that activities that entail little or no physical exertion may also be beneficial" (86, p. 480). From an occupational perspective this finding is particularly interesting, because it recognizes that the benefits of engaging in occupation are not merely physical (87), and that a "range of mechanisms, both physiological and psychosocial, may be involved in the association between activity and mortality" (86, p. 480).

In summary, this section has introduced occupational science by considering the definition of the field first presented in the literature. It has been argued that understanding "what is occupational science" is relatively straightforward; it is the study of humans as occupational beings including the nature and structure of occupation and the relationship between occupation and health, viewed broadly to include optimal well-being and equitable participation in the everyday life of a society by all citizens. Based on this definition, this section also presented a sampling of occupational science research, including examples of research on occupation that have not previously been broadly cited within occupational science. By reflecting on the definition and some research, it can be seen that occupation takes center stage in occupational science.

THE RELATIONSHIP BETWEEN THE SCIENCE AND THERAPY

Although the relationship between occupational science and occupational therapy was outlined in the first paper on occupational science, that relationship is still developing, and the boundaries continue to be negotiated. For example, at the outset in the 1980s, occupational science was proposed as a basic science, and occupational therapy has been a profession based on applied science for over 100 years. Some critics of occupational science agreed with that distinction, and argued for a complete separation of the two fields so that each could become independent (42, 43). Other critics have argued that a basic science that focuses on occupation is unnecessary, given the large knowledge of occupation generated by already existing academic disciplines (88). Although it is true that other fields contribute valuable information that can be used to understand human occupation, such research does not adopt occupation as the central or organizing concept for research (37, 44, 89–92).

For example, psychologists might undertake research that examines the nature of identity, but they are unlikely to move on to consider how individuals and groups construct, express, and change their identity through engaging in occupation. This "magpie approach" to picking up ideas about occupation from various fields to build a knowledge base about humans as occupational beings and the relationship between occupation and health is considered by some to be a problem. The main argument against the "magpie-approach" is that it has long been recognized that the profession of occupational therapy has lacked coherence in using knowledge of occupation, despite widespread belief that such knowledge should be central to practice in a profession labeled *occupational* therapy (93). Furthermore, a profession must be able to distinguish its theoretical foundations, and if it cannot, others may begin to question the profession's uniqueness and utility (94). Humans are much more than the sum of their parts, and so a field of research that takes an explicitly occupational perspective is important to society.

The other significant debate about the relationship between occupational science and occupational therapy has focused on the ways in which knowledge is generated.

It was first raised by Mosey (42), but has been taken up by Kielhofner and colleagues (95, 96). In brief, their argument is that for knowledge to be useful to practitioners, a concern for its application in practice must be present from the outset of the research, and in their view this can be achieved by using a conceptual model of practice to structure knowledge generation about occupation. This author's view is that this approach underestimates the ability of occupational therapists to use knowledge from many fields to inform their own practices, rather than being obliged to follow recipes or the tools offered in various texts (see, for example, 97, 98).

Given that occupational therapists are engaged in professional practice, a technical, rational approach to practice, such as that described by Fish (99), is inappropriate. In the method advocated by Fish, the boundaries of professional knowledge are finite, and the role of the practitioner is to apply known facts and procedures to well-defined situations. For example, if a recipe states that people with rheumatoid arthritis benefit from a kitchen cart to assist them in performing cooking/eating occupations, the implication is that an occupational therapist should prescribe a kitchen cart for each person with rheumatoid arthritis. The differences inherent in working with individuals, families, groups, or communities, however, makes such prescriptive approaches problematic. Indeed occupational therapists, like other professionals, must be able to develop creative strategies for action, given that many practice situations will be unstructured, complex, uncertain, and have many possible solutions (100). For example, what if the occupational therapist's client with rheumatoid arthritis had a stroke several years earlier and has left-sided weakness or lives in a small flat with others where there is no room for a trolley? In the algorithm of rheumatoid arthritis and kitchen-based occupations, a kitchen trolley is unlikely to be applicable because there are so many environmental, personal, and occupation factors to consider. The particularity of situations requires occupational therapists to create a unique therapeutic approach specific to every client, and so use professional artistry (99). When working with the complexity of human experience, as occupational therapists do, professional practice is not reducible to a finite list of skills and knowledge. As authors have long acknowledged, there is both an art and science to occupational therapy practice (101, 102), and as such a true occupational therapy professional must be able to apply knowledge to practice without restriction to particular protocols, rules, recipes or tools.

In an attempt to contribute to this debate, the author's perspective on the relationship between occupational science and occupational therapy is offered. First, given that both occupational science and occupational therapy are concerned with human occupation, Molineux can see no logical argument why occupational science would not be useful for occupational therapy, or vice versa. His view of the link between the two fields draws on Kielhofner's (8) view of professional knowledge.

Kielhofner (8) argued that occupational therapy's professional knowledge comprises three components: the paradigm, related knowledge, and conceptual practice models. The paradigm is the knowledge that sits at the heart of the profession and provides a particular perspective from which to view the world, understand the "problems" professionals address, and guide action. The paradigm provides unity to the profession as it encompasses the knowledge that is shared by all and distinguishes the field from others. For occupational therapy, the paradigm includes knowledge about humans as occupational beings and the relationship between occupation and health. Related knowledge is that which, although not unique to the field, is nonetheless useful for members of the profession. The related knowledge of occupational therapy draws on a range of areas, such as psychology, sociology, politics, anatomy, anthropology, and physiology. Finally, conceptual practice models provide a means by which knowledge is organized so that it can be used by practitioners. They generally include theories that explain order, disorder, and therapeutic intervention. Furthermore, conceptual practice models include technology for application in the form of tools and methods for assessment and intervention.

Given the description of occupational science presented earlier, it is this author's contention that, in Kielhofner's view of professional knowledge, occupational science sits firmly within the profession's paradigm. It belongs there because occupational science contributes to the profession's particular perspective, namely an occupational perspective, which dictates how occupational therapists view the world, the "problems" of their clients, and how they act in practice. An occupational perspective is ideally shared by all members of the profession and distinguishes the profession from all others.

CHAPTER SUMMARY

This chapter has presented an overview of occupational therapy and occupational science and considered the relationship between the two. It has shown that occupational therapy, when it is practiced in a manner consistent with the profession's philosophy, has an explicit concern with occupation. It is true, however, that the practice of individual occupational therapists in particular settings varies. That notwithstanding, it is this author's view that occupational therapy is without doubt concerned with human occupation and the relationship between occupation and health. Similarly, occupational science has been introduced, and it has been shown that, by definition, occupation is the key construct of that developing field of study. Examples of research from within the field have been presented to show how occupational science research has contributed to the understanding of occupation and health.

While acknowledging some of the debates about the relationship between occupational science and occupational therapy, this chapter has argued that although the two fields are different, they are closely related. They are both concerned with human occupation and the relationship between occupation and health. Although occupational science was first named nearly 20 years ago, the debates about the relationship between it, occupational therapy, and other fields continue. These debates should, in fact, be encouraged so that both occupational science and occupational therapy can develop into robust fields that continue to make valuable contributions to the key issues relevant to society and particular groups within society. Whether occupational science would develop as an interdisciplinary field without its strong link to occupational therapy is another question for debate.

STUDY GUIDE

Study Guide Author: Kristine Haertl

Summary of Main Points

Occupational therapy predates the naming of occupational science, yet both fields hold central the concept of "occupation" and view humans as "occupational beings." As the profession of occupational therapy has evolved, practitioners have stressed the importance of establishing an underlying theoretical foundation. Emphasis on expanding research contributes to an understanding of occupational perspectives, which in turn has helped to formulate a professional paradigm and clarify the professional identity with occupation at center stage.

Occupational science is a field of study in its own right that also provides the central foundation of occupational therapy. Both the field of occupational science and the profession of occupational therapy share a central interest in understanding human occupation and the relationship between occupation and health, broadly defined to include optimal and equitable participation by all in everyday life. Although occupational science is viewed as a basic science that contributes to the understanding of occupational therapy, the field is distinct in developing theories and research that are multidisciplinary and related to other fields of study.

Application to Occupational Therapy

The profession of occupational therapy and the research field of occupational science are distinct yet share core values in which occupation is the center stage. Core assumptions of occupational therapy include (a) the central role of occupation in human life, (b) the mind-body link and the environmental or contextual influences that shape and are shaped by engagement in occupations, (c) the belief that a lack of occupation may contribute to poor health and dysfunction, and (d) that occupational participation may restore health and function. An understanding of the nature and social structure of occupation and its therapeutic properties helps to guide occupational therapists through the process of practice, which in this chapter is summarized in relation to assessment, planning, intervention and evaluation. Continued study of occupation will facilitate the development of conceptual models of practice that guide occupational therapy practice because they integrate core knowledge about occupation and other concepts and link this knowledge to processes of practice that can be applied with various types of individual, family, group, community, organizational and population clients.

The chapter distinguishes occupational science from occupational therapy by claiming that occupational science is a basic science focused on the nature and structure of occupation and its relationship to health, whereas occupational therapy is an applied science. Therefore, the underlying theories and research in occupational science provide an understanding of the therapeutic agent "occupation" used within the occupational therapy profession. Continued research in occupational science may also further establish empirical support for the occupational therapy profession. Conversely, continued research in occupational therapy may further clarify and test how knowledge of occupation can be applied by a profession with occupation at center stage.

Individual Learning Activities

1. Divide a piece of paper into two columns. On one side write "occupational science" and on the other, "occupational therapy." Brainstorm a list of words that describes each. Following your list, write a definition for occupational science, and another for occupational therapy. Write a three- to four-page paper comparing and contrasting occupational science and occupational therapy and the relationship between the two.
2. Go to the following link: http://www.isoccsci.org/ (International Society for Occupational Science) and read the PDF titled *The Way Forward Plan.*

   In a two- to three-page reflection paper, consider the following: (a) In reviewing this document, what contribution do you see occupational science having for occupational therapy? (b) How can it contribute to other disciplines? (c) Where do you envision the field of occupational science in 5 years, and in 10?

Group Learning Activity

Form two to four groups of three to five individuals. Each group should be assigned either "occupational therapy" or "occupational science." As a group, design and create an artistic representation of your topic. Prepare a 10-minute description of how your group chose to represent occupational science or occupational therapy. Following your "occupational engagement" in artistic representation, each group will present their creation to the large group. Once all groups have had a chance to share, consider the following questions in a large-group discussion:

a. What collective process occurred in each group to complete the occupation of creating your artistic example?
b. How did the process of engaging socially in this occupation differ from an individual that were to complete this project alone?
c. How did the artistic pieces representing "occupational science" differ from those representing "occupational therapy?" What were the similarities and how do you see the relationship between the two?
d. Summarize the experience.

Study Questions

1. Which of the following are core assumptions of occupational therapy?
   a. Occupation is an essential feature of human life.
   b. There is a link between mind and body.
   c. Participation in occupation may contribute to health and well-being.
   d. All of the above
2. The reductionist approach
   a. Is focused on the mind-body link
   b. Emphasizes the unique role of occupation in therapy
   c. Focuses on individual body structures and functions
   d. None of the above

3. Occupational science
   a. Predates occupational therapy and provides the foundation for the discipline
   b. Like occupational therapy, has the focus of occupation as its roots, yet though largely birthed in occupational therapy, is interdisciplinary in nature
   c. Both of the above
   d. None of the above
4. "*Homo Occupatio*" is a term coined by Yerxa to denote
   a. The similar structure and functions of all occupation
   b. The fact that all life forms have occupation
   c. Humans are intrinsically occupational in nature
   d. All of the above
5. True or False: Occupational therapy is a basic science, whereas occupational science is considered an applied science
   a. True
   b. False

REFERENCES

1. Wilcock, A. (1998). *An occupational perspective of health.* Thorofare: Slack.
2. Wilcock, A. (2002). *Occupation for health. Volume 2: A journey from prescription to self health.* London: College of Occupational Therapists.
3. Wilcock, A. (2001). *Occupation for health. Volume 1: A journey from self health to prescription.* London: College of Occupational Therapists.
4. Peloquin, S. (1991). Occupational therapy service: Individual and collective understandings of the founders, Part 1. *American Journal of Occupational Therapy, 45*(4), 352–360.
5. Peloquin, S. (1991). Occupational therapy service: Individual and collective understandings of the founders, Part 2. *American Journal of Occupational Therapy, 45*(8), 733–744.
6. Reed, K. (1993). The beginnings of occupational therapy. In H. Hopkins & H. Smith (Eds.), *Willard and Spackman's occupational therapy* (8th ed., pp. 26–43). Philadelphia: J. B. Lippincott.
7. Schemm, R. (1994). Bridging conflicting ideologies: The origins of American and British occupational therapy. *American Journal of Occupational Therapy, 48*(11), 1082–1088.
8. Kielhofner, G. (2004). *Conceptual foundations of occupational therapy* (3rd ed.). Philadelphia: F. A. Davis.
9. Reilly, M. (1962). Occupational therapy can be one of the great ideas of 20th century medicine. *American Journal of Occupational Therapy, 16*(1), 1–9.
10. Rogers, J. (1984). Why study human occupation? *American Journal of Occupational Therapy, 38*(1), 47–49.
11. West, W. (1984). A reaffirmed philosophy and practice of occupational therapy for the 1980s. *American Journal of Occupational Therapy, 38*(1), 15–23.
12. Yerxa, E. (1991). Occupational therapy: An endangered species or an academic discipline in the 21st century? *American Journal of Occupational Therapy, 45*(8), 680–685.
13. Yerxa, E. (1967). Authentic occupational therapy. *American Journal of Occupational Therapy, 21*(1), 1–9.

14. Kielhofner, G. (1992). *Conceptual foundations of occupational therapy.* Philadelphia: F. A. Davis.
15. Kielhofner, G. (1997). *Conceptual foundations of occupational therapy* (2nd ed.). Philadelphia: F. A. Davis.
16. Whiteford, G., Townsend, E., & Hocking, C. (2000). Reflections on a renaissance of occupation. *Canadian Journal of Occupational Therapy, 67*(1), 61–69.
17. World Federation of Occupational Therapists International Advisory Group: Occupational Science. (2004). *Definition of occupational therapy.* Unpublished document produced for the World Federation of Occupational Therapists.
18. World Health Organization. (2001). *International classification of functioning and disability: ICF.* Geneva: Author.
19. Turner, A., Foster, M., & Johnson, S. (Eds.). (2002). *Occupational therapy and physical dysfunction: Principles, skills and practice* (5th ed.). Edinburgh: Churchill Livingstone.
20. Trombly, C. (1995). Occupation: Purposefulness and meaningfulness as therapeutic mechanisms. *American Journal of Occupational Therapy, 49*(10), 960–972.
21. Rogers, J. (2004). Occupational diagnosis. In M. Molineux (Ed.), *Occupation for occupational therapists* (pp. 17–31). Oxford: Blackwell Publishing.
22. Hocking, C. (2001). Implementing occupation-based assessment. *American Journal of Occupational Therapy, 55*(4), 463–469.
23. Neistadt, M., & Crepeau, E. (Eds.). (2003). *Willard and Spackman's occupational therapy* (10th ed.). Philadelphia: J. B. Lippincott.
24. Canadian Association of Occupational Therapists. (1991). *Occupational therapy guidelines for client-centered practice.* Toronto: CAOT Publications.
25. Stanton, S., Thompson-Franson, T., & Kramer, C. (2002). Linking concepts to a process for working with clients. In E. Townsend (Ed.), *Enabling occupation: An occupational therapy perspective* (Rev. ed., pp. 57–94). Ottawa: Canadian Association of Occupational Therapists.
26. Reed, K., & Sanderson, S. (1992). *Concepts of occupational therapy.* Baltimore: Williams & Wilkins.
27. Mattingly, C. (1998). *Healing dramas and clinical plots: The narrative structure of experience.* Cambridge: Cambridge University Press.
28. Mattingly, C., & Fleming, M. (1994). *Clinical reasoning: Forms of inquiry in a therapeutic practice.* Philadelphia: F. A. Davis.
29. Schell, B. (2003). Clinical reasoning: The basis of practice. In E. Crepeau, E. Cohn, & B. Schell (Eds.), *Willard and Spackman's occupational therapy* (10th ed., pp. 131–139). Philadelphia: Lippincott, Williams & Wilkins.
30. Yerxa, E., Clark, F., Jackson, J., Parham, D., Pierce, D., Stein, C., & Zemke, R. (1989). An introduction to occupational science, a foundation for occupational therapy in the 21st century. *Occupational Therapy in Health Care, 6*(4), 1–17.
31. Wilcock, A. (2001). Occupational science: The key to broadening horizons. *British Journal of Occupational Therapy, 64*(8), 412–417.
32. Wilcock, A. (2003). Occupational science: The study of humans as occupational beings. In P. Kramer, J. Hinojosa, & C. Royeen (Eds.), *Perspectives in human occupation: Participation in life* (pp. 156–180). Baltimore: Lippincott, Williams & Wilkins.
33. Larson, E., Wood, W., & Clark, F. (2003). Occupational science: Building the science and practice of occupation through an academic discipline. In E. Crepeau, E. Cohn, & B. Schell (Eds.), *Willard and Spackman's occupational therapy* (10th ed., pp. 15–26). Philadelphia: Lippincott, Williams & Wilkins.

34. Clark, F., & Larson, E. (1993). Developing an academic discipline: The science of occupation. In H. Hopkins & H. Smith (Eds.), *Willard and Spackman's occupational therapy* (8th ed., pp. 44–57). Philadelphia: J. B. Lippincott.
35. Yerxa, E. (2003). *The infinite distance between the "I" and the "It"*. Invited keynote presentation at the Society for the Study of Occupation: USA Second Research Conference, Park City, Utah.
36. Yerxa, E. (2000). Confessions of an occupational therapist who became a detective. *British Journal of Occupational Therapy, 63*(5), 192–199.
37. Clark, F., Parham, D., Carlson, M., Frank, G., Jackson, J., Pierce, D., Wolfe, R., & Zemke, R. (1991). Occupational science: Academic innovation in the service of occupational therapy's future. *American Journal of Occupational Therapy, 45*(4), 300–310.
38. Wilcock, A. (1991). Occupational science. *British Journal of Occupational Therapy, 54*(8), 297–300.
39. Hinojosa, J. (2003). Therapist or scientist—How do these roles differ? *American Journal of Occupational Therapy, 57*(2), 225–226.
40. Rey, D. (2001). Resources and research priorities [Letter]. *British Journal of Occupational Therapy, 64*(10), 518–519.
41. Forsyth, K. (2001). Occupational science as a selected research priority [Letter]. *British Journal of Occupational Therapy, 64*(8), 420.
42. Mosey, A. C. (1992). Partition of occupational science and occupational therapy. *American Journal of Occupational Therapy, 46*(7), 851–853.
43. Mosey, A. C. (1993). Partition of occupational science and occupational therapy: Sorting out some issues. *American Journal of Occupational Therapy, 47*(8), 751–754.
44. Zemke, R., & Clark, F. (Eds.). (1996). *Occupational science: The evolving discipline.* Philadelphia: F. A. Davis.
45. Pierce, D. (2003). *Occupation by design: Building therapeutic power.* Philadelphia: F. A. Davis.
46. Kramer, P., Hinojosa, J., & Royeen, C. (Eds.). (2003). *Perspectives in human occupation: Participation in life.* Baltimore: Lippincott, Williams & Wilkins.
47. Molineux, M. (Ed.). (2004). *Occupation for occupational therapists.* Oxford: Blackwell Publishing.
48. Watson, R., & Swartz, L. (Eds.). (2004). *Transformation through occupation.* London: Whurr.
49. Whiteford, G., & Wright-St. Clair, V. (Eds.). (2005). *Occupation and practice in context.* Sydney: Churchill Livingstone.
50. Hasselkus, B. (2002). *The meaning of everyday occupation.* Thorofare: Slack.
51. Molke, D., Polatajko, H., & Laliberte-Rudman, D. (2004). The promise of occupational science: A developmental assessment of an emerging academic discipline. *Canadian Journal of Occupational Therapy, 71*(5), 269–280.
52. Hocking, C. (2000). Occupational science: A stock take of accumulated insights. *Journal of Occupational Science, 7*(2), 58–67.
53. Clark, F. (2006). One person's thoughts on the future of occupational science. *Journal of Occupational Science, 13*(3), 167–179.
54. Iwarsson, S., Samuelsson, G., & Hagberg, B. (1999). Occupation: Construct validity and empirical testing of predicting factors in an ageing population. *Occupational Therapy International, 6*(2), 77–89.
55. DeKuiper, W., Nelson, D., & White, B. (1993). Materials-based occupation versus imagery-based occupation versus rote exercise: A replication and extension. *Occupational Therapy Journal of Research, 13*(3), 183–197.
56. Yoder, R., Nelson, D., & Smith, D. (1989). Added-purpose versus rote exercise in female nursing home residents. *American Journal of Occupational Therapy, 43*(9), 581–586.

57. Rice, M., Alaimo, A., & Cook, J. (1999). Movement dynamics and occupational embeddedness in a grasping and placing task. *Occupational Therapy International, 6*(4), 298–310.
58. Thomas, J., Vander Wyk, S., & Boyer, J. (1999). Contrasting occupational forms: Effects on performance and affect in patients undergoing phase II cardiac rehabilitation. *Occupational Therapy Journal of Research, 19*(3), 187–202.
59. Ross, L., & Nelson, D. (2000). Comparing materials-based occupation, imagery-based occupation, and rote movement through kinematic analysis of reach. *Occupational Therapy Journal of Research, 20*(1), 45–60.
60. Hsieh, C., Nelson, D., Smith, D., & Peterson, C. (1996). A comparison of performance in added-purpose occupations and rote exercise for dynamic standing in persons with hemiplegia. *American Journal of Occupational Therapy, 50*(1), 10–16.
61. Thomas, J. (1996). Materials-based, imagery-based, and rote exercise occupational forms: Effect on repetitions, heart rate, duration of performance, and self-perceived rest period in well elderly. *American Journal of Occupational Therapy, 50*(10), 783–789.
62. Hartman, B., Kopp Miller, B., & Nelson, D. (2000). The effects of hands-on occupation versus demonstration on children's recall memory. *American Journal of Occupational Therapy, 54*(5), 477–483.
63. Zimmerer-Branum, S., & Nelson, D. (1995). Occupationally embedded exercise versus rote exercise: A choice between occupational forms by elderly nursing home residents. *American Journal of Occupational Therapy, 49*(5), 397–402.
64. Rudman, D., Cook, J., & Polatajko, H. (1997). Understanding the potential of occupation: A qualitative exploration of seniors' perspectives on activity. *American Journal of Occupational Therapy, 51*(8), 640–650.
65. Duncan-Myers, A., & Huebner, R. (2000). Relationship between choice and quality of life among residents in long-term-care facilities. *American Journal of Occupational Therapy, 54*(5), 504–508.
66. Laliberte-Rudman, D. (2002). Linking occupation and identity: Lessons learned through qualitative exploration. *Journal of Occupational Science, 9*(1), 12–19.
67. Rebeiro, K., & Allen, J. (1998). Voluntarism as occupation. *Canadian Journal of Occupational Therapy, 65*(5), 279–285.
68. Law, M., Steinwender, S., & Leclair, L. (1998). Occupation, health and well-being. *Canadian Journal of Occupational Therapy, 65*(2), 81–91.
69. Fanchiang, S. (1996). The other side of the coin: Growing up with a learning disability. *American Journal of Occupational Therapy, 50*(4), 277–285.
70. Magnus, E. (2001). Everyday occupations and the process of redefinition: A study of how meaning in occupation influences redefinition of identity in women with a disability. *Scandinavian Journal of Occupational Therapy, 8*(3), 115–124.
71. Rebeiro, K., Day, D., Semeniuk, B., O'Brien, M., & Wilson, B. (2001). Northern Initiative for Social Action: An occupation-based mental health program. *American Journal of Occupational Therapy, 55*(5), 493–500.
72. Braveman, B., & Helfrich, C. (2001). Occupational identity: Exploring the narratives of three men living with AIDS. *Journal of Occupational Science, 8*(2), 25–31.
73. Jackson, J. (1998). The value of occupation as the core of treatment: Sandy's experience. *American Journal of Occupational Therapy, 52*(6), 466–473.
74. Clark, F. (1993). Occupation embedded in a real life: Interweaving occupational science and occupational therapy. *American Journal of Occupational Therapy, 47*(12), 1067–1078.
75. Rebeiro, K., & Cook, J. (1999). Opportunity, not prescription: An exploratory study of the experience of occupational engagement. *Canadian Journal of Occupational Therapy, 66*(4), 176–187.

76. Price-Lackey, P., & Cashman, J. (1996). Jenny's story: Reinventing oneself through occupation and narrative configuration. *American Journal of Occupational Therapy, 50*(4), 306–314.
77. Unruh, A. (2004). "So ... what do you do?" Occupation and the construction of identity. *Canadian Journal of Occupational Therapy, 71*(5), 290–295.
78. Unruh, A., Smith, N., & Scammell, C. (1999). The occupation of gardening in life-threatening illness: A qualitative pilot project. *Canadian Journal of Occupational Therapy, 67*(1), 70–77.
79. Thoren-Jonsson, A., & Moller, A. (1999). How the concept of occupational self influences everyday life strategies of people with poliomyelitis sequelae. *Scandinavian Journal of Occupational Therapy, 6*(2), 71–83.
80. Vrkljan, B., & Miller-Polgar, J. (2001). Meaning of occupational engagement in life-threatening illness: A qualitative pilot project. *Canadian Journal of Occupational Therapy, 68*(4), 237–246.
81. Taylor, L., & McGruder, J. (1996). The meaning of sea kayaking for persons with spinal cord injuries. *American Journal of Occupational Therapy, 50*(1), 39–46.
82. Ludwig, F. (1997). How routine facilitates well-being in older women. *Occupational Therapy International, 4*(3), 215–228.
83. Hunter, E. (2006). *Occupation toward the end of life: Women's creation and transmission of personal legacy.* Paper presented at the Society for the Study of Occupation: USA Fifth Research Conference, St. Louis, Missouri, United States of America.
84. Hasselkus, B. (1998). Occupation and well-being in dementia: The experience of day-care staff. *American Journal of Occupational Therapy, 52*(6), 423–434.
85. Iwarsson, S., Isacsson, A., Persson, D., & Schersten, B. (1998). Occupation and survival: A 25-year follow-up study of an aging population. *American Journal of Occupational Therapy, 52*(1), 65–70.
86. Glass, T., De Leon, C., Marottoli, R., & Berkman, L. (1999). Population based study of social and productive activities as predictors of survival among elderly Americans. *British Medical Journal, 319*(7208), 478–483.
87. Molineux, M. (2000). Activity (occupation) is important for survival [Letter]. *British Medical Journal, 320*(7228), 184.
88. Kielhofner, G. (2002). *Challenges and directions for the future of occupational therapy.* Invited keynote presentation at the World Federation of Occupational Therapists 13th World Congress, Stockholm, Sweden.
89. Carlson, M., & Dunlea, M. (1995). Further thoughts on the pitfalls of partition: A response to Mosey. *American Journal of Occupational Therapy, 49*(1), 73–81.
90. Clark, F., Zemke, R., Frank, G., Parham, D., Neville-Jan, A., Hedricks, C., Carson, M., Fazio, L., & Abreu, B. (1993). Dangers inherent in the partition of occupational therapy and occupational science. *American Journal of Occupational Therapy, 47*(2), 184–186.
91. Haggard, L. (2002). Broadening horizons [Letter]. *British Journal of Occupational Therapy, 65*(2), 98–99.
92. Polatajko, H. (2004). The study of occupation. In C. Christiansen & E. Townsend (Eds.), *Introduction to occupation: The art and science of living* (pp. 29–46). Upper Saddle River, NJ: Prentice Hall.
93. Kielhofner, G. (1983). A paradigm for practice: The hierarchical organisation of occupational therapy knowledge. In G. Kielhofner (Ed.), *Health through occupation: Theory and practice in occupational therapy* (pp. 55–91). Philadelphia: F. A. Davis.

94. Mailloux, Z., Mack, W., & Coper, C. (1983). Knowing what to do: The organisation of knowledge for clinical practice. In G. Kielhofner (Ed.), *Health through occupation: Theory and practice in occupational therapy* (pp. 281–294). Philadelphia: F. A. Davis.
95. Braveman, B., Helfrich, C., & Fisher, G. (2001). Developing and maintaining community partnerships within "A Scholarship of Practice." *Occupational Therapy in Health Care, 15*(1/2), 109–125.
96. Forsyth, K., Summerfield Mann, L., & Kielhofner, G. (2005). Scholarship of practice: Making occupation-focused, theory-drive, evidence-based practice a reality. *British Journal of Occupational Therapy, 68*(6), 260–268.
97. Forsyth, K., & Kielhofner, G. (2002). Section II master table. In G. Kielhofner (Ed.), *A model of human occupation: Theory and application* (3rd ed., pp. 346–355). Baltimore: Lippincott Williams & Wilkins.
98. Hansen, R., & Atchison, B. (Eds.). (1993). *Conditions in occupational therapy: Effect on occupational performance.* Baltimore: Williams & Wilkins.
99. Fish, D. (1995). *Quality mentoring for student teachers: A principled approach to practice.* London: David Fulton.
100. Higgs, J., & Hunt, A. (1999). Rethinking the beginning practitioner: Introducing the "interactional professional". In J. Higgs & H. Edwards (Eds.), *Educating beginning practitioners: Challenges for health professional education* (pp. 10–18). Oxford: Butterworth-Heinemann.
101. Peloquin, S. (1989). Sustaining the art of practice in occupational therapy. *American Journal of Occupational Therapy, 43*(4), 219–226.
102. Mosey, A. C. (1981). *Occupational therapy. configuration of a profession.* New York: Raven Press.

Endnotes

[1]Occupational therapists may work with individuals, groups, or whole communities but in the interests of readability, this discussion will refer to individual clients, although the principles can be applied to all categories, whether groups or individuals.

[2]It remains unclear how participating in imagery-based occupations compares with these two conditions.

CHAPTER 15

Globalization and Occupation: Perspectives from Japan, South Africa, and Hong Kong

Eric Asaba, Alfred T. Ramukumba, Annah R. Lesunyane, and Simon Kam Man Wong

OBJECTIVES

1. Recognize the important role that culture plays in occupational choice and the assignment of meaning.
2. Understand how technology has influenced occupation throughout the world.
3. Appreciate occupation as a dynamic social process.
4. Appreciate how history and sociocultural practices shape occupation.
5. Appreciate the unique yet universal presence of ritual, ceremony, and celebration in different cultural contexts.
6. Recognize cultural differences in the meanings of independence and interdependence.

KEY WORDS

Africa
China
Culture
Eastern societies
Globalization
Fifth wave
History
Hong Kong
Japan
Language
Meanings

(continued)

www.prenhall.com/christiansen

The Internet provides an exciting means for interacting with this textbook and for enhancing your understanding of humans' experiences with occupations and the organization of occupations in society. Use the address above to access the interactive Companion Website created specifically to accompany this book. Here you will find an array of self-study material designed to help you gain a richer understanding of the concepts presented in this chapter.

Occupation
Occupational science
Ritual
Routine
Social structure
South Africa
Technology
Time use

CHAPTER PROFILE

Globalization is transforming everyday life. This closing chapter in the 2nd edition of *Introduction to Occupation* offers three occupational perspectives on globalization and occupation from Japan, South Africa, and China, specifically Hong Kong. One purpose of the chapter is to remind the student of *occupation* that the sociocultural, geographic, technological, political, and economic contexts of everyday experiences vary greatly around the world. We are reminded to consider culture, not as a static set of habits or competencies, but rather as a dynamic, social process. The other purpose of this chapter is to spark discussion about the different and common features of occupational experience worldwide. Readers will find that different histories, conditions, and sociocultural practices produce different occupational lives. Yet, the three perspectives show us that in the fundamental and profound realm of everyday life, people need to develop routines, habits, rituals, and satisfactory lifestyles to survive. We need to find meaning, connect with others, honor those who are important to us, celebrate important events, and participate as citizens in the economy and society. To spark discussion on the question of how occupations differ yet create human bonds of shared experience, each author raises issues about culture and social structures, profiles typical occupations, considers the impact of new technologies, and projects possible futures in their part of the world.

INTRODUCTION

Globalization is both a trade-related and cultural phenomenon that Nussbaum (1) defines as "the social process in which the constraints of geography on social and cultural arrangements recede" (2, cited in Whiteford, p. 47). Cultural, communication, work, and related occupations are changing rapidly under the effects of global trade, media images, and corporate agendas. One outcome of change is a growing recognition of the global resource of human *capabilities,* known as *social capital,* which is not easily measurable and is not calculated in measures of economic capital. Social capital is generated by what people do in everyday occupations and can be directed toward (or away from) global justice (1). Another outcome is a growing awareness that time and place greatly shape occupations differently across the lifespan for men and women. People know, for instance, that there are major gender differences in occupations, and in social and economic capital, in different parts of the world (3). Globalization is, thus, recognized by scholars as having a huge impact on the everyday lives of people everywhere. Technology is particularly powerful in changing occupational routines and relationships. With technology people learn, interact, and act so differently now than in the past that old cultural patterns are disrupted, and one can hardly predict what everyday life will be like in the future (4). Technology creates new power relations and identities (5). Research by McCoy, Labonte, and Orbinski indicates that people increasingly recognize the need for global initiatives to make use of technological advances and to advocate for the kind of world that supports healthy living (6). They suggest that we may need a global health watch; perhaps we also need a *global occupation watch.*

This chapter presents perspectives on occupations from three parts of the world: Japan, South Africa, and Hong Kong, China. The authors introduce readers to occupational routines, cultural practices, and the rapid transformation of everyday life in light of technology in the occupational lives of ordinary people.

AN OCCUPATIONAL PERSPECTIVE FROM JAPAN By Eric Asaba

Introduction

This segment begins with an assertion that addresses the very dilemma of many cultural discourses on occupation. As a result of an increasingly multilayered and conceptual complexity surrounding experiences of culture around the world, one needs to be skeptical about attempts to condense "culture" into simplistically communicated characteristics pertaining to different ways of living daily life in different geographic regions of the world. One might argue that providing a textbook version of *the* Japanese lifestyle or culture in a scholarly manner is virtually not feasible today. This difficulty stems only partly from generic notions of multiple subcultures within a broader *culture;* the more profound dilemma is that discussions of culture tend to present simplistic, all-encompassing examples that are then perpetuated by future generations. The argument here is that concrete definitions of *culture* tend to be static, which is the precise antithesis of what it means to critically think about culture in relation to what we call *occupation* within occupational therapy and occupational science. This opening statement introduces an exploration of ways of putting topics of occupation and culture into dialogue with many colleagues around the world.

Subsequent segments will draw from examples and data gathered in Japan. Although these examples represent specific data from Japan on a descriptive level, the relationship between culture and occupation should be understood through an analytic abstraction of the material. Literature will be used from occupational science, occupational therapy, social sciences, and personal research. A description will be incorporated from two national surveys: Time Use and Leisure Activities (7) and Communications Usage Trend 2005 (8), published by the Japanese Ministry of Internal Affairs and Communications.

Because culture has been defined in myriad ways over the years and across disciplines, it is important to briefly situate the conceptual use of the term *culture* here. Some occupational therapy scholars have devoted attention specifically to the exploration of cultural aspects affecting knowledge production and use of *occupation* concepts in Japan (9–12). Citing from this literature, culture has been defined as: "shared experiences and common spheres of meaning, and the (collective) social processes by which distinctions, meanings, categorizations of objects and phenomena are created and maintained" (12, p. 12). To prevent the reduction of culture to race or ethnicity, Iwama (9, 12) and others have made an attempt to explore culture as part of a more dynamic process. However, culture constitutes multiple facets of meaning that are in flux, rather than only maintained. Moreover, in an attempt to continue an international dialogue already begun about culture and occupation, the aim is to challenge the reader to consider the implications of communicating about culture as a concept related to globalization and occupation.

Observations from Japanese Psychiatry

The following example is based on an analysis of what some might generically call a type of assembly work within psychiatric rehabilitation programs in Japan. Using a case of *hashi-ire* (packaging chopsticks), issues of interdependence as experienced through occupation are explored among a group of individuals living with mental illness in Japan (13). This material is introduced here for two reasons. First, concerns have been voiced about the future of Japanese occupational therapy (13). "An epistemological crisis is emerging as both academics and clinicians (exceeding 20,000) are involved in a movement in which its core constructs, such as *occupation,* are problematically left unreconciled to the Japanese experience of the social. Social theories that reflect foreign ideals, such as individualism, monotheism, future temporal orientation, independence, and self-determinism, are studied rote in Japan, stripped of meaning and the power to explain" (9, p. 587). In an attempt to both address the "unreconciled" Japanese experience and provide data from which to understand cultural phenomena, *hashi-ire* is introduced (see Figure 15-1 ■). Second, *hashi-ire* serves as a springboard for critically exploring aspects of a culture in relation to an occupation being carried out. Reiterating from the introduction, what is intended to convey here is not that *hashi-ire* is *Japanese culture.* Rather, there are aspects of the experience of *hashi-ire* shared here that speak to a more abstract Japanese experience often associated with what is often considered Japanese culture. A brief introduction to *hashi-ire,* begins with an excerpt from a paper presented by the author at the 2004 Society for the Study of Occupation meeting in Warm Springs, Oregon.

When I attended my first hashi-ire *group, I felt somewhat odd, sitting at a table with a few patients assembling chopstick packets. As I looked around the room, I was fascinated by how much it felt like a group of workers engaged in the micro-tasks of assembly. Although placing a pair of chopsticks into a paper slip looked easy, I soon learned that this was much more difficult than I expected. I also came to see that* hashi-ire *was not only about placing chopsticks in paper slips, but was actually a series of interdependent occupations. Assembly was not only about inserting chopsticks into the paper slips, but also involved packaging the completed sets into a plastic bag. The plastic bags were placed toward the corners of the tables. About two to three participants would continually migrate through the aisles surveying the tabletops, delivering the ready plastic bags to a table at the front of the room. A group of participants sitting toward the front of the room would tape and seal each bag after*

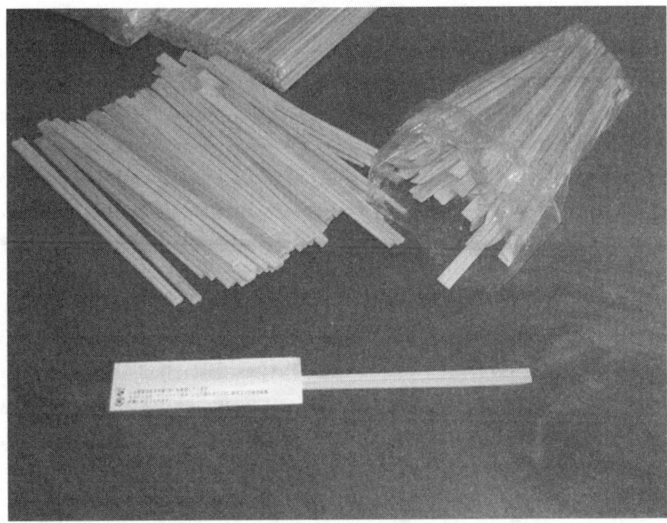

FIGURE 15-1 *Hashi-ire* group packaging chopsticks as an interdependent occupation.
(Courtesy E. Asaba. Used with permission)

checking the contents. All of the completed packages were funneled over to one person who placed 50 packages in one box.

Simply stated, hashi-ire *might be seen as a network of interconnected occupations in which a participant is invested, experiencing valued work and interdependence. As I reflected on my observations of* hashi-ire, *I thought about the monotony and wondered why participants eagerly returned each day. Moreover, the ideology of a program such as* hashi-ire *strikes many as outdated and misplaced in the more contemporary health-care climate. Many occupational therapists want to distance themselves from something that seems to lack the therapeutic virtues of meaning as well as addressing the individual and his or her independence.*

Considering the *hashi-ire* program through the lenses of social history and scholarship about what often characterizes Japanese experiences reveals that participation enables sharing in a common goal and becoming part of a whole, or broader collective. This shared experience of occupation is perhaps similar to what Ramukumba and Lesunyane refer to as *Ubuntu* (togetherness) later in this chapter. Many of the participants have a long history of disconnect and lack of family support. As part of their illness, many find it difficult to *fit in* a society where *fitting in* is a requisite for survival (14,15). The *hashi-ire* group exemplifies a group habitus, to borrow Bourdieu's (16) term, a certain rhythmic, embodied, harmonious engagement in the respective occupations of assembly, delivery, packaging, and boxing. In this way *hashi-ire* provides a venue for harmonious and active participation, and for interdependence among a group of individuals who do not otherwise have easy access to such experiences. The importance of group habitus in the Japanese workplace has already been recognized (15). Japanese culture has been said to be permeated with a need to "fulfill and create obligation, and in general become part of various interpersonal relationships . . . to have a constant concern for belongingness, reliance, dependency, empathy, occupying one's proper place, and reciprocity" (14, pp. 227–228), what Lebra described as *social relativism of the Japanese ethos* (17, p.1). The idea of interdependence in this sense does not mean a merging of self and other, nor does it imply a lack of agency. Rather, the relationship between self and other remains complex, as it is constantly in flux depending on context; moreover, exercising and expressing restraint and adjusting to others to maintain harmony within the collective is seen as highly agentic (i.e., lacking individual human agency) (14).

Some might feel a nostalgic affinity to the collective work ethics of chopstick assembly. Others might feel that *hashi-ire* represents an *old* Japan and symbolizes outdated ideologies that they would rather brush aside. Lenz has commented on this dichotomy of nostalgia for the old yet a desire to get rid of the old in his research on the Japanese women's movement.

> Some observers see a rightist and neo-patriarchal turn of Japanese political culture, but I think they underestimate the profound value changes in present-day Japanese society and tend to conjure up stereotyped specters of the past. Instead, the notion of a "vacuum" in the middle of society, which formed from the structural and social changes resulting from globalization may be useful (18, p. 100).

That this is not only a "turn of Japanese political culture," but is also a matter of culture in relation to occupational engagement. *Hashi-ire* is a powerful illustration of the "turn of Japanese political culture." So, too, is a walk through the city of Kyoto. Kyoto is the old capital of Japan, and those who have visited know the magnitude of the contrast between the renovated Kyoto Station ("the cube") and the temples, shrines, and other ancient sanctuaries tucked away at the basin of the valley.

Activity, Time Use, and Technological Trends

Time Use and Leisure Activities

In contrast to philosophical walks among Kyoto sanctuaries and interdependent performances of occupations to pack chopsticks, Japan has also seen a rapid increase in the use of technology to communicate and access information. The following numbers give a brief overview of a few of the major categories of activities that respondents named in a 2001 survey (7) and the changes in this category since 1996: Internet use 46.4%, not surveyed in 1996; full-time paid employment 62%, –1.5%; full-time homemaking 16.5%, +0.5%; hobbies and amusement 85.9%, –4.6%; travel 80.9%, –1.9%; sports 72.2%, –3.8%; studies/research 36.2%, +5.6%; and, volunteer activities 28.9%, +3.6%. These results might suggest that the Japanese population is spending less time engaging in leisure activities, travel, and sports and instead is spending more time at a computer communicating with others or looking up information. One might also infer that many of the occupational categories represented by a negative change are also occupations in which people are more physically active. Thus the introduction of the Internet, as well as the increase in time spent on studies/research on the Internet, might suggest a more sedentary lifestyle.

Communications Usage Trend Survey

The pervasiveness of computer use in Japanese society today requires further exploration. The steady increase of such technology usage inevitably has an impact on the repertoire of occupations that constitute daily lifestyle patterns in Japan. Consider briefly some highlights of the consumer trends based on the Communications Usage Trend Survey (8), which has been conducted annually since 1990 on a national level by the ministry of internal communications. The survey sample is divided into three cohorts consisting of "household," "companies (enterprises with more than 100 employees)," and "offices (establishments with more than five employees)." Informants within each cohort are selected randomly and receive the survey via postal service.

Based on the 2005 Communications Usage Trend Survey, the number of broadband subscribers rose by 10.8% between 2004 and 2005. Broadband is represented by a number of different high-speed lines such as digital subscriber lines (DSL), cable, and optic fiber lines. In 2005, an estimated 65% of Japanese households had broadband at home, and 68.1% of corporate Internet users had access to broadband. However, when looking at the Internet penetration rate, reports indicate an astounding estimate of 99% for large companies, 87% for households, and 85% for small companies. In comparison, at the end of 2000, Internet penetration rates were 95%, 44%, and 34%, respectively, for large companies, households, and small companies. Internet penetration does not mean that people are actually using Internet services. However, in 2005, an estimated 85.29 million people accessed the Internet in Japan, which represents a 7.3% increase from the year prior. Furthermore, in 2005, Internet access via a mobile phone increased by 10.98 million users since 2004 and surpassed access via a computer terminal for the first time recorded. A substantial proportion of the Japanese population is undoubtedly "logged on!"

Impact of Demographics Factors

Another aspect of interest is the impact of the demographics factors of household users on occupations that use information technology (IT). Based on the 2005 survey, age had the greatest impact on Internet use: Those in the categories *12 years or younger* and *50 years or older* were much less likely to use the Internet in relation to the overall population. Household income, city size, and gender also had an impact, albeit to a lesser degree. Households with an annual income of less than 6 million yen had a negative impact on IT occupations, whereas households with an annual income of over 6 million yen had a positive impact. Living in a major city had a positive impact on IT occupations, whereas living in a rural area had a negative impact. Men were more likely to use the Internet than women.

Reflections on Past, Present, and Future

It might be concluded that a large part of the adult population less than 65 years old in Japan are working, either in or outside of the home. Although many people travel and engage in leisure occupations, there has been a downward trend since the late 1990s. On the other hand there has been an upward trend in the use of technologies to facilitate communication. These figures provide us only with certain raw materials from which to describe specific aspects of everyday life and trends in Japan. What is more interesting, perhaps, is how these technologies are used in occupations and for what purpose. Considering a generally supported idea that social belonging and positioning is important during most occupational engagement in Japan, the simultaneous embracing of next-generation, communications technology and more traditional contexts for work are not difficult to understand. Without claiming scholarly expertise on all things *occupational* in Japanese contexts or *Japanese* about occupations, the claim here is that social theory on culture as dynamic, as introduced earlier, can be of some help in thinking about culture and occupation.

Drawing from the classic works of social scientists, such as Geertz and Johnson (19, 20), it seems that from a Western perspective, people inherently view themselves as independent from others, separate from one another (14); in other words, "independence requires construing oneself as an individual whose behavior is organized and made meaningful primarily by reference to one's own internal repertoire of thoughts, feelings, and action, rather than by reference to the thoughts, feelings, and actions of others" (14, p. 226). Conversely, in non-Western cultures, particularly from a Japanese perspective, people may experience interdependence as "seeing oneself as part of an encompassing social relationship and recognizing that one's behavior is determined, contingent on, and, to a large extent organized by what the actor perceives to be the thoughts, feelings, and actions of *others* in the relationship" (14, p. 227). The tensions between values attributed to the individual and their independence and values attributed to the collective and interdependence in occupations is a concern echoed in occupational therapy and occupational science research (10, 21–23).

In occupational science and occupational therapy, the idea has frequently been expressed that occupations should be individually meaningful and tailored to the unique needs of the individual in hopes of fostering a sort of independence. In Japan, interdependence has been found to be valued over independence and sameness over uniqueness. The different views of independence and interdependence prompt one to ask: What if the concept of *individually meaningful occupations tailored to the unique needs for independence of the individual* is reframed to recognize the equally valid concept of *collectively meaningful occupations tailored to the unique needs of the group for sameness and interdependence?* This question is posed rhetorically for the purpose of discussion.

In conclusion, the perspective presented is not an us/they dichotomy, a singular Japanese issue, or even an ethnic culture issue, but rather a call to consider that occupation may be guided by collective as well as individual values. The interests expressed here contribute to an ongoing discourse around occupation, as a way to create, reinterpret, express, and perhaps most important, relate evolving understandings. The occupational nature and language of a collective cultural dynamic remains something for readers to ponder.

AN OCCUPATIONAL PERSPECTIVE FROM SOUTH AFRICA By Alfred T. Ramukumba and Annah R. Lesunyane

Most countries in the African continent, including South Africa, are characterized by diverse cultural contexts. The consequence is multiple worlds' experiences ranging from typical First to Third World realities (24). African countries present varied sociocultural, economic, and political contexts. Factors contributing to different realities include globalization, diverse communities, integration of different cultural groups, and accessibility of information. The impact is further influenced by traditional, sociocultural, religious, survival, political, and educational needs. These variations pose challenges in defining occupational experiences and patterns. This section will attempt to provide insights regarding everyday occupations in the South African context with awareness that the landscape of occupations in South Africa is one of diversity. Rather than attempt to represent all South Africa, the authors have chosen to focus on the occupational profiles of Black African cultures.

Diverse Cultural Contexts

South Africa is situated in the southern part of the African continent with a heterogeneous population of approximately 45 million people (25). A large proportion of people fall in younger age categories (< 20 years of age) and a relatively small proportion in the older age categories (> 65 years of age). The breakdown of the population is Black African (79%), Coloured (8.9%), Indian/Asian (2.5%), and White (9.6%). The majority of White, Coloured, and Indian/Asian people speak English or Afrikaans (languages of European origin). Among the Black African people, nine indigenous African languages are used as home languages. A small (about 5%) percentage of Black South Africans has acquired English or Afrikaans as a second spoken language. Recognition for official usage of all eleven languages has made information more accessible to most previously disadvantaged communities (26).

South Africa is recognized worldwide as a country rich in experiences of people from different cultural backgrounds and traditions. Certainly one needs to understand the history and the diverse perspectives of the country to appreciate the occupational experiences of people in South Africa. As captured in most literature, a history of oppression, fostered by the apartheid laws of the time, led to one grouping of people dominating all other groups (27–29). Consequently, one culture had a major influence over the visibility and opportunities of other cultures; that is to say that Western- and European-inclined cultures had an influence over African traditional cultures. Although there have been changes in government laws, the impact on everyday occupations of historical events is still a reality facing the country today. Examples of such challenges include poor socioeconomic circumstances, unemployment (about 25% are unemployed and looking for work) with 42.2% of the population not economically active (15–65 years; among them are students, seniors, disabled persons, homemakers, etc.). As the South Africa Census (25) reveals, formal employment can be categorized as mining and quarrying (4.4%); financial, insurance, real estate, and business services (10. 4%); as well as agriculture, hunting, forestry, and fishing in some provinces as high as 28.3%. The lower the education, the greater the likelihood is that people work as labourers. Conversely, the higher the education, the greater the likelihood is that people work in the community, social services, financial services, insurance, real estate, and business services.

A remarkable percentage (21.9%) of people with no education work mainly as domestic workers and gardeners in private households. Other challenges include limited access to decent housing (14.8% of houses are traditional and informal), and limited transport and recreational facilities. Some face challenges to secure running, piped, clean water on site and electricity (firewood is still the main source for cooking among Black African households). Challenges, such as family disorganization as a result of migration from rural areas to major cities (i.e. migration from less to more urbanized provinces to look for better job opportunities) are still very prevalent (25).

Occupational Choices

Although a discussion on occupation may seem straightforward, in the South African context with its heterogeneous population, this is not the case. What complicates this matter is the fact that this country has diverse cultural groups and it is still going through the transformation period after major political changes in 1994 (from apartheid to democratic government). In light of great diversity, the authors claim no attempt to equally discuss occupations associated with all cultural groups. Limited representative studies as well as limited references on occupations across different cultural and racial groups are some of the factors that make it inappropriate to generalize in discussing occupation in the context of South Africa.

Furthermore, most African cultural experiences are not documented, given that traditional Black South Africans relied on preserving the oral method of passing information from one generation to another (24, 29). The focus here is particularly on the communities that are influenced by Black African cultures to highlight influences that may have an impact on occupational choices in developing countries.

Occupational experiences and patterns in the South African context, and possibly in other contexts, are influenced by factors that vary from region to region. The extent of the influence of these factors differs and is dependent on the response of communities and individuals. These factors may include available resources, values, norms, cultural diversity, beliefs, technological development, political factors, government policies, environmental factors, and individual choices and preferences. All these contextual factors influence occupational choices and engagement, as noted by Watson and Fourie (30). Context is said to influence the choice, range, and execution of occupations. This view is also widely acknowledged in literature on occupational science and occupational therapy (31–33). Because language is part of the context for occupations, one result of South Africa's language policy (that of 11 official languages) is that the language spoken at home may be different from the one at work, school, and in some instances, the community in which one lives. Understandably, some people are unable to participate in certain occupations due to language barriers.

Bührmann (34) is of the view that "the African continent is in a . . . dilemma because of the extreme pressure on its Black inhabitants to develop a Western-oriented society, a Western type of ego consciousness with Western goals and measures of achievement. This may lead to anxiety, confusion and a search for identity" (p. 100). To appreciate what influences occupational choices, Bührmann (34) further stated that one needs to "understand, respect fully or enter in the inner world of another, be that other a person of his own culture or from another culture" and to know "the history of his people and their world view, or how that person experiences and interprets personal and historical events" (p. 24).

The authors know from personal experiences that the factors that influence occupational choices change from time to time depending on the challenges and needs of communities. Harsh realities such as poverty, hunger, disease, lack of resources, unemployment, and political instability seem to be considered first in informing occupational choices. For example, the need to survive by providing income for the family may be a deciding factor when choosing the type of occupation. As a result, income-generating occupations seem to be occupations of choice for underprivileged communities, as well as for communities with high rates of unemployment. In other words, socioeconomic realities influence choices.

In instances where individuals and communities have more choices because of less pressure to choose available paid occupations to survive, beliefs and values may play a greater influence in occupational choices. The majority of occupations in African communities are *culturally associated expressions.* As Sonn stated (35), *culturally associated occupations* face a challenge of being undervalued and not recognized as contributing to economic development. A classic example is that some communities and individuals still perceive Europeans as better than Africans and believe that Western and European occupations are better than traditional African occupations. Communities and individuals that value Western and European cultures tend to participate in occupations associated with these cultures, even though they have spent most of their lives living in the African context. This observation is supported by Helms (36) who stated that "White people's adherence to White culture has allowed White people to survive and thrive" (p. 14). Sonn, Helms, and the authors' own observations are that a preference by some people for Western and European occupations extends to all areas of life, including work, recreation, social, and survival occupations.

These observations confirm that the majority of people who belong to and/or those who adopt the Western and European cultures tend to participate in occupations valued in such cultures. Such occupations are done in a more "formal" and "commercialized" fashion. Common examples of formal, commercialized recreational occupations include camping, hiking, mountain climbing, swimming, athletics, performing arts, and sports such as cricket, rugby, netball, and soccer. Similar occupations are done in an informal noncommercialized fashion among the people in African cultures. Those who choose Western occupations tend to choose individualized, group, and organized occupations that are more meaningful to individuals than to groups.

In addition, income, the type of employment, and level of education influence occupational choices. Those with lower income tend to do elementary, blue-collar occupations, whereas those with higher incomes are likely to be in managerial, white-collar, and professional occupations (25). Full-time employment has been observed to impinge on time spent on occupations of choice.

Common Occupations Among South Africans

The majority of people from South African cultures still participate in African traditional occupations (37). These include traditional dances, music ceremonies, wedding celebrations, and family get-togethers. Acknowledgment should be given to the reality that, although the focus here is on the majority of the population, each minority group has a well-established culture and customs which, in addition to other factors, influences the choice of occupations.

Coincidentally, both authors of this section grew up in Limpopo Province, which is situated in the northern part of South Africa. Even though they belong to two different indigenous groups (i.e., Ndebele and Venda), the environments and backgrounds under which they grew up are very similar. This area was and is still characterized by limited resources, traditional houses, poor infrastructure, and limited educational facilities (i.e., classical rural areas with most of the harsh realities experienced in classical Third World communities).

Ordinary people in these communities make their livelihood from the land, however small their land plots may be. They plow fields, do laundry, and fetch water from the rivers or water holes; they fetch wood from the veldt to make an open fire for cooking; they spend time building, decorating, and cleaning their traditional houses as well as cleaning their yards. They plant and water vegetable gardens in their yards; they participate in traditional pottery to construct cooking pots, bowls, and water containers; they look after those who are elderly, people with disabilities, children, and livestock, like goats, cattle, sheep, and donkeys. Even though some of these occupations are perceived as gender specific, for example, cooking is mainly done by women, everybody could participate, depending on the need. On a social level, adults get together for traditional music and dances. During such events, they may drink traditional beers.

Adults, particularly men, migrate to cities and farms for formal employment. They also visit their families from once a month to once or twice a year, or for a short time for holidays or to attend to family matters. Women tend to be left at home looking after children, elderly persons, and those who need care.

Families and individuals may participate in rituals such as circumcision for boys, ancestral worship ceremonies, and religious activities, depending on their belief. Children are observed to mainly use natural materials such as clay, stones, and wood when playing. They also play with scrap materials such as old tins and wires to construct toys. Some participate in traditional music and dances under the guidance and supervision of adults. *Make-believe* and role-plays as well as *hide and seek* are some of the most common games they play.

Furthermore, children in these communities are expected to attend school irrespective of limited resources and facilities as laid down by South African legislation. The majority of students (93.9%) in Limpopo Province have to walk long distances to school on a daily basis. In addition, they are expected to participate in adult roles such as doing household chores, for instance, fetching water and wood, cleaning the house, cooking, and doing laundry, as well as planting and watering vegetable gardens in their yards. They are also expected to look after their younger siblings as well as those who are elderly and those with disabilities.

Evening and weekend occupations include listening to the radio and watching TV, where such facilities are available. The majority tend to use this time for fairy tales, storytelling, and riddles. Information and history are passed from one generation to another by word of mouth. Informal education on cultural matters also takes place while engaging in such occupations.

The highlights in these communities include wedding ceremonies as well as traditional music *competitions*. Common contests involve the horn dance, playing drums, and singing of traditional songs. Some of these get-togethers take place in the chiefs' kraals, (traditional fenced villages). Once a month the elders come together to meet their chief to discuss matters of interest to the community. The chief also uses this opportunity to address his subjects.

Relocation to an area that is more urbanized, in one of the main cities in South Africa, exposed the authors to communities and individuals in transition. Here, the dilemma of the influence of different backgrounds and cultures becomes more apparent. In urban communities, on a social level, the majority of Black Africans love sport; during weekends they pack stadiums to watch their favorite soccer teams (38). Young people in urban areas are observed to spend time after school playing games, such as soccer and computer games, or watching movies, attending parties, visiting friends, playing music, listening to the radio, and watching television. Reading newspapers, magazines, and books are common occupations among professionals and those who are literate. Other occupations include participating in political or church occupations, jazz festivals, choral musical, and social recreational occupations, investing in *stokvels* (a type of credit union in which a group of people contribute a fixed amount of money periodically for mutual financial assistance) (39), and gathering with friends at *shebeens* (informal drinking places).

Communities in rural areas seem to be satisfied by simple things as they engage in everyday occupations. On the contrary, communities in urban areas seem to want more than they have already acquired. They also appear to want to adopt the influence of Western and European cultures when choosing their occupations (40, 41).

Communities in both rural and urban settings carry on with their daily lives, irrespective of the harsh realities of their context and backgrounds. They make the best of what they have and from the resources available. Those in rural areas tend to share, improvise, and make plans to survive poverty, hunger, and diseases. They strive to improve their lives by looking for employment and generating income. People in both settings make curio crafts like beadwork, wood, clay, and woven articles as well as traditional dresses to sell to both locals and tourists. Fresh produce like vegetables and fruit from small gardens in the backyard and from the market/farms are also sold to generate income. In urban areas both formal and informal marketplaces are used to sell products, whereas in rural areas most of the markets are informal. Some people prepare meals to sell to workers and travelers as street vendors (food stalls are common at train stations and bus and taxi ranks). Irrespective of the hardships they face on a daily basis, with smiles in their faces, people bargain prices with their customers, some of whom are tourists, by trying to get the highest price for their handmade crafts. Irrespective of language differences, they seem to communicate successfully with their customers.

Occupations Creating Communities

The subtitle "occupations creating communities" refers to occupations that develop and sustain communities and families as well as individuals. The fact that the South African population is multiracial, multilingual, and of multicontinental origin results in a population with varied customs and lifestyles. Consequently, the population has to engage in "various rituals and ceremonies" to give "meaning and validity to life and existence" (24, p. 213).

Culturally associated occupations are also regarded as occupations creating communities. They are influenced by myths, rituals, and cultural ceremonies (34). These include wedding ceremonies, initiation celebrations, ancestral worships, religious ceremonies, and celebrations related to significant days like Heritage Day. During these ceremonies and celebrations, appropriate songs and dances are used to mark the occasion. Other activities associated with family responsibilities such as caregiving to children, and people who are aged, sick, or disabled can also be regarded as culturally associated occupations.

Occupations creating communities for the majority of African populations in South Africa can be categorized as those that offer support to individuals, families, and communities. Many occupations are performed in groups and are influenced by the African concept of *Ubuntu* (togetherness), the main purpose being participation in occupations that are more meaningful to groups than individuals. Families, friends, and colleagues tend to interact during their free time. These may be occupations that are seen to make a major contribution in community development and identity (29, 41).

To address challenges faced by the majority of the population in South Africa, community development projects, particularly those related to survival and livelihood, appear to be the priority occupations of choice. This is more so for people who do not have formal employment because they lack training, skills, education, and employment opportunities. According to a Labour Force Survey published in 2005 (42), 67.2% of people who start a business give unemployment as a reason. The rate of unemployment among different groups in 2005 was 31.5% (Africans), 22.4 % (Coloured), 15.8 % (Indians), and 5.1% (White). Starting a business poses a number of challenges, such as limited access to funding and poor sustainability. The Labour Force Survey indicated that 96.8% of those with businesses that yielded a maximum turnover (gross sales) of less than R300 000.00 (approximately U.S. $39,000) had not accessed a loan or grant.

Community Development Occupations

To provide some insights about community development occupations for this chapter, the authors interviewed Mr. Pitswane (43), branch general manager of a nonprofit organization (NPO) that has branches in several provinces in South Africa. The highlights of the interview are summarized as encompassing the following principles:

- Community development occupations should include those that address the mind, body, and spirit.
- The physical body should be addressed by physical activities such as aerobics, karate, soccer, netball, music, and dance.
- The mind should be addressed through educational programs such as life skills and leadership training.
- Establishment of recreational parks and other recreational facilities enhance community participation in various occupations (e.g., games, get-togethers).
- Job creation and poverty alleviation programs should focus on projects such as those that recycle or reuse resources, and reduce waste.

Community development in South Africa, and probably in most developing countries, is negatively affected by the HIV/AIDS pandemic. This results in major psychosocial and economic problems, such as the increased rate of orphans and child-headed households, many community members having to look after those affected, people losing their employment and income, multiple deaths and funerals in the community, as well as the rising costs of medical treatment. Grandmothers, using their social and foster care grants, assume the role of surrogate parent in most of these households. Undoubtedly, such challenges influence occupational choices. The manager told us that "the real impact of the pandemic is often down-played by those who do not have first hand experiences."

Limited funding, skills, and access to information are some of the challenges encountered when embarking on community development projects. The manager is of the view that poverty is very prevalent in the community and forces people to do certain occupations for survival and livelihood. In the manager's words, "Income generation is very important to our people." Although people are aware of technology and how it could improve their lives, the challenge is that they cannot afford it. The principles outlined by the manager are supported by Swanepoel and De Beer (44), who emphasized the importance of adhering to ethical (human orientation, participation, ownership, empowerment, and release) and practical principles (learning, adaptiveness, and simplicity).

Community development occupations include self-help projects, home-based projects, small businesses, income-generating projects, and informal employment, as briefly described next.

Self-help projects are projects done by individuals or groups of people to generate income and provide livelihood. Common projects include vegetable gardening, small-scale farming, recycling of used materials (empty cans, bottles, and paper) as well as arts and crafts using natural materials.

Home-based projects are projects run from homes with common activities being sewing, cooking, and baking, particularly among the low socioeconomic class communities.

Small businesses include shoe repair, street vendors (fruits, vegetables, secondhand clothing, etc.), repair of electrical appliances, *spaza* shops (small convenience stores often run from homes), and hair and beauty salons.

Other income-generating projects include trades like carpentry, plumbing, and small-scale building constructions. Informal employment (commonly referred to as "piece jobs") also fall in this category, with common examples being casual labor, domestic work, child minding, and gardening.

Influences of Modern Technology on Occupations

Modern technology like radio, television, cell phones (mobile phones), e-mail, Internet, and computers lead to exposure to different cultures worldwide. According to the 2001 census (25), 42.4 % of households had access to a telephone, which was a large increase from 28.8 % in 1996. During the same year (2001), 73.0% possessed at least one radio, whereas 53.8% possessed at least one television set. Technologies also give access to international perspectives and new occupations. Improved literacy and a decrease in the proportion of people with no education (from 19.3% in 1996 to 17.9% in 2001) have made information more accessible to most previously isolated or disadvantaged communities. In addition, individuals have more opportunities to participate in occupations such as sports and games on their own, for instance, electronic games. Modern technology is currently extending to the most rural communities and communities in informal settlements and has made access to information easier. This is mainly due to the improved electricity supply to previously disadvantaged communities. However, access to technology is still limited for the majority of unemployed people because they lack the required funds. Although technology is perceived to have improved the lives of individuals, negative consequences are associated with technological developments. Such realities include alienation (as a result of limited creativity in what people are expected to do), deskilling and increased unemployment (due to automation), and reduced direct social interaction as family members spend more time on computers and watching television. Children tend to participate in passive, less physically active play, such as electronic games (45). Consequently, some of the interactive connections that made families and communities strong are being destroyed. Young people are being diverted from participating in occupations that traditionally lead to the successful assumption of adult responsibilities in later life.

Current and Possible Future Occupations in the South African Context

Communities and individuals participate in varied occupations that are influenced by culture, religion, traditional practices, and acquired cultures. The influence of outside cultural practices seems to be more affirmed now than during the apartheid era. This is possibly due to the democratic government allowing cross-cultural interaction, freedom of association, and freedom of movement. The international community is more accessible since the abolition of the Apartheid Laws. Irrespective of acculturation, some communities and individuals appear to prefer traditional, culturally meaningful occupations. This trend is a strong influence on occupational choices now and possibly in the future.

The influence of globalization will undoubtedly continue to inform occupational choice. Television, movies, and the Internet are the main new influences as communities are exposed to different occupations and lifestyles from around the world. The exposure influences choices as well as engagement in the traditional, cultural occupations. The younger generations, white-collar earners, and professionals are observed to display the tendency to abandon their traditional occupations in favor of the acquired ones (46).

Similarities regarding the backgrounds, contexts, and types of occupations for Black African communities were observed in other developing countries in the African continent, namely Uganda, Kenya, Swaziland, and Tanzania (47). An overall conclusion that can be drawn is that in developing countries, both cultural influences and survival needs (as a result of poverty, unemployment, poor socioeconomic status, and limited resources) are some of the main factors that influence the choice of occupations.

Continuous changes and developments worldwide influence cultural adjustments necessary for survival, thus factors influencing occupational choices are evolving continuously. Theories on motivation seem to provide answers that could be regarded as general reasons for people to choose certain occupations, as are theories about communities and social structures. The tendency to give greater value to addressing basic needs before paying attention to self actualization or community building is apparent among individuals and the communities observed.

AN OCCUPATIONAL PERSPECTIVE FROM HONG KONG, CHINA By Simon Kam Man Wong

Introduction

Hong Kong is a place of vast occupational diversity. It is not just a place where East meets West; rather, it is the place where East and West are successfully integrated (48). Diversity and inclusiveness are definitive traits of the Hong Kong lifestyle (49). Hong Kong's existence as a British colony for over 150 years brought along more exposure and opportunity to extract the best from both the East and West to form a new Hong Kong culture. That means there is a great multitude of different occupations and lifestyles within the same context of Hong Kong. For example, people practice Tai Chi and aerobic exercise in the park, and local flavor is added to the hamburger sold by McDonald's.

Hong Kong culture should not be regarded as the traditional Chinese culture. The education during the time of the colony did not reinforce the traditional Chinese values, so traditional Chinese roots are shallow. Nevertheless, although colonial education did not emphasize ancient Chinese values, these have been transmitted through family and social influence. People in Hong Kong still cling to their Chinese roots, to their traditional beliefs and religions. They continue to pray and make offerings at more than 600 old and new temples, shrines, and monasteries scattered across the country. Celebrations of festivals, which served religious and ethnic as well as moral functions, are still taking place in the community. Moreover, the daily life in Hong Kong is influenced by the philosophical traditions of Confucianism (50, 51). Under such ethical principles, humanity and piety are still two important social values for Hong Kong citizens.

The mixture of Chinese and Western culture may lead to conflict. The younger generations have better chances than older generations to receive more education, especially in science and democracy. This may induce conflicts with the older generation because of the clash of values. Traditional Chinese families are more hierarchical, and the elders may not accept the Western way of communication of the young people. When extended to the political arena, there are disputes on public policies, which are all due to the conflict of interest or clash of values in different ethnic or social groups.

Typical Occupations in Hong Kong

Yamcha or Morning Tea

Yamcha (drinking tea), is what Guangdong and Hong Kong people in particular do if they go out for breakfast in the early morning. Dimsum (touching heart) is a generic term for a variety of small food items that are usually savory or sweet and are consumed together with Chinese tea. In Hong Kong, yamcha is an occupation that has been integrated into many people's lives. Some people do this occupation as part of their morning routine, perhaps going to yamcha after having a morning walk or doing Tai Chi in the park. It is not uncommon that people spend a long time, even the whole morning, doing yamcha.

Yamcha is also an occupation that maintains and promotes family ties. As Hong Kong is a small place with a dense population, it is hard to find a big house to accommodate an extended family with two or more generations. If they are influenced by Western culture, young married couples prefer not to live with their parents. Moreover, Hong Kong people are so busy working and studying that they may not have a chance to get together with parents or siblings every day. Therefore, yamcha becomes a good occupation in which family members can get together for a longer time, sharing what has been happening among them in the past week.

Serving tea has a long tradition in the Chinese culture. It is a means of politeness for the host to extend to the guests, especially foreign friends from overseas. Dimsum items are made in bite-sizes that are appealing to the senses and are judged accordingly in three aspects, namely, look, smell, and taste. So dimsum is also a means for the Chinese to express their aesthetic sense. Some people regard having a cup of tea in a leisurely fashion as a reflection of one's quality of life. In a World Health Organization study on quality of life, the local research team added a national question on "eating" to the questionnaire, reflecting that *food* and *appetite* is an important category of quality of life for Hong Kong Chinese (52).

Playing Mahjong

Mahjong is another occupation based in Chinese roots. On weekends, many household members like to play mahjong after having the morning tea. During a Chinese wedding banquet, guests will play mahjong during the waiting time. A count-down mahjong before the Chinese New Year is also very common. So mahjong can be regarded as a cultural occupation that serves to bring family members or friends to a small table, which provides a perfect social distance for communication.

Mahjong is a traditional Chinese game with 144 dominos and played by four persons. The bamboo, dots, and flowers are mainly pictorial, whereas the characters in mahjong are simple, so even those who are unable to read can learn to play the game quickly. While simple to learn, mahjong has far more combinations than bridge (144 tiles versus 52 cards) to be remembered or controlled. It is a perfect family leisure occupation, given that the elders are equally competitive with the young irrespective of education and intellectual difference. The challenge-skill combination of the game can also bring an experience of harmony, competence and enjoyment, what Csikszentmihalyi (53) described as "flow." Many people regard mahjong as a form of training for patience and self-control in times of adversity. So mahjong can break through the challenge of finding a common occupation for family leisure because, as Shaw found, it is sometimes hard to find an occupation that suits the mixture of ages, sexes, interests, and the complexity of the rules of the game (54).

An occupational analysis, as done by occupational therapists, would show that mahjong is an occupation rich in therapeutic values. Physically, trunk, shoulder, elbow, and hand movements are required in getting and shuffling tiles; grip strength is required in stacking tiles; and where scar tissue after hand injuries reduces hand use, desensitization of finger scars may occur when picking up mahjong tiles. Cognitively, attention, short-term memory, organization, and judgment are essential components to participate in and win the game. Perceptually, distinguishing bamboo, dots, Chinese characters, winds, and special honors involves perception of color, shape, and size. Socially, it provides an opportunity for family members, relatives, and friends to get together for an entire day to share recent happenings or to gossip. The mahjong table is also a place for practicing social skills when meeting new friends. Emotionally, it is socially acceptable to hit the tiles onto the table as a means of expressing anger or relieving emotion; mahjong is also a good way to test one's temper and patience in times of adversity or bad luck. Culturally, the game has been played in China for hundreds of years. Psychologically, winning the game may bring great pleasure and a sense of achievement; one may become more confident in doing other things if the person playing thinks about mahjong as a sign of good luck.

Mahjong has been used in geriatric rehabilitation services in Hong Kong for over 20 years (see Figure 15-2 ■). Cheng (55) showed that mahjong is a viable treatment for dementia. The subjects of the study showed consistent gains across all cognitive

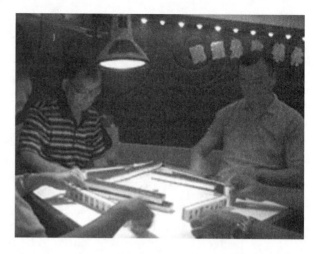

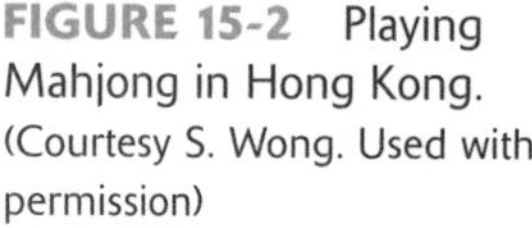

FIGURE 15-2 Playing Mahjong in Hong Kong. (Courtesy S. Wong. Used with permission)

performance measures, such as the Mini Mental State Examination (MMSE), the Digit Span test, and observation of verbal memory. The effects lasted after mahjong had been withdrawn for a month, suggesting that constant practice is not necessary to achieve therapeutic effect once an initial threshold is attained.

Technology and Occupation

Hong Kong is a metropolis with a very good infrastructure for information technology (IT). As the Global Information Technology Report noted, this is reflected in the high ranking of 11th in 2005 on the Networked Readiness Index (NRI) (56). The NRI is defined as the degree of preparedness of a nation or community to participate in and benefit from information and communication technology. Other global rankings for Hong Kong related to IT indicators include: 3rd in cellular telephones, 4th in telephone subscribers, 9th in personal computers, and 4th in Digital Subscriber Line (DSL) Internet subscribers. Hong Kong also had the first cellular phone system that can be used on underground trains. All the preceding data indicate that Hong Kong is highly susceptible to globalization and is highly successful in embracing the latest in information technology.

The advances of technology do affect people's ways of living, however. Computers are making typewriters out of date. Similarly, the design of the digital camera has nearly extinguished the photography industry. It is more convenient to take and print digital photographs than it is to develop film. People will take pictures as freely and as often as possible because they can delete unfavorable ones. Money and space are saved from not printing and storing photographic prints. Photographs can be stored in electronic form and are highly portable for sharing on the Internet. However, some people mourn the loss of the old way of taking photographs that exercised their skills in photography, especially if they experienced the artistic sense of taking black-and-white photographs.

The invention of cell telephones also has pros and cons in daily living. The cell phone feels like it shortens the distance for connecting people because it makes it much easier and affordable to contact friends from far away. For those who have a camera feature on their phone, the cell phone is not just limited to voice; you can see the faces of your friends. Nevertheless, one may be annoyed by the noise of people talking on cell phones on public transportation, such as buses and railway cars, where it can be hard to find a quiet place to rest or read. Sometimes, there are strange sights. Someone may look as if they are arguing to the air but in fact they are using earphones for talking on their cell phone. Writers and poets sometimes mourn the loss of the traditional way of writing letters. Through words, concerns for some may be expressed more thoroughly and in depth in writing than by talking. It can also be more artistic, particularly for those who use calligraphy, to express themselves on paper. Though people can connect faster by using a cell phone, the level of connection seems more superficial. Similarly, junk calls and spam email have become an annoyance associated with cell phone, e-mail, Internet, and other modern information technologies. Some people may even regard the ring of a cell phone as unnatural; they prefer to hear birds singing or streams flowing rather than phones ringing. Moreover, the increased pressures of life to participate in so many forms of information technology can make people feel that it is difficult to take a breath, relax, or think. It is hard to delay answers or decision making because one can be reached anytime, anywhere through network connections.

Globalization and Occupation

Kwong and Miscevic noted that Hong Kong is universally lauded for hard work, flexibility, and the rule of law, and its success has been largely attributed to its willingness to transform itself and its ability to harness rather than resist the forces of globalization (57). Another favorable factor for globalization development in Hong Kong is that the speed and freedom of obtaining information from all over the world can be supported by its good IT infrastructure.

In the process of globalization, the mass media play an important role in affecting the culture of the community. The mass media are like another set of eyes to filter what is received from the world and to integrate information into local values and new cultural expressions. Unfortunately, few people really learn to be selective and critical when receiving messages from the mass media. To develop the ability to select and critique media messages and cultural forms, the Hong Kong government has included the General Education or Liberal Arts as mandatory subjects to balance the highly instrumental focus of most Hong Kong education. Some schools have even introduced the subject of mass media literacy in primary education to teach the younger generation to be critical in receiving information from the mass media.

Globalization is not a one-way process of receiving information from outside Hong Kong. Hong Kong is also exporting the values of Chinese culture. The Hong Kong people have the advantage of having roots to understand both Eastern and

Western values. Hong Kong's role as a bridge between East and West should be regarded as a great asset to improve global understanding.

For example, Hong Kong and its Asian neighbors are educating the West about Chinese medicine. A study by Chan et al. found that Chinese medicine has become more popular in Western communities because of its gentle effects and its ability to eradicate the roots of some diseases (58). Hong Kong can play a role in bringing Western and Chinese medicine together to improve the health of human beings. The Chinese advocate a balance of yin and yang to maintain health through balance. Daily occupations such as food preparation and mealtime gatherings are affected by the time and seasons, or even the weather, as those factors greatly influence balance as the principle through which people interweave their occupations into daily routines. The yin and yang concept is also in line with the concept of occupational balance in the literature of occupational science and occupational therapy (see Chapter 9 on occupational balance). The occupational scientist or occupational therapist may use the idea of balance to classify occupations into yin or yang categories and to study the effects of various occupational combinations.

The lack of meaning in life is possibly one of the causes of depression and substance abuse in Hong Kong. If meaning, form, and function are three pillars of occupation (59), traditional Chinese ideologies may enhance occupational experiences by offering wisdom to help people discover their sense of meaning in life. For example, Confucianism promotes a harmonious family structure and a model of maintaining relationships among different circles of people. It recognizes that the degree of closeness decreases from nuclear family members to relatives, to friends, to colleagues and finally to strangers. This sense of a family network provides pragmatic guidance for daily occupations. The *benevolence principle* and the *doctrine of the mean* in Confucianism are useful mottos to guide behavior. Followers of Taoism are advised to follow nature in life. That means one should not be too serious about success or failure. Looking at things from different perspectives may be a solution to difficult situations in everyday occupations. Buddhism provides another view to perceive the world. A Buddhist understanding of the meaning of life may help an individual to build up resilience to adversities and sufferings.

Political, Socioeconomic Environment, and Occupation

In the '80s and early '90s, Hong Kong people lacked confidence about the reunion of Hong Kong and mainland China. With fear of the unknown, many people migrated to foreign countries, like the United States, Canada, or Australia. Murphy reports government figures, which show that about 30,000 people left Hong Kong in 1988, 40,000 in 1989, and 62,000 in 1990 (60). Migration affected the social structure and opportunities for occupations. When families emigrated, many elderly were left behind in Hong Kong because they believed that they would not adapt well to a foreign country. Now they may live in a home for seniors with limited social support. This affects their quality of life, because they cannot enjoy the sense of meaning that they would potentially gain from engaging in occupations with their children and grandchildren. Those who have migrated have been deprived of occupations, for instance, in which they would have taken care of their parents or participated in family funerals when their parents pass away.

Given that many people left Hong Kong around the '80s and '90s, there are many occupational opportunities in the workforce and in land development. Many people have experienced a dramatic rise in their socioeconomic status through this golden opportunity. Others have experienced financial turmoil and hardship. Any change in socioeconomic status certainly affects one's occupations and lifestyle. Some may need more knowledge and academic qualifications to prepare themselves for promotion in their occupations, so they attend evening courses to obtain better qualifications, such as a higher degree.

In the first few years after the reunion with China, Hong Kong experienced financial turmoil and the effects of the worldwide, severe acute respiratory syndrome (SARS) outbreak, which in turn affected the morale and quality of life of the Hong Kong people. The downturn in the economy certainly affected people's choice of paid occupations. Many people were laid off or even bankrupted, so they were very cautious in spending money. They were unable to afford to live at the standard they had previously enjoyed. With improvements in the performance of Hong Kong's economy in the last few years, people are happier and more willing to spend money in recreational activities and on more expensive goods. As Asaba, and Ramukumba and Lesunyane highlighted, economic, socio-cultural and political environmental influences are strong factors in occupational choice and selection.

One final comment is important in considering occupations in Hong Kong. The change in demographics due to an aging population is universal. Hong Kong's population was 6.8 million in 2003, and 11.7% were aged 65 or older. The older population is projected to rise to 27% by 2033 (61). Males are ranked higher than females on life expectancy. With people living longer, there will be increases in the socioeconomic burden of older people on society. The effect of the earlier migration may worsen in the next 15 years when parents, who may be living alone, age and lose the ability to take care of themselves. The low birth rate in Hong Kong will present another problem in the future. As young couples have only one child or even no children, the small family structure will leave those who are old or in adversity to rely on the government and friends. People may find that they have no relatives to support them when they are in need.

The advancement of technology will continue to affect the everyday occupations of Hong Kong people. It will affect the way people perform work, communication, and even human relationships. The border between Hong Kong and Mainland China will disappear gradually. With the development of the economy on the Mainland, Hong Kong will lose its leadership role in finance and human capital. More people will be forced to find jobs on the Mainland, and the differences in values and cultures between the two places will decrease.

Hong Kong is unique in the world in absorbing aspects of both Eastern and Western cultures. With this advantage, the occupations of the Hong Kong people are rich in forms, function, and meaning (59). It has been illustrated that occupations are deeply affected by traditions, technology, and the political and socioeconomical environment. With the existing good infrastructure and flexibility, the people of Hong Kong will not just passively receive the impact of globalization, but will play a more active role to contribute to global values. With the increase in international trade, there will be more opportunities for Western countries to learn about Chinese wisdom.

The everyday life of Hong Kong citizens will become more comfortable with the advancement of technologies that reduce travel time, create faster communication channels, improve TV qualities, and offer more fashionable cell phones with various integrated functions. The Chinese ethical structure and dynamic will still be maintained because these deep-rooted meanings will not be easily changed. People will likely treasure more time and greater relationships with their family members. Social occupations, like yumcha and mahjong, will not be made extinct by the forces of globalization. Using the language and concept of occupation, the form and function of Hong Kong occupations may be more susceptible to change with advancing technologies, but the meanings inherent in everyday Hong Kong life do not seem likely to change.

CHAPTER SUMMARY

Chapter 15 has portrayed diverse perspectives on occupation from Japan, Black South Africa, and Hong Kong. It has been illustrated that occupations are deeply affected by traditions, technology, and the political and socioeconomical environments. The same technological advances that might create social disparities in everyday occupations also enable people to work together. The occupation of electronic collaboration to write a chapter involved the authors in sharing perspectives and enabled them to challenge their own views, arguably a vital feature of discussions about occupation and culture.

The chapter described real-life experiences that, like culture, are not static. What influences occupation may change over time. Culture plays a major influence on choices. An understanding that culture is dynamic and changing, and that an acquired culture is maintained until there is a crisis or a significant life event may help to explain how occupations change as individual or community need arises.

Challenges in life tend to drive individuals and communities back to their roots. Therefore, dialogues on occupation plant seeds to probe further on related subjects. Discussions of occupation make people more inquisitive about everyday life and what influences choices. The breadth and complexity of occupation make it challenging to remain objective and fair when writing about culturally complex societies, such as Japan, or culturally diverse societies, such as South Africa. Yet culturally complex or diverse societies may offer freedom and opportunity to choose from great varieties of occupations, as in the richness of intermingling Eastern and Western occupation with diverse forms, function, and meaning in Hong Kong.

Many factors influence occupations, including tradition, technology, health, socioeconomic development, political climate, and globalization. Their influences may be sudden, subtle, gradual, microscopic, or macroscopic. It is difficult to know the exact mechanisms through which factors exert their influence. Therefore, ongoing dialogues about occupation may inform us about the importance to everyone of everyday occupations and the diverse and complex mechanisms that influence occupations around the world.

This final chapter is compelling because it touches on the heart of global issues. The three occupational perspectives, from Japan, South Africa, and Hong Kong, offered portraits of everyday life that differ in many ways. Although each author's portrayal of everyday life illustrates how occupations within lives differ profoundly, readers will recognize common elements in living. Every society seems to develop routine, group occupations, like *hashi-ire* in Japan, that give people a sense of place, shared decision making and belonging in society. Every society seems to need innovative, local economic occupations, such as the locally owned credit union *stokvels* developed in South Africa. And every society seems to need ritualized occupations, like yamcha tea drinking and mahjong in Hong Kong, to bring communities together.

STUDY GUIDE

Study Guide Author: Kate Barrett

Summary of Main Points

Each contributor to this chapter discusses in concrete terms the complex connections between culture, occupation, and meaning. Whether playing a game of mahjong in Hong Kong or haggling with tourists over the price of vegetables in South Africa, one learns that seemingly simple occupations are imbued with complex meanings and associations. Without an understanding of culture and context, the rich complexity of seemingly simple occupations is easily overlooked or misconstrued. This chapter also highlights the diversity of cultural assumptions, thereby encouraging students to explore their own. Often these assumptions are experienced as values shared and understood by all. As Eric Asaba observed in his exploration of *hashi-ire* (packaging chopsticks), one can not apply the typical Western assumptions about the value of independence over interdependence.

History and tradition are central to understanding meaning but this chapter also highlights how technology is rapidly changing what people do around the world. Integration of and accessibility to technology have emerged in unique ways around the world as key factors shaping community and connection. Technology has created, for some, new opportunities for communication, education, and connection to a wider world. It has created new communities, new opportunities for entertainment, and new ways to play and work. At the same time, technology is replacing or subjugating old, traditional ways of doing, being and becoming. Readers can see that technology has created new divides between people, new opportunities for alienation and isolation largely influenced by age, income, education, and infrastructure. In Japan, as access to the

Internet has steadily increased, participation in certain leisure occupations has declined. In South Africa children playing computer games don't participate in occupations that lead to later assumption of adult responsibilities.

Application to Occupational Therapy

This final chapter provides a global occupational perspective for bringing cultural and socio-political awareness to occupation-based practice. Without an understanding of culture and context, the rich complexity of seemingly simple occupations could be easily overlooked. Opportunities to employ common, meaningful occupations for their therapeutic value may not be maximized. Also, ignoring culture may result in individuals, groups or populations being asked to participate in occupations that are unnecessarily confusing or offensive. Rather than encouraging participation and connections, practitioners may unwittingly alienate or create additional barriers to participation in everyday occupations. Understanding the norms, values, and assumptions of cultures other than one's own requires recognition that each person has unique norms, values, and assumptions that are significantly influenced by culture. The challenge is to think about culture as dynamic in shaping the everyday routines, habits, rituals, celebrations, relationships and social structures in particular contexts. One way to explore the assumptions one holds is through contrast. The contrasting portrayals of occupations in Japan, Black South Africa, and Hong Kong, China provide examples for students to explore their own values and assumptions.

Meaning is culturally defined. Since occupational therapy needs to be rooted in an awareness of and respect for cultural differences, this chapter provides many examples of occupations that have meanings only fully comprehended by understanding their cultural significance. Occupational therapists' awareness of culture as a dynamic force shaping occupations will increase the likelihood that they will deliver services in ways that are meaningful, relevant, and respectful to the recipients of service. The lessons to draw from this chapter are that occupational therapists and others are encouraged to explore the assumptions they hold about meaningful occupations, about the nature of culture, and the impact of technology.

Individual Learning Activities

Think about a holiday or celebration that is meaningful to you. How would you explain this celebration to someone who has never participated in it? What activities and occupations are performed? What foods do you eat? Who participates? Is there music involved? Are there roles assigned or rituals performed? How are the roles and rituals assigned? What do they mean? Do most of the people in your community celebrate in the same way?

Think about an occupation that is meaningful to you. Now, imagine someone in Japan, South Africa, or Hong Kong engaging in the same occupation. What might be different about how they participate? Describe similarities and differences about how the occupation might be performed, the meaning it may hold, the economic and socio-cultural context, and how the occupation contributes to a sense of belonging.

Self-Reflection

You are encouraged to discuss with friends, students, colleagues, family, and others the questions that this chapter raises for you. Here are a few suggestions.

a. How is your everyday life different from that of your parents?
b. What differences are there between the way your mother lives every day, and the way your grandmother—or her grandmother would have lived? Why are their lives different?
c. What are the differences for your father—and his father or his grandfather?
d. What do you do to be part of a community? How often? Where? Why?
e. What occupations express your individual identity? Why is this important to you?
f. What occupations make you fit into and belong to a community? Why is this important to you?
g. What technologies do you use each day? How has technology changed your own occupations in your lifetime? What is the worst and best influence of global technology on your everyday life? What might you do about your technology and your occupations if you want to live a happy and healthy life with others?

Group Activity

Within your small group, you will play the North American game of Monopoly, a game that may be familiar to many readers in the West. Readers in the East might play mahjong. Readers in Africa might play *hide and seek*. As you play the game, think about what values are communicated. What knowledge might you have that helps you to understand the game? How would you play the game differently if an even distribution of money were the goal in Monopoly? Or if a quick win by the 'new person in town' was the goal in mahjong? Or if some players in *hide and seek* were aggressive in holding others from being found, or willing to tell others where to find everyone? How would these games be played differently by individuals? Or if other players were considered members of your clan, and you were required to assist them?

Study Questions

1. Of the following, which is NOT listed by Eric Asaba as a possible desirable outcome of participation in a *hashi-ire* (chopstick packaging) group?
   a. Fostering a sense of independence
   b. Experiencing valued work
   c. Sharing a common goal
   d. Providing a venue for interdependence
2. Which of the following demographic factors had the greatest impact on Internet usage rates in Japan?
   a. Gender
   b. Household Income
   c. Age
   d. City size

3. Which of the following do Ramukumba and Lesunyane list as a result of the HIV/AIDS pandemic in South Africa?
   a. Loss of employment and income
   b. Increase in number of child-headed households
   c. Increase in the cost of medical treatment
   d. All of the above
4. All of the following are listed as having an impact on occupational choices EXCEPT:
   a. Democracy
   b. Apartheid
   c. Homogenous population
   d. Language
5. The Chinese advocate a balance of yin and yang to maintain health through balance by:
   a. Chinese people emphasize collective food preparation and mealtime gatherings
   b. Time is measured daily
   c. Weight loss is practised to stay healthy
   d. Everyone plays mahjong
6. Quoting the Global Information Technology Report, Simon Wong indicated that Hong Kong was ranked 11th in 2005 on the Networked Readiness Index (NRI)
   a. True
   b. False

REFERENCES

1. Nussbaum, M. C. (2004). Beyond the social contract: Capabilities and global justice. *Oxford Development Studies, 32*(1), 3–18.
2. Whiteford, G. (2005). Globalisation and the enabling state. In G. Whiteford, & V. Wright-St. Clair (Eds.), *Occupation and practice in context* (pp. 349–361). Merrickville, NSW: Elsevier Australia.
3. Waring, M. (1988). *If women counted: A new feminist economics.* San Francisco: Harper and Row.
4. Scanlon, E., Jones, A., Barnard, J., Thompson, J., & Calder, J. (2000). Evaluating information and communication technologies for learning. *Educational Technology & Society, 3*(4), 10.
5. McLaughlin, J., & Webster, A. (1998). Rationalising knowledge: IT systems, professional identities and power. *The Sociological Review, 46*(4), 781–802.
6. McCoy, D., Labonte, R., & Orbinski, J. (2006). Global health watch Canada? Mobilizing the Canadian public health community around a global health advocacy agenda. *Canadian Journal of Public Health, 97*(2), 142–152.
7. *Survey on time use and leisure activities.* (2006). In Ministry of Internal Affairs and Communications.
8. *Communications usage trend survey in 2005.* (2005). In Japanese Ministry of Internal Affairs and Communications.

9. Iwama, M. (2003). The issue is . . . toward culturally relevant epistemologies in occupational therapy. *American Journal of Occupational Therapy, 57*(5), 582–588.
10. Kondo, T. (2004). Cultural tensions in occupational therapy practice: Considerations from a Japanese vantage point. *American Journal of Occupational Therapy, 58*(2), 174–184.
11. Odawara, E. (2005). Cultural competency in occupational therapy: Beyond a cross-cultural view of practice. *American Journal of Occupational Therapy 59*(3), 325–334.
12. Iwama, M. (2006). *The Kawa model: Culturally relevant occupational therapy.* Edinburgh: Churchill Livingstone-Elsevier Press.
13. Asaba, E. (2004). Hashi-ire: Where mental health, chopsticks, and occupation intersect. In *Society for Study of Occupation: USA 3rd annual research conference.* Warm Springs, Oregon, Retrieved August 2008, from conference Abstracts http://www.sso-usa.org/SSO%20-%202004%20Abstracts.pdf
14. Markus, H. R., & Kitayama S. (1991). Culture and the self: Implications for cognition, emotion, and motivation. *Psychological Review, 98*(2), 224–253.
15. Kondo, D. K. (1990). *Crafting selves: Power, gender, and discourses of identity in a Japanese workplace.* Chicago: University of Chicago Press.
16. Bourdieu, P. (1977). *Outline of a theory of practice.* Cambridge, UK: Cambridge University Press.
17. Lebra, T. K. (1976). *Japanese patterns of behavior.* Honolulu: University of Hawaii Press.
18. Lenz, I. (2006). From mothers of the nation to global civil society: The changing role of the Japanese woman's movement in globalization. *Social Science Japan Journal, 9*(1), 91–102.
19. Geertz, C. (1973). *The interpretation of cultures.* New York, NY: Basic Books; 1973.
20. Johnson, F. (1985). The Western concept of self. In A. Marsella, G. De Vos, & F. L. K. Hsu (Eds.), *Culture and self.* London: Tavistock.
21. Borell, L, Asaba, E., Rosenberg, L., Schult, M., & Townsend, E. A. (2006). Exploring experiences of "participation" among individuals living with chronic pain. *Scandinavian Journal of Occupational Therapy, 13,* 76–85.
22. Bonder, B. R., Martin, L., & Miracle, A. W. (2004). Culture emergent in occupation. *American Journal of Occupational Therapy, 58*(2), 159–168.
23. Yerxa, E. J. (1993). Occupational science: A new source of power for participants in occupational therapy. *Journal of Occupational Science, 1*(1), 3–10.
24. Afoloyan, F. (2004). *Culture and customs of South Africa.* Westport, CT: Greenwood Press.
25. Census 2001: Achieving a better life for all, Progress between Census '96 and Census '01. (2001). *Statistics South Africa.* [Report No.03-02-16 (2001)]
26. Thomson, L. (1995). *A history of South Africa* (Rev. ed.). London: Yale University Press.
27. Worden, N. (1995). *The making of a modern South Africa: Conquest, segregation and apartheid.* Oxford: Blackwell.
28. Saunders, C., & Southey, N. (1998). *A dictionary of South African History.* Cape Town. David Philip.
29. Broodryk, J. (2005). *Ubuntu management philosophy.* Randburg: Knowres Publishing.
30. Watson, R., & Fourie, M. (2004). International influences and African influences on occupational therapy. In R. Watson & L Swartz (Eds.), *Transformation through occupation.* London: Whurr Publishers.
31. Hagedorn, R. (2001). *Foundations for practice in occupational therapy.* Edinburgh: Churchill Livingstone.

32. Hasselkus, B. R. (2002). *The meaning of everyday occupation.* Thorofare: Slack.
33. Kielhofner, G. (2002). *The model of human occupation: Theory and application* (3rd ed.). Baltimore: Williams and Wilkins Publishers.
34. Bührmann, M. V. (1986). *Living in two worlds: communication between a white healer and her black counterparts.* Wilmette: Chiron Publications.
35. Sonn, J. (1996). Rewriting the "white-is-right" model: Towards an inclusive society. In M. E. Steyn & K. B. Motshabi (Eds.), *Cultural synergy in South Africa: weaving strands of Africa and Europe.* Randburg: Knowledge Resources.
36. Helms, J. E. (1992). *A race is a nice thing to have—a guide to being a white person or understanding the white persons in your life.* Topeka: Content communication.
37. *Time Use Survey 2000.* (2007). Retrieved March 9, 2007, from www.statssa.gov.za/publications/TimeUse/TimeUse2000.pdf
38. World Book International. (2003). *South Africa in the World Book Encyclopedia, 18,* 55–87.
39. Lukhele, A. K. (1990). *Stokvels in South Africa: Informal savings schemes by blacks for the black community.* Johannesburg: Amagi Books.
40. *Class Mobility Gauteng.* (2007). Retrieved March 7, 2007, from www.sundaytimes.co.za/TheVault/Documents/ClassMobilityGauteng.ppt
41. Mbigi, L., & Maree, J. (1995). *Ubuntu: The spirit of African transformation management.* Randburg: Knowledge Resources.
42. *Labour Force Survey 2005.* (2007). Retrieved March 9, 2007, from http//www.statssa.gov.za/publications/PO210March2006.pdf
43. Pitswane, L. (2007). Interview about community development projects by A. T. Ramukumba & A. R. Lesunyane. 7 March 2007.
44. Swanepoel, H., & De Beer, F. (2006). *Community development: Breaking the cycle of poverty* (4th ed.). Lansdowne: Juta & Co Ltd.
45. Mooney, L. A., Knox, D., & Schacht, C. (2005). *Understanding social problems* (4th ed.). Australia: Thomson Wadsworth.
46. *Defining the emerging black middle class.* (2007). Retrieved April 12, 2007, from www.redinkpublishing.co.za/ezines/african_response/online/african_response_9.htm
47. Makhene, M. M. (1996). The morning after uhuru: Music, rhythm and the performing arts. In M. E. Steyn & K. B. Motshabi (Eds.), *Cultural synergy in South Africa: weaving strands of Africa and Europe.* Randburg: Knowledge Resources.
48. Baher, G. (1997). Hong Kong is where the East meets West. *FOCUS, 44*(3), 33–35.
49. Tam, S. M. (1997). Eating metropolitaneity: Hong Kong identity in yumcha. *The Australian Journal of Anthropology, 8*(3), 291–306.
50. Aryee, S., Fields, D., & Luk, V. (1999). A cross-cultural of a model of the work-family interface. *Journal of Management, 25*(4), 491–502.
51. Chan, H. M., & Lee, R. P. L. (1995). Hong Kong families: At the crossroads of modernism and traditionalism. *Journal of Comparative Family Studies, XXVI*(1), 83–99.
52. Leung K. F., Wong W. W., Tay M. S. M., Chu M. M. L., & Ng, S. S. W. (2005). Development and validation of the interview version of the Hong Kong Chinese WHOQOL-BRIEF. *Quality of Life Research, 14,*1413–1419.
53. Csikszentmihalyi, M. (1997). *Finding flow: The psychology of engagement with everyday life.* New York: Basic Books.
54. Shaw, S. M. (1992). Family leisure and leisure services. *Parks & Recreation, 27*(12), 13–17.

55. Cheng, S. T. (2006). An exploratory study of the effect of mahjong on the cognitive functioning of persons with dementia. *International Journal of Geriatric Psychiatry, 21,* 611–617.
56. Dutta, S., Lopez-Claros, A., & Mia, I. (2006). *The Global Information Technology Report 2005–2006: Leveraging ICT for development.* New York: Palgrave Macmillan.
57. Kwong, P., & Miscevic, D. (2002). Globalization and Hong Kong's future. *Journal of Contemporary Asia, 32*(3), 323–327.
58. Chan, E. A., Cheung, K., Mok, E., Cheung, S., & Tong, E. (2006). A narrative inquiry into the Hong Kong Chinese adults' concepts of health through their cultural stories. *International Journal of Nursing Studies, 43,*301–309.
59. Clark, F., Wood, W., & Larson, E. A. (1998). Occupational science: Occupational therapy's legacy for the 21st century. In M. E. Neistadt & E. B. Crepeau (Eds.), *Willard & Spackman's occupational therapy* (9th ed.). Philadelphia: Lippincott.
60. Murphy, C. A. (1991). Culture of emigration; destination: Canada, Belize, the Federal Republic of Corterra. *The Atlantic. 267*(4). 20–23.
61. Chong, A. M. L., Ng, S. H., Woo, J., & Kwan, A. Y. H. (2006). Positive ageing: The views of middle-aged and older adults in Hong Kong. *Aging & Society, 26,* 243–265.

Glossary

Achievement motivation: Psychological need to succeed or attain mastery.

Active participation: Concept that views humans as active agents in their own development.

Activity (ies): An observable unit of behavior, and recognizable sequence of actions taken together in a particular context; beyond tasks yet without the complexity of occupations in the simple to complex hierarchy of tasks, activities and occupations.

Adaptation: Genetic changes in species necessary for survival within given environmental circumstances; or in intentional behaviors, designing, planning and building changes in social organizations or in the built or natural environment.

Affordance: Any characteristic of a place or thing that enables or influences interactions with a living creature; an actionable property between the environment and individual.

Agency: Capacity, condition, or state of acting or exerting power; a transaction between a human and objects or people within their environments; willful acts.

Allee effect: A term used in sociobiology that is synonymous with cooperation.

Allostasis: A physiological term for the body's response to stressors. This concept is now measured through various objective indictors, such as the body mass index, levels of serum cortisol and serum cholesterol, among others.

Altruism: A type of group cooperation characterized by active donation of resources to others at cost to the donor.

Amae: Japanese term for the emotion of attachment that draws people together in a common social bond of interdependence and mutual concern.

Archetypal places: An approach to classifying places by the type of societal or individual function they serve; basic settings necessary to sustain human existence.

Assistive technology: Technological inventions (devices) designed to enable active engagement or participation in occupations through energy conservation, accommodation for diverse physical abilities, or compensation for functional limitations or disabilities.

Attributions: The explanations people give to the outcomes of their own behavior or that of others.

Automaticity: A characteristic of behavior that is done automatically and repeatedly without direct or conscious attention or awareness.

Avatar: A representation of the self that is used in virtual environments.

Behavioral area: Groups of activities, which usually can be considered occupations.

Committed occupations: Occupations that are productive but typically unpaid, such as household work, meal preparation, shopping, child care, elder care, and home and vehicle maintenance.

Committed time: Time spent in committed occupations.

Community: A geographic or virtual connection between groups that engenders relationships based on proximity, interactions, or the development of shared values and experiences.

Community animation: Processes that foster the building of community spirit.

Compartmentalization: The idea in leisure theory that leisure and work exist in different spheres and that there is no discernible relationship between choices and experiences in one area and the other.

Compensation: In leisure theory, the idea that forms of leisure are chosen to meet human needs that are not met through paid work.

Competence: A match between the environmental demands or challenges of an occupation and the knowledge and/or skills of persons.

Competition: The rivalry or struggle between and within species for survival or other desired ends.

Context: The circumstance, situation, or environment within which an occupation is performed, including geographic, economic, sociocultural, political and regulatory contextual forces.

Continuity theory: A perspective of the life course that views humans as developing continuously from birth until death.

Contracted occupations: Engagement in formal occupations such as work or education that are often governed by explicit contracts or expectations.

Contracted time: Time spent in contracted occupations.

Cooperation: Acting together to facilitate survival or other shared goals.

Cultural norms: The expected behaviors or practices within a social group.

Culture: Shared experiences of meaning and social processes that create meanings.

Disability: A social construct of perceived limitation for particular individuals or social groups in the workplace, community or home, or an individual cognitive, emotional, intellectual, mental (disorder) physical, or psychological limitation, or a combination of both that restricts full social participation in society.

Discretionary: Liberty or power of deciding, or of acting according to one's own judgment or as one thinks fit.

Dislocation: The displacement of something from its usual or customary location.

Displacement: Loss of place; movement from familiar places; involuntarily occupying a lodging other than one's customary home.

Division of labor: Specialization of occupations or roles within a society.

D-needs: Term given to unmet needs by Abraham Maslow in his theory of human motivation.

Drive theory: A view of motivation that identifies compensatory behaviors as predictable responses to needs (such as hunger, thirst, or pain).

Eastern Societies: Referring to cultures of the globally defined East, typically in Asia or Southeast Asia; characterized by complexity, diversity, and social and religious practices that differ historically and in modern times from those in Western Societies.

Ecological niche: Environmental conditions that enable successful adaptation for a group.

Embedded occupations: Those occupations done concurrently with others (for example, talking on the telephone while watching children). Other terms for this concept are secondary activities and nested occupations.

Empowerment: A complex, participatory process of individual, group and social change aimed at achieving greater societal justice and equity through enabling groups who are disempowered or otherwise disadvantaged or oppressed to exercise greater power, entitlement, privilege and overall influence as citizens.

Enablement: The positive form of the term *disablement;* Use of processes such as adaptation, advocacy, collaboration, coordination, education, and design in mutual, reciprocal relationships with others to create opportunities, policies, legislation, and economic conditions, while also prompting others to develop the personal factors to participate to their potential in the occupations that they need and want to do as citizens, to promote health, well-being and social inclusion irrespective of physical or mental impairment or environmental challenges.

Engaging occupation: According to Jonsson, an occupational pursuit that has the characteristics of having positive meaning, being intense or absorbing, coherent, representing more than personal pleasure, enabling social connectedness, and having some characteristics analogous with work.

Environmental press: A term credited to United States psychologist Henry Murray to describe any environmental condition that works in combination with an individual's need to influence behavior. In more current use, the term refers to any environmental characteristic that influences behavior.

Environmentalist viewpoint: View that human development is influenced exclusively by the environment, or through human experiences.

Epistemology: The study of knowledge.

Everyday Life: The customary routines of occupation that characterize a person's daily use of time and energy.

Exaptation: Functional evolved traits that emerge not as genetic changes but as opportunistic consequences of genetic changes.

Flow: Term given by United States psychologist Mihalyi Csikzentmihalyi to the experience of engagement that occurs when an individual is deeply interested in a task or occupation and his or her skills are at a level that matches or exceeds the challenges of the task.

Folk taxonomy: A lay classification created through convention or popular discourse.

Free rider problem: Situation created when members of a group take advantage of altruism without reciprocation, otherwise known as "gaming the system" (from sociobiology).

Free time: Time available that is not consumed by necessary, contracted, and committed occupations.

Free-time occupations: Occupations done during discretionary or uncommitted time.

Freedom: Absence of structure, control, constraint, and restriction, able to choose without limitations.

Game theory: An approach to understanding strategies of competition and cooperation that enhance the survivability of species.

Gender roles: Roles traditionally, culturally, or socially associated with being male or female (such as child rearing, or hunting).

Globalization: The processes through which social and organizational practices (such as corporate organization) become adopted on a worldwide scale.

Habit: A repetitive pattern of occupation or time use; a disposition to act in a certain way, without conscious attention.

Habitus: Term credited to French sociologist Pierre Bourdieu to describe the unconscious patterns of doing, thinking, speaking, and perceiving that people exhibit in the personal or subjective worlds they occupy.

Homeostasis: Term credited to United States physiologist Walter Cannon pertaining to the adaptive processes used by physiological systems to maintain a balance necessary for survival.

Human occupation: Groups of culturally-defined everyday tasks and activities with individual and cultural meaning, and with diverse purposes for looking after the self, enjoying life, expressing spirituality, being a member of various communities, or participating in building (or negatively disrupting) the social and economic production of a particular society.

Incarceration: Being confined in a controlled or limited environment against one's will in consequence to behaviours considered in a particular context to be deviant, undesirable, or dangerous to others.

Interactionist viewpoint: A perspective that considers occupational, environmental and individual factors as interacting in human development across the lifespan.

Interdependence: The reliance that people have on one another as a natural consequence of group living.

International Standard Classification of Occupations (ISCO): A hierarchical scheme or taxonomy of occupations developed in 1988 and adopted for use by several nations.

Justice of difference and social inclusion: A concept of justice to recognize and take into account all forms of diversity among humans and sociocultural conditions that influence participation in everyday life; a justice concerned with social inclusion in everyday occupations, despite human and sociocultural differences; a justice to examine occupational rights to meaning, participation, choice and balance in cases of occupational alienation, occupational deprivation, occupational marginalization, and occupational imbalance in conditions that inequitably restrict some groups from participation in the everyday life of a society, for instance because of normative views that may be disabling for people with bodily impairments.

Labor: Physical, mental, and spiritual exertion directed toward meeting the material wants of a community; the specific productive services rendered by a worker or artisan, and the sense of purpose for occupational engagement.

Leisure: Free or uncommitted time or opportunity to do something.

Leisure pursuits: Occupations or activities that are freely chosen.

Life satisfaction: One's overall satisfaction with the experiences of life.

Life transitions: Periods in life where occupational participation, roles and expectations change significantly, as, for example, advancing from childhood to adolescence and adulthood, or changing from being single to being married, from employment to retirement, or from formal study to commencing a career, etc.

Life balance: A consistent and desired pattern of occupations that enables people to manage stress and promote health and well-being. Patterns may be viewed on several dimensions, including time allocation, fulfillment of social roles, and meeting psychological needs. (Synonyms or closely related terms include role balance, work-related balance, work family balance, lifestyle balance, work-life balance, and occupational balance).

Life-world: A phenomenological model of the world of the individual that sees behaviors in situations as the result of a person's culture, experiences, social relationships, beliefs, and attitudes.

Mastery: Proficiency in dealing successfully with the challenges of living that occur at any point in time.

Maturationist viewpoint: A developmental view characterized by the belief that heredity (genetic makeup) determines the life course.

Meaning: Having symbolic or explicit significance.

Meaningful occupations: Occupations that are chosen and performed with reference to a sociocultural context to generate experiences of personal and collective meaning for individuals, groups, or communities.

Meme: An idea that is replicated through transmission in a culture or group.

Memetics: The science that studies the process and impact of idea generation and adoption.

Metacognition: Higher-order thinking representing the combination of types of thought processes considered together.

Multiple determinicity: Being influenced by many factors, as in the many factors that influence human occupational development.

Multiple patternicity: Having many patterns, as in the richness of patterns of occupational engagement in human development.

Multiple variation: The idea that growth and development show different patterns of change at different times.

Narrative methodology: An approach for studying human action that relies on a careful analysis of the themes found in personal accounts or stories. (See *Qualitative research.*)

Narrative plot: An analysis of how people organize, understand, and interpret their experience as revealed in their narratives, or storied accounts of their lives. How experience is interpreted from the standpoint of its meaning to the participant.

Narrative slope: The direction, progressive or regressive, of a series of events as interpreted by the individual giving a personal account of what they experienced in a segment of their life story.

Narratives: The personal and collective stories through which individuals, families, groups, communities, organizations, and populations construct meaning through reflection and participation in occupations.

Naturalistic paradigm: A qualitative or experiential way of knowing and understanding phenomena, which recognizes that a researcher's biases and values are part of the research process and emphasizes observation in naturalistic or "real-world" settings and conditions.

Necessary occupations: Term for describing those human endeavors aimed at meeting basic physiological and self-maintenance needs constituting necessary time.

Necessary time: Term credited to D. Aas (1980) for time spent doing necessary activities [occupations].

Obligatory time: Term credited to D. Aas (1980) for time spent doing that which must be done.

Occupation: Engagement or participation in a recognizable everyday life endeavor.

Occupational adaptation: Adjustments and changes in the methods, tools, locations, and other forces that determine participation in occupations by individuals, groups, and communities.

Occupational alienation: Experiences devoid of meaning or purpose, a sense of isolation, powerlessness, frustration, loss of control, or estrangement from society or self that results from engagement in occupations that do not satisfy inner needs related to meaning and/or purpose.

Occupational analysis: Analysis of the occupations according to features (e.g., meaning, choice, personal demands, purposes), environment (e.g., built, classification, economic, geographic, political, sociocultural), demands/press (e.g., effort, performance requirements, mental and spiritual demands); occupational analysis is a core competency of occupational therapy; also known to occupational therapists and others as activity analysis, task analysis.

Occupational apartheid: Term credited to Kronenberg and Algado (2005) to describe the deliberate, political exclusion of some populations from some occupational opportunities and resources.

Occupational balance: A concept referring to the distribution of time for engagement in the habits and routines of everyday occupations; an interpretive concept for assessing time use with reference to health, well-being, and quality of life when the patterns of occupation are taken into account for individuals, groups, and communities; perceived state of satisfactory participation in valued, obligatory, and discretionary activities; occurs when the impact of occupations on one another is harmonious, cohesive, and under control. (See *Life balance*)

Occupational behavior: Human action produced by the combined efforts and expressions of mind, body, and spirit.

Occupational capacity: Ability (actual or potential) for occupational performance or engagement.

Occupational citizenship: Participation with choice and decision-making opportunities to realize one's potential in the typical occupations of a society.

Occupational classification: Any systematic approach to describing or categorizing intentional human time use.

Occupational competence: Ability, skill, knowledge, and attitudes for engagement in occupations.

Occupational culture: A set of technical, social, and cultural characteristics and attributes associated with one's place in the social division of labor and perception of one's self in the system.

Occupational deprivation: A term credited to Wilcock and Whiteford (2000) referring to a state of prolonged preclusion from engagement in occupations of necessity or meaning due to factors outside the control of an individual, such as through geographic isolation, incarceration, or disability.

Occupational development: Change over the life span; development may be a systematic progression of growth and maturation for participation in a repertoire of occupations related to age; or development may be shaped by life circumstances that require a unexpected developmental path.

Occupational disruption: A transient or temporary condition of being restricted from participation in necessary or meaningful occupations, such as that caused by illness, temporary relocation, or temporary unemployment.

Occupational engagement: Full participation in occupations for purposes of doing what one needs and wants to do, being, becoming who one desires to be, and belonging through shared occupations in communities.

Occupational enrichment: Enhanced environmental resources to enable optimal participation in occupations.

Occupational grouping: An interconnected set of occupations.

Occupational habits: Recurring, largely automatic patterns of time use within the context of daily occupations.

Occupational history: The historical narrative of occupational development and engagement over the life span; a documented record of occupational participation.

Occupational identity: The socially constructed image of self as a participant in occupations.

Occupational imbalance: An individual or group experience in which health and quality of life are compromised because of being overoccupied or underoccupied.

Occupational issues (OI): Experiences that are challenging, problematic, exceptional, or otherwise profiled about engagement in occupations.

Occupational justice/injustice: Term credited to Townsend (Canada) and Wilcock (Australia) (2000) referring to justice related to opportunities and resources required for occupational participation sufficient to satisfy personal needs and full citizenship.

Occupational life course: The accumulated occupational repertoire of experiences, events, and conditions over the life span.

Occupational marginalization: Experiences of inequity from being outside the dominant or mainstream discourse and events of everyday occupations in a particular context; invisible, silent, on the edge of privilege and entitlement to occupational opportunities and resources.

Occupational mastery: Excelling in competence for participation in an occupation.

Occupational participation: The engagement of the individual's mind, body, and soul in goal-directed pursuits.

Occupational pattern: Habits or routines in occupational engagement over time and in particular places.

Occupational performance: The task-oriented, completion, or doing aspect of occupations; often, but not exclusively, involving observable movement.

Occupational potential: A vision of future possibilities for engagement in occupations, or for structuring society to enable people to participate as fully as possible.

Occupational reasoning: Processes of thinking about, reflecting on, analyzing, and understanding occupations and participation in everyday life; includes conditional reasoning about the context for occupations, narrative reasoning about occupational experiences, and positivist reasoning based on empirical data on occupations.

Occupational repertoire: A person's or community's interwoven composition or patterns of occupations.

Occupational rhythm: The temporal pace or pattern of action or experience within a given occupation.

Occupational right: The idea that one has a moral entitlement to choose or have access to occupational pursuits that are necessary for health, well-being and social inclusion regardless of differences in ability, age, social class and other characteristics.

Occupational role: Socioculturally defined expectations for participation in occupations.

Occupational routines: Recurring sequences of time use, such as the regimen repeated upon waking each day.

Occupational satisfaction: Contentment with occupations.

Occupational science: The study of the experiences and factors pertaining to human occupation; also known as *occupationology*.

Occupational therapist: A regulated professional who has special knowledge in understanding the influence of occupation on health and well-being.

Occupational therapy: A profession practiced in many nations. Occupational therapy is based on knowledge about humans' intrinsic needs and desires to explore the world and engage in occupational pursuits that are necessary, engaging, meaningful, and purposeful, and that the social, spiritual, physical, and psychological benefits of occupational engagement are essential to health, well-being and equitable social inclusion.

Occupational therapy support personnel: Persons who work as assistants with supervision by registered/licensed professional occupational therapists.

Occupational transitions: Circumstances creating a change in the nature or type of occupational engagement pursued by or available to an individual. Such transitions may be the result of choice, changes in physical or mental status, life transitions, geographical change, geopolitical strife, or other factors. (See *Life transitions* and *Occupational deprivation.*)

Occupational well-being: Experiences of satisfaction and meaning derived from participation in occupations.

Occupationally just world: A utopian vision of a world that is governed in such a way as to enable individuals, families, communities and populations to flourish by doing what they decide is most meaningful, useful and environmentally sustainable to promote health, well-being and social inclusion for individuals, their families, communities, and nations.

Occupationology: A term attributed to Polatajko (Canada) to refer to the study of occupation (occupational science).

Occupations: Things that people do to occupy life for intended purposes such as paid work, unpaid work, personal-care, care of others, leisure, recreation, or subsistence. Includes groups of activities and tasks of everyday life, named, organized, and given value and meaning by individuals and a culture. Categories used by researchers and governments to track human participation in the labor market and society.

Ontology: In philosophy, the study of being or existence and diverse ways of knowing.

Overemployment: A form of occupational deprivation that occurs when people are overoccupied either in the paid workforce or in other aspects of daily life.

Paradigm: A model or way of viewing the world or a given phenomenon.

Places: The physical surroundings or environments that are natural or built in which people occupy themselves and create shared meaning, and the meanings and cultural constructions that create a sense of 'home,' 'community' or other place in the mind, in actual reality, or in virtual reality.

Play: Occupations selected for amusement, recreation, diversion, sport, or frolic.

Political environments: Situations or places where sanctions by those in control influence behavior or opportunity.

Positivistic paradigm: A view of the world based on the belief that phenomena can be best understood through observation and measurement.

Postmodernism: In general, a term referring to ways of thinking that reject hierarchical or empirical explanations of phenomena in favor of views that acknowledge complexity, ambiguity, and interconnectedness.

Preformationist viewpoint: An early historical view of human development, dating to the Middle Ages, that considered children as miniature adults.

Prisoner's dilemma: A specific example of game theory used for teaching purposes.

Purposive view of motivation: Emphasis on goal-directed or intentional action caused by anticipated benefit or a desire to avoid harm.

Qualitative research: Methods for understanding phenomena that allow an investigator to experience events, identify themes on the basis of that experience, and formulate theories.

Reductionistic: Reducing to parts; a way of explaining based on understanding the parts that make up a whole.

Refugeeism: The state of being forced to evacuate one's home and community as the result of war, violence, natural disaster, famine, or fear of communicable disease.

Regulatory motivators: Physiological influences on behavior that resist conscious control such as hunger, pain, and fatigue.

Relativism: The idea that concepts about phenomena vary according to differences in situations and cultures.

Rest: The natural repose or relief from daily activity or occupation that is obtained by sleep or reduced physical activity.

Retirement: A sociological term referring to the period of life following completion of paid or unpaid work as a career or extended employment or participation in a worker role.

Ritual: An established pattern of actions in a prescribed or ordered manner often performed as part of a ceremony or observance and typically having an associated meaning beyond the action itself.

Role balance: Satisfactory fulfillment of all valued roles.

Role overload: Having too much to do in the amount of time available; feeling time crunched and busycrazy.

Role strain: Distress or burden arising from excessive demands or insufficient capacity to fulfill the role; capacity includes personal knowledge and skills as well as available resources (financial, educational, social support).

Routine: A regular or customary pattern of time use through activity and occupation.

Social Structure: Pertaining to patterns of behavior or relationships within a society, particularly as these pertain to groups.

Spillover: The influence or effect of work on other life domains.

Stress: The effect of challenge or threat on the body or the perception of threat or challenge. Increasingly, distinction is made between the sources of threat or challenge (stressors) and their effects, now increasingly referred to as allostasis or allostatic load.

Sustainability: Use of natural resources in a manner that does not compromise the survival of future generations.

Symbolic interactionism: School of thought in psychology derived from the work of G. H. Mead. It views behavior as influenced by one's consideration of the image or thought of the self in relationship to others.

Tabula rasa: Concept credited to English philosopher John Locke in the 18th century, who viewed humans at birth as a blank slate whose life course would be written by life's experiences.

Tasks: A means of accomplishing an activity.

Taxonomy: A classification used to distinguish between ideas, objects, events, or things based on their defined properties.

Technology: The study, development, or use of inventions for practical purposes.

Tele-immersion: The creation of virtual environments that facilitate scientific collaboration over distances.

Temporal: Pertaining to time.

Theory of occupational justice: A theory to define beliefs, principles, and other features that distinguish occupational from social justice. (See *Occupational justice.*)

Time pressure: The experience of expectation to perform or accomplish more within a defined or inadequate segment of time.

Time use: How humans allocate time through activity and occupation.

Traits: Tendencies to behave or act in particular ways.

Uchi: Japanese term for the inner group, or circle of immediate friends and acquaintances, which dictates customs of language and deference that guide social interaction with visitors or outsiders of the "soto," or out-group. (See *Soto.*)

Underemployment: A form of occupational deprivation that occurs when people are underoccupied either in the paid workforce or in other aspects of daily life.

Unemployment: A form of occupational disruption (if short term) or occupational deprivation (if long term) caused by forces outside the individual, although individual responses to unemployment are important to consider.

Universalism: In general, applying to all persons and/or all things for all times and in all situations. The term has different meanings in different fields.

Virtual places: Any nonphysical representation of a location, such as an electronic or digitally simulated environment created on the Internet.

Volition: Choice or will; intentionality.

Well-being: The affect or emotion about one's psychological, emotional, or physical state as perceived at a given moment.

Work: Labor or exertion; to make, construct, manufacture, form, fashion, or shape objects; to organize, plan, or evaluate services or processes of living or governing; committed occupations that are performed with or without financial reward.

Work-leisure relationship: The study of how a person's choices and experiences of work influence their leisure and vice versa.

Work-life balance: Perceived ability to manage individual and family time, and perceived conflict in doing so. (see *Life balance, Occupational balance*)

Work-life conflict: A condition characterized by demands of work and personal/family life. Occurs when the cumulative demands of work and nonwork roles are incompatible such that participation in one role is made more difficult by participation in the other. At least three subsets of work-life conflict have been articulated: role overload, interference from family demands to work life, and interference from work demands to family life (see *Spillover*).

Study Guide Answers to Multiple-Choice Questions

Chapter 1

1. b. Seize (*Occupatio* is from the latin word meaning to Seize).
2. a. Simultaneous participation in more than one occupation.
3. d. Habits are relatively automatic repeated patterns of behavior.
4. a. True—Habits allow humans to conserve energy, but they can reduce vigilance and create difficulties when typical conditions change and such changes go unnoticed so that behaviors are not modified appropriately.
5. c. Personality is not a biological factor, but rather a psychological influence on occupation.

Chapter 2

1. b. The Western world often adheres to objectivity and the scientific method in seeking knowledge.
2. a. Relativism holds to the viewpoint that truth and criteria of judgment are relative to the circumstances, people, and contexts involved.
3. b. False—The Japanese uphold a hierarchical structure within their society.
4. b. Occupation and environment are considered together from the collective integrated unity of the whole.
5. c. Postmodernism often takes a relativist view.

Chapter 3

1. c. Ways of understanding. This definition of epistemological positions is based on the work of Perry.
2. a. Ways of knowing are always unique to the discipline. Ways of knowing are often specific to the discipline, but not necessarily unique to the discipline.
3. b. Qualitative research. The naturalistic paradigm is also described as qualitative research.
4. c. Grounded theory studies. Grounded theories studies are associated with the naturalistic paradigm or qualitative research.
5. d. When. Understanding "when" focuses on how occupations and time are related to each other.

Chapter 4

1. a. All occupations are viewed equally. Viewpoints agree that some occupations are viewed more highly within a society than others.
2. d. Sociology. Durkheim is known as an important French sociologist.

3. d. Job. The International Standard Classification of Occupations shows that at the top level are broad categories of employment, while at the bottom are very descriptive and more detailed descriptions of jobs or duties and responsibilities.
4. b. Employers. The focus of this chapter did not include the perspectives of employers.
5. c. Turning right in a stressful situation. This option described a suboccupation directly related to driving.

Chapter 5

1. b. Formal education would be considered contracted time.
2. a. True.
3. b. Roles are socially expected behaviors that are often situation specific.
4. b. Social support and income are extrinsic factors; in comparison, physical and psychological traits would be considered intrinsic factors.
5. a. Options b. (control over an area or domain) and c. (constraints related location timing and resources) respectively refer to authority and coupling constraints.

Chapter 6

1. a. The maturationist viewpoint believes a person's genes dictate human development and that heredity alone influences the course of development.
2. b. The Interactional Model of Occupational Development is based on the three variables of (1) occupational behavior, (2) time, and (3) interaction.
3. b. The meso level of occupational development is at the level of the individual.
4. c. Bronfenbrenner identified four aspects of the human environment to include the microsystem, mesosystem, exosystem, and macrosystem. More recently, the chronosystem was added to his General Ecological Model.
5. d. None of the above. The principle of multiple variation states that development is neither smooth nor unidirectional; it involves both growth and decline.

Chapter 7

1. a. Rubin did not include sharing. Rubin's five structural characteristics include size, focus, stability, social structure, and participation.
2. c. McMillan and Chavis did not include social skills. They described the following four ways to generate a psychological sense of community: sense of belonging, fulfillment of member needs, provide influence, and offer shared connections.
3. d. Composting, recycling, and using natural resources are all behaviors consistent with a sustainable community.
4. c. The definition of interdependence includes mutual dependence, aid, moral commitment and responsibility to recognize and support difference.
5. b. An ecological niche is one in which a particular species can successfully adapt.

Chapter 8

1. a. Minor changes in occupational repertoire of activities. Occupational transitions focus on major changes.
2. b. False—Retirement involves a process of adaptation over time.
3. c. Social contact and fellowship. This factor was identified as the most positive aspect of work.

4. a. Going from an imbalance of too many demands in work to an imbalance of too few demands in retirement. The paradox is that there is imbalance in both work and retirement.
5. a. True—The loss of the work routines increases awareness of the meaning of time and day.

Chapter 9

1. d. Occupational balance is multifaceted and dynamic, but there is agreement that it is beneficial to health and well being.
2. a. True—Increasing numbers of peope are working more than 40 or less than 30 hours weekly.
3. c. According to the author, depth of lifestyle refers to the need for an individual to create meaning in life.
4. b. False—Leisure and work in some contexts may be considered overlapping concepts.
5. d. Occupational balance. Other listed terms refer to an aspect of balance across a person's daily activities, but may be more limiting depending on how they are defined.

Chapter 10

1. c. Place does shape how occupation is performed. Occupations shape the meaning of a place. Place influences why occupations are performed. Place shapes the meaning of occupations, therefore occupations performed in different places do have different meanings.
2. b. An archetype is any object that is deeply rooted in human history and serves as a symbol or model for other objects. The term *semiotics* refers to the study of anything in social life that stands for something else. Habitus describes the behaviors of people.
3. a. Habits are reinforced by the place in which they are performed on a regular basis, not new environments. New places can provide a sense of refreshing change, may disrupt habits and routines, and can create a sense of stress.
4. d. All are true. Meanings of places are socially constructed in a variety of ways.
5. c. Habitus describes the unconscious patterns of doing, thinking, speaking, and perceiving that people exhibit in familiar circumstances.

Chapter 11

1. a. True, according to the authors and research as cited by Kabanoff.
2. a. The spillover hypothesis suggests a congruent relationship between work and leisure.
3. b. The W-O-L paradigm emphasizes that the effects of work on leisure participation is often mediated by cognitive processes or personality traits.
4. c. This is the definition for occupational culture as provided by the author.
5. a. True.

Chapter 12

1. a. The contributing factors are typically beyond one's control.
   Occupational deprivation, in contrast, is defined as usually associated with "factors or situations over which the individual has some control, such as moving to a new town, or changing jobs."
2. d. Geographic. Although geography has been recently discussed in case examples of occupational deprivation, it was not proposed as one of the three determinants identified in Stadnyk, Townsend, and Wilcock's exploratory theory of occupational justice. It is likely that geography infuences occupational engagement, but less likely that it determines this.

3. d. Both of the above statements a. and b. are considered essential features of occupational deprivation.
4. b. Motivation for work. The primary factors influencing unemployment were identified as environmental or contextual factors, rather than internal factors.
5. c. Recidivism. Occupational deprivation was not identified as a factor increasing risk for recidivism.

Chapter 13

1. c. Social justice involves the fair distribution of resources and opportunities in general. Occupational justice describes fair access to opportunity for engagement in occupation.
2. d. In the same way that social injustice is combated through many strategies, so too is occupational injustice addressed through activism and other strategies for increasing social awareness, policy changes, and enablement strategies (such as information and education).
3. a. Occupational preference is not an outcome of occupational injustice.
4. c. Obviously, physical abilities cannot be distributed, since they are personal rather than social resources. However, they can be developed through improved access to resources.
5. b. The concept of occupational justice owes its origins to many people, but the impetus behind its development must be attributed to Elizabeth Townsend and Ann Wilcock.

Chapter 14

1. d. All of the above. Each of the listed ideas is a core assumption of occupational therapy.
2. c. The reductionist approach is less holistic and more component based, emphasizing structure and function of the body.
3. b. Occupation is the core of occupational science, and is interdisciplinary in nature. As a formal discipline, occupational science did not predate occupational therapy.
4. c. The latin translation of *homo occupatio* is "human who occupies"; as in seizing the day through purposeful action.
5. b. False—Occupational therapy is the applied science, as it uses information from occupational science in an applied way within the profession. Occupational science is devoted to understanding the nature and complexity of occupation as it engages and influences the lives of people.

Chapter 15

1. a. Packaging chopsticks is a communal activity. Experiencing valued work, sharing a common goal, and providing a venue for interdependence are all outcomes of participation in chopstick packaging. Fostering a sense of independence is not a trait associated with packaging chopsticks.
2. c. Age was described as the biggest indicator for Internet usage; the younger the population, the more they use the Internet.
3. d. The HIV/AIDS pandemic in South Africa has caused loss of employment and income, increase in number of child-headed households, and an increase in the cost of medical treatment.
4. c. Democracy, apartheid, and language all shape occupational choices. Homogeneous population was not named as a factor shaping occupational choice in South Africa, as the population is quite heterogeneous.
5. a. The emphasis is on shared meal preparation and eating instead of on individualistic occupations.
6. a. True—Hong Kong has made a huge commitment to technological development.

Index